Basic Clinical
Massage Therapy:

INTEGRATING ANATOMY AND TREATMENT

11

Basic Clinical Massage Therapy:

INTEGRATING ANATOMY AND TREATMENT

JAMES H. CLAY, MMH, NCTMB

DAVID M. POUNDS, MA, BS

Photographs by Vicki Overman
Illustrations by David M. Pounds, Certified Medical Illustrator

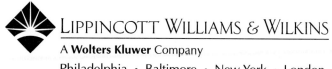

LIPPINCOTT WILLIAMS & WILKINS
A **Wolters Kluwer** Company

Philadelphia • Baltimore • New York • London
Buenos Aires • Hong Kong • Sydney • Tokyo

Editor: Pete Darcy
Developmental Editor: Kathleen Scogna
Marketing Manager: Christen DeMarco
Production Editor: Jennifer D. Weir
Compositor: Graphic World
Printer: Quebecor World
Designer: Karen Quigley

Library of Congress Cataloging-in-Publication Data

Clay, James H.
    Basic clinical massage therapy : integrating anatomy and treatment / James H. Clay,
 David M. Pounds ; photographs by Vicki Overman.
        p. ; cm.
    Includes bibliographical references and index.
    ISBN 0-683-30653-7
    1. Massage therapy. 2. Human anatomy. I. Pounds, David M. II. Title.
    [DNLM: 1. Massage—methods. WB 537 C619b 2002]
    RM721 .C53 2002
    615.8'22—dc21

                                                              2001050743

To purchase additional copies of this book, call our customer service department at **(800) 638-3030** or fax orders to **(301) 824-7390**. International customers should call **(301) 714-2324**.

Visit Lippincott Williams & Wilkins on the Internet: *http://www.LWW.com*. Lippincott Williams & Wilkins customer service representatives are available from 8:30 am to 6:00 pm, EST.

02 03 04 05 06
1 2 3 4 5 6 7 8 9 10

For
Jacque and Tim Pennell
and
Anne and Dick Clay
—James Clay

To my wife Kathleen for her support and patience,
and to my parents Arthur M. and Jean T. Pounds
—David Pounds

Preface

Basic Clinical Massage Therapy: Integrating Anatomy and Treatment is primarily a textbook for advanced massage therapy students who have already acquired the basic skills of Swedish massage and are now pursuing additional training in clinical massage therapy. In this book, I define "clinical massage therapy" as the use of manual manipulation of the soft tissues to relieve specific complaints of pain and dysfunction. As its title implies, our book integrates detailed anatomical information with basic clinical massage therapy techniques. By imbedding illustrations of internal structures into photographs of live models, we are able to show exactly what muscle is being worked on, where it is, where it attached, how it can be accessed manually, what kind of problems it can cause, and one or more basic techniques for effectively treating it. The student can clearly see the involved structures in relation to surrounding structures, surface landmarks, and the therapist's hands. This book, therefore, offers a truly innovative visual and tactile understanding of anatomical spatial relationships integrated with the learning of treatment technique, which has not been possible with traditional approaches. Our approach is possible only through teamwork. Although I have had chief responsibility for the text and Dave Pounds for the illustrations, we are truly co-authors, in that this project has been planned and executed by both of us working closely together from its very inception. Vicki Overman, an outstanding photographer, has also worked with us and shared our enthusiasm from the beginning.

In addition to its use as a textbook, Basic Clinical Massage Therapy: Integrating Anatomy and Treatment can also serve in the following roles:

- A palpatory and muscle anatomy reference for practitioners. The anatomy of muscles and bones

is complex, and an accurate knowledge of it is essential to effective treatment. The practitioner must have reliable reference sources to consult. In the past, practitioners have used atlases of anatomy designed chiefly for surgeons. This book is tailored specifically to the needs of the clinical massage therapist. By presenting the anatomy of muscles and bones in the context of the living human body, it bridges the gap between internal muscular and external surface anatomy and allows students and practitioners to see through the surface to the internal structures.

- A client education tool. One of the biggest difficulties facing a therapist in dealing with clients is explaining where a problem may lie, what structures may be involved, and what type of work is proposed. Currently, practitioners must turn to traditional anatomy references, or to whole or partial skeletons or other educational aids to make such explanations. The therapist can use this book to present necessary information to clients in a way that is easily comprehensible.

ORGANIZATION AND STRUCTURE

This book is divided into two parts. Part I, Foundations of Clinical Massage Therapy, presents essential information about the basic principles on which clinical massage therapy is based. The first chapter explains the place of clinical massage therapy in the health field and reviews the essentials about muscle structure and function, body mechanics, basic techniques, and draping.

The second chapter is a guide to examination: interviewing, observation, photography, and palpation. It also presents examples of forms to use and covers communication with physicians and other health professionals.

Part II, Approaching Treatment, constitutes the "meat" of the book. We have organized the chapters in this part into body regions that have functional, topographical, and clinical coherence. These regions are:

- head, face, and neck
- shoulder, chest, and upper back
- arm and hand
- vertebral column
- low back and abdomen
- pelvis
- thigh
- leg and foot

Each Part II chapter has the same internal structure. This rigorous internal consistency is deliberate: learning is based on repetition, and a repetitive organization allows the reader to more easily process and internalize information. Each chapter, therefore, has the following components:

- Overview of the Region. Here, we review the muscular and skeletal components of the region under discussion, and offer observations on conditions that typically cause pain and dysfunction in that region. Extensive anatomy plates, presented in a horizontal ("landscape") format, depict in detail the internal anatomy. Labels point out each pertinent structure and are keyed to the text discussion.
- Muscle sections. Each muscle of that region is then discussed. These sections are distinguished by their use of various icons that highlight key pieces of information:
- Pronunciation. As communication between massage therapists and other members of the health care community continues to increase, it's important to know how to pronounce each muscle name correctly. We use a phonetic pronunciation key that is easy to decipher.
- Etymology. A brief derivation of each muscle name is given. Etymologies are extremely helpful in learning and remembering anatomical structures.
- Overview. Here, we give a succinct but thorough overview of the structure and function of the muscle. We also review potential causes of pain and dysfunction that may affect the muscle.

- Comments. Where appropriate, interesting or esoteric comments about the muscle are included. For instance, we point out that biceps brachii resides on the humerus but has no attachments to it, and that in addition to being a flexor it is the most powerful supinator of the forearm.

The following icons are then used to highlight particular information:

Attachments

The attachments of the muscle are cited. Because the tradition of describing muscle attachments as origins and insertions can be confusing and misleading, we refer to attachments as proximal and distal, superior and inferior, or lateral and medial, as appropriate.

Actions

The principal functions of each muscle are listed.

Caution

Client safety is a primary concern for the massage therapist. Where appropriate, cautionary notes that alert the massage therapist to potential contraindications to specific techniques, as well as precautions to take while performing particular techniques for all clients are included.

Referral Areas

The areas to which the muscle typically refers pain are listed.

Other Muscles to Examine

Other muscles are listed that may refer pain to the same area.

Manual Therapy.
One or more basic techniques for treating the muscle are described and illustrated. In order of frequency, these techniques are stripping massage, compression, cross-fiber stroking, stretching, and myofascial stretching, all of which are discussed in Chapter 1.

DESIGN

The design of this book is intended to facilitate its use during hands-on practice sessions. Students are encouraged to use the book as a tabletop resource while practicing the techniques on a fellow student or other volunteer. Design features that will help students in their practice sessions are as follows:

- A specially designed lay-flat binding keeps the book open to the page a student wants to study.
- The colorful icons in the muscle sections focus the reader's attention and help prevent the reader from losing his or her place in the narrative.
- The technique illustrations include arrows ➡ that show the direction of the moving strokes. A second kind of arrow ▥ denotes static compression, and a third ◀●▶ indicates myofascial stretching. These devices help take the guesswork out of performing the techniques.

ADDITIONAL CONTENT

Anatomical structures are shown in the anatomy plates and are boldfaced in the text. Other boldfaced terms are defined in the glossary. There are also the following appendices:

- Latin and Greek prefixes and suffixes, and a brief explanation of the structure of Latin words
- Illustrations of terms for body planes, relative location in the body, and positions and movements
- A list of muscles according to their pain referral zones
- A list of other suggested books and resources

IMPORTANT COMMENTS

- The illustrations in this book feature paid models (not clients) who are shown nude or with minimal draping (child models are in underwear) to show clearly both internal structures and external body landmarks. This approach should not be taken as a suggestion for clinical practice. Suggestions for draping are given wherever appropriate, with reference to corresponding illustrations of the draping techniques in the first chapter.
- Due to the demands of photography and the need to show landmarks and internal structures clearly, many compromises had to be made in the positioning of the therapist and client; as a result, the body mechanics in the illustrations may not always be ideal. Likewise, the prone subject is usually, though not always, shown in a face cradle. I urge you to look to Chapter 1, not the individual therapy illustrations, for models of body mechanics.
- Myofascial stretching as a preparatory technique before specific muscle work is highly recommended. We describe and illustrate myofascial stretching for all regions of the torso, but not for the limbs. The technique is fairly simple and straightforward, and the student should be able to transfer the technique to the arms and legs without difficulty.
- I use the word "compression" in this book to indicate any pressure exerted in a direction deep to the body surface, whether over firm structure (such as bone) or not.
- It is always challenging to know how to organize material about the human body, since the body is an integrated whole, and a book is necessarily linear. Within each chapter, we have organized the muscles into logical groups (flexors together, extensors together, etc.). Within each group, the muscles are presented in no particular order.

SUMMARY

In short, this book is intended to bridge the wide gap between the anatomy book and the living body on the massage table especially for students, but also for practitioners. As your hands rest on the body, your eyes can move back and forth between the illustrations and the subject, allowing you to incorporate the anatomical information with both visual and tactile senses. It will also allow you to find essential information about any muscle quickly and easily either for the first time as a student or to refresh your memory as an experienced practitioner. It is flexible enough to be used in any massage class. Since the material is presented in a format that is easily referenced, instructors may assign as little or as much of the material as they choose.

We wish every reader success, and we hope this book finds a prominent place in your treatment room for many years to come.

CALL FOR COMMENTS

I welcome criticisms, corrections, suggestions, and, yes, even compliments, any of which may be sent to:

James H. Clay, MMH, LMBT
2723 Stockton Street
Winston-Salem, NC 27127
Email: **doc@clinicalmassage.info**

Acknowledgments

Nancy Evans, Editorial Director for Lippincott Williams & Wilkins, first saw the potential of our book and presented it to Rina Steinhauer, at that time an Acquisitions Editor for LWW. Rina negotiated our contract and supplied an enormous amount of encouragement and enthusiasm from the beginning, and Nancy has continued to give much support to the project. We are deeply grateful to them both.

Since that time, many others at Lippincott Williams & Wilkins have worked hard for the project, including Acquisitions Editor Pete Darcy and Editorial Assistants Katie Cooke, Lisa Manhart, and Joseph Latta. Our thanks to them.

This book has been reviewed chapter by chapter by professionals in the massage therapy field during its development, and they have offered many extremely helpful comments and suggestions. These reviewers are:

Cassandra E. Orem, RN, MS, MA, CMT
Samantha Hens
Annie Henson, LMT, NCTMB, CIMI, RM/T, TTT(TM), ABMP, CD(DONA)
Clifford Korn, LMT, NCTMB
Sharon Long, BFA, CMT, NCTBM
Whitney Lowe, LMT
Alexandra Hamer, LMBT
Donald Webb, CMT, NCTMB

We thank each of them for their time, effort, and contributions.

A special thanks to Walter J. Bo, PhD, Professor, and Mr. Robert Lee Bowden, Instructor in Gross Anatomy of the Department of Neurobiology and Anatomy, Wake Forest University School of Medicine, for access to cadavers in the Gross Anatomy Lab.

Thanks to David G. Simons, MD, for consultation and clarification of issues concerning myofascial trigger points and posture.

We thank Lisa Meloncon Posner for early assistance with organizing materials for the text. We also thank the staff of the Silas Creek Parkway PhotoLab, where all of our photos were processed, for consistently professional and courteous service.

We want to thank those who served as volunteer models when the book was still the germ of an idea: Sarah Kelly, Shanda Smith, Debbie Garner Transou, and M.D.

We thank our very first "official" model, Elizabeth Shuler, who probably appears more often in the book than any other model, and all of the wonderful models who followed: Anna Bigelow, Joe Cox, Jack Edmonds, Lindsay Fisher, Amanda Furches, Sabrina Hertel, Olivia Honeycutt, Evan Johnson, Sarah Kelly, Jason Kittleberger, Kate Merritt, Helen Naples, Mike Orsillo, Bronwyn Queen, Nike Roach, Shanta Rudd, Shana Schwarz, Emily Sparkman, Matt Swaim, Katie Swords, and Yvonne Truhon.

James Clay would particularly like to thank Linda Laughrun; John and Sally Foushee; Stacie Queen; David Barabe, DDS; Kim Heath; Ladd Freeman; Wallace and Melba Sidden; Rebecca Ashby; the Brodkin family, Philip and Roberta Powell; D.A. and Patricia Oldis; and Travis Jackson, MD.

And the best for last: Kathleen Scogna, our Managing/Developmental Editor at Lippincott Williams & Wilkins, has served for 4 years as our editor, counselor, mediator, advocate, psychotherapist, teacher, champion, and friend. Her name should be on the cover. Thank you, Kathleen. You're the best.

James H. Clay
David M. Pounds

Contents

Expanded Contents

Foundations of Clinical Massage Therapy

1

"Is there not such a thing as a diffused bodily pain, extending, radiating out into other parts, which, however, it leaves, to vanish altogether, if the practitioner lays his finger on the precise spot from which it springs? And yet, until that moment, its extension made it seem to us so vague and sinister that, powerless to explain or even to locate it, we imagined that there was no possibility of its being healed."

Marcel Proust, The Remembrance of Things Past
(The Guermantes Way, *1920)*

Approaching Clinical Massage Therapy

A young girl has pain that does not go away. Her mother has heard from a friend that there is a healer not far away who can get rid of such pain. One day the mother takes the girl to see this healer. The healer asks a few questions; then, rather than giving her something to swallow, the healer places skilled hands on her and presses and rubs in various places. When the healer is finished, the girl's pain is diminished. The mother pays the healer and they leave. A day or two later, the pain is completely gone.

These events may very well have taken place in China in 1000 BCE. They could have occurred in India at least as early as the 3rd century BCE. The healer in question could have been Herodicus or his pupil, Hippocrates, in 5th-century (BCE) Greece, or Asclepiades, who brought the practice to Rome in the 1st century BCE. And the story can often be told today, thanks to the rediscovery and development of **clinical massage therapy,** the use of manual manipulation of the soft tissues to relieve specific complaints of pain and dysfunction.

The practice of massage therapy lay dormant in the Western world from the decline of Rome until the 18th century, when the Enlightenment fostered renewed interest in exploring the frontiers of medical knowledge. In the early 19th century, Per Henrik Ling developed a system of medical exercises and massage that his followers disseminated throughout the western world in subsequent years. This system profoundly influenced the birth and development of physical therapy, and the massage elements of his system became what is known today as **Swedish massage.** This type of massage has been continuously practiced in health clubs and spas over the past century, but was largely considered a luxury available only to the wealthy, and was not generally viewed as a health-related procedure until the gradual resurgence of massage therapy over the last 30 to 40 years.

In conjunction with massage therapy, the term *bodywork* has come into common use. This term arose from two principal sources: first, the psychiatrist Wilhelm Reich, originally a disciple of Freud, postulated the expression of the personality through body structure and formulated an approach to the simultaneous treatment of the body and the emotions. His work has been carried on by Alexander Lowen in the system called bioenergetics. Other practitioners, such as Ron Kurtz, have continued to work along similar lines.

Second, Ida Rolf developed a system that she called structural integration, but which has come to be called **Rolfing**™ in her honor. Her approach emphasizes the restructuring of the fascia. When we join the terms "massage" and "bodywork," as in the name of the **National Certification Board for Therapeutic Massage and Bodywork,** we reflect the fact that these two streams are in the process of merging, and many therapists consider themselves the heirs and practitioners of both traditions.

Two other approaches to health care in the last two centuries have also made significant contributions to the formation of clinical massage therapy and bodywork. Osteopathy (see further in the chapter) developed as a medical field that sought to relieve health problems through the manipulation of both joints and soft tissues, and many osteopathic practices have found their way into clinical massage therapy with the help of such osteopaths as Leon Chaitow. In medicine, the late Janet G. Travell, MD, and David G. Simons, MD, have explored the phenomenon of referred pain from **trigger points,** tender points in soft tissue that radiate or refer pain to distant areas.

Thus, at a time when many people are looking beyond the traditional medical offerings of pharmacological and surgical intervention, the confluence of these multiple influences has produced the field of clinical massage therapy, which is both one of the oldest and one of the newest health professions.

THE PLACE OF CLINICAL MASSAGE THERAPY IN HEALTH CARE

Because of the complexity of the human organism, a variety of approaches to the manual treatment of the soft tissues have evolved. Other health disciplines take the following approaches to pain and dysfunction:

- *Traditional western medicine* employs three principal means of treatment: pharmacology, surgery, and referral to an allied therapeutic specialties practitioner. One of the problems with the traditional medical approach to muscular problems is that no medical specialty focuses primarily on muscles. Aside from the primary care physician (family practitioner, pediatrician, internist, gynecologist, etc.), a patient with soft-tissue pain or dysfunction is likely to see a neurologist or neurosurgeon (specializing in the nervous system), an orthopedist (specializing in bones), or a rheumatologist (specializing in joints). Depending on the particulars of the case, such a patient is most likely to receive either surgery, drugs, or a referral to a physical therapist.
- *Osteopathy* began as an approach to health that focused on the manipulation of bones and joints, but has since moved in the direction of classical Western medicine. It tends to be heavily represented in certain areas of this country (British osteopathy is significantly different in education and practice from American osteopathy). Certain representatives of osteopathy, such as Leon Chaitow and Philip Greenman, have maintained the tradition of examining and treating pain problems through joint manipulation, and they have had a profound effect on recent developments in clinical massage therapy.
- *Chiropractic* focuses on treatment of the joints, particularly those of the vertebrae. These prac-

titioners attribute pain and other health problems to misalignments (subluxations) of the vertebral joints that impinge on nerve roots.

- *Physical therapy* uses physical exercise and movement as a means of restoring healthy function to muscles and joints. Although today physical therapists take advantage of many technological advances, such as hydrotherapy, ultrasound, and electrical stimulation of muscles, their emphasis remains on exercise and movement. Also, physical therapists tend to focus on more severe conditions, such as rehabilitation following surgery, serious injury, or congenital deformities.
- The remaining approach is *direct manipulation of the soft tissues.* This approach is the special territory of the clinical massage therapist and is what this book is about.

THE PRINCIPLES OF CLINICAL MASSAGE THERAPY

Clinical massage therapists operate according to certain assumptions that are so self-evident that they might be considered axioms of the field.

1. *The individual is a whole organism: everything is connected and related.* Complex systems are more than the mere sum of their parts; that is, it is essential to see the forest and the trees. Although this book is necessarily reductionist to some degree—we cannot understand the whole without a knowledge of the parts, and they must be examined in a linear way—the therapist should remember that the part must also be seen in the context of the whole. For example, a client with a sprained ankle will favor the injured leg, causing muscles in the hip and low back to tighten. The resulting imbalance in the back can affect the neck muscles, causing a headache. Treating the neck muscles alone will not solve the problem.
2. *Shortened muscle tissue can do no work.* Muscle tissue does its work by contracting and, therefore, can do no further work if shortened. What we are concerned with as therapists is persistently or pathologically shortened tissue; in other words, tissue that has shortened, in all likelihood for defensive reasons, is unable to work, and resists lengthening.

   A muscle may be shortened actively or passively. Examples of chronic passive shortening are the shortening of the biceps brachii when

the arm is kept in a sling for a period of healing, and the flexed position of the iliopsoas muscles (hip flexors) in a baby who is not yet standing and walking. Postural misalignment always involves habitual passive shortening of many postural muscles.

Active shortening, on the other hand, is muscular contraction, and may be either the intentional contraction that is the work of the muscle, or defensive contraction representing the muscle's response to a threat such as overload, repetitive motion, or excessive stretch. When a portion of muscle tissue is contracted in this way, it cannot contract further, and is unavailable to do the work of the muscle.

3. *The soft tissues of the body respond to touch.* There are many theories as to why this is so. One of the most persuasive is that myofascial pain is caused by a self-perpetuating neuromuscular feedback circuit in which the stimulation of touch interferes, thus restoring normal function. Depending on the choice of technique, manual intervention in the dysfunctional tissues interrupts this feedback process, forcing some change in the neural response and, therefore, in the functioning of the affected tissue itself. The intervention may take the form of **ischemic compression, passive stretching, passive shortening,** or any simultaneous or sequential combination of these.

Clinical massage therapy, and therefore, this book, is based firmly on these three principles. The clinical massage therapist is one who approaches persistently shortened soft tissues and attempts to restore their natural, pain-free function through touch, while keeping the whole client in mind.

STRUCTURE AND FUNCTION OF MUSCLES

Although we treat muscles as distinct entities for anatomical convenience, we must remember that the neuromuscular system does not activate muscles in that way. The nervous system stimulates portions of contractile tissue to contract in patterns that will produce the desired effect, and this activation usually involves parts of several muscles acting in fine coordination. No action recruits all of a muscle, and no action recruits only one muscle. When we say, for example, that biceps brachii flexes the arm at the elbow, we are making a broad generalization. Depending on the position of the arm when we make the movement, certain portions of biceps brachii will be activated. In addition, portions of brachialis will also contract, as well as portions of certain muscles in the forearm. Portions of triceps brachii will be recruited to temper the movement and keep it smooth. As the movement occurs, there is a shift in weight, and parts of muscles throughout the torso and legs respond to maintain balance. Therefore, it is not so much individual muscles that do the work of the body as it is patterns of portions of muscle tissue. In order to gain an understanding of these broad patterns of muscular action over the whole body, we must first acquaint ourselves with the elemental parts of muscle tissue and how they work.

The Muscle Cell

The contractile filaments that perform the work of the muscle are called **myofilaments.** Two basic types of myofilaments perform the work of the muscle. One type is the thick **myosin** filament, the other is the thin **actin** filament. The myosin filament has molecular "heads" that extend to attractor sites on the adjacent actin filament and bend to bring about contraction. These myosin and actin filaments lie parallel to each other in an overlapping pattern that produces the characteristic striped (striated) appearance of skeletal muscle. Several of these myofilaments together form a **sarcomere,** which is considered the "unit" of contraction in a muscle cell.

A string of **sarcomeres** lined up in sequence form a **myofibril** (muscle thread) (Fig. 1-1). Surrounding and penetrating the myofibrils is a system of microscopic tubes called **transverse tubules** and the **sarcoplasmic reticulum.** These tubules carry the chemical trigger, calcium, necessary to initiate contraction at the molecular level. A muscle cell is composed of several myofibrils.

The expression **"muscle cell"** is equivalent to the expression **"muscle fiber."** The number of

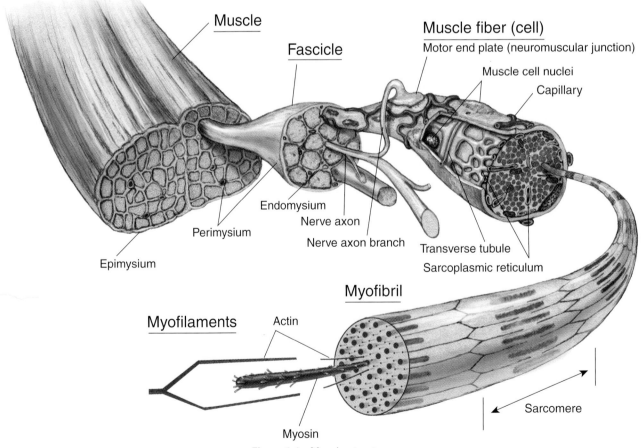

Figure 1-1   Muscle structure

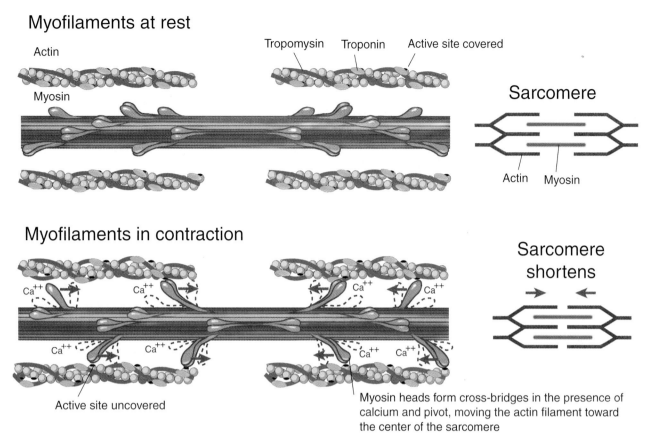

Figure 1-2 Crossbridge theory of muscle contraction

muscle cells in the body is believed to remain constant; when we strengthen muscles or increase their size and bulk, it is the contractile content, not the number, of the cells or fibers that is changed. Unlike most cells, muscle cells contain many nuclei scattered along the length of the cell. Multiple nuclei are necessary because muscle cells can be quite long, and their internal needs, which must be assessed and met by the nuclei, vary from one part of the cell to the next. Muscle cells are second only to nerve cells in length and can be over 11 inches long in some muscles.

The Cross-Bridge Theory

The most commonly accepted theory of muscle function is the cross-bridge theory. It attempts to explain the contractile action of muscle tissue—that is, how muscle tissue shortens when stimulated by a motor neuron.

When a nerve impulse excites the neuromuscular junction, calcium is released from the sarcoplasmic reticulum into the fluid surrounding the myofilaments. This causes a molecular response in which attractor sites on the actin filaments are exposed, attracting "heads" from the myosin filaments, which cross the gap between the filaments, attach themselves to their sites on the actin filaments and bend, propelling the actin filaments into a more deeply overlapped and interlocked position in relation to the myosin filaments. This shortens the sarcomere and, as all the sarcomeres in many muscle cells shorten, muscle contraction occurs (Fig. 1-2). Muscle tissue is capable of shortening by about 40% of its length.

When nerve stimulation ceases, the calcium is actively transported back into the transverse tubules, the myosin heads release and contraction stops. The muscle, however, cannot lengthen on its own. The contractile units (sarcomeres) must be stretched back to their starting position by an outside force, such as the pull of gravity or an opposing muscle, before it can again shorten in contraction.

If you imagine the myosin and actin filaments in fully overlapped position, then you can see how muscle tissue that is shortened in this way can do no further work.

The Neuromuscular Junction

The point of contact between the nervous system and the muscular system is the **neuromuscular junction. Synapses,** which are the points at which nerve cells communicate chemically with each other, also exist between the motor nerve cell and the muscle. Since muscles cover a lot of territory and since different parts of them must function in different ways, a nerve made up of many neurons can innervate, or have nerve endings (neuromuscular junctions) with, many different locations on a muscle. Although each muscle cell (fiber) is innervated by only one neuron, each neuron may innervate many muscle cells. A particular neuron and all of the muscle cells that it innervates is known as a **motor unit.** This neuron extends an individual axon branch to each muscle fiber. Each muscle fiber has a single neuromuscular junction, approximately at its middle, composed of a cluster of axon terminals. These are the points at which the impulse to contract is communicated from the nervous system to the muscle.

Individual muscles are comprised of **fascicles,** or bundles, of muscle cells (fibers). These smaller bundles are held together to form larger bundles and are separated from each other by connective tissue (deep fascia, myofascia).

The source of energy within muscle cells is called adenosine triphosphate (ATP), derived from the metabolism of glycogen (a form of glucose) stored in the muscle. When muscle tissue is excited by the nervous system, it **recruits** a number of motor units based on the strength of the excitation. If the excitation and, therefore, the contraction are sustained, then some motor units may experience **exhaustion;** that is, they deplete their supply of ATP. As this occurs, other motor units are recruited to relieve them. As the excitation increases, additional motor units are recruited.

Muscle Architecture

Muscle architecture is the arrangement of muscle fibers relative to the axis of force generation. It is one of the most important aspects of muscle anatomy for massage therapists for two reasons:

1. The arrangement of the muscle fibers determines the kinesiological function of the muscle or that particular part of the muscle.
2. The direction of the fibers in a particular section of a muscle will often determine the direction and type of the work to be done. For these

reasons, it is important to learn the architectural characteristics of each muscle.

The term used to describe the angle of the fibers to the force-generating axis is *pennation,* and muscles fall into several general categories: (Fig. 1-3)

- *Pennate*
  - *Unipennate:* Fibers lie at a single angle to the force-generating axis. (Examples: vastus lateralis and medialis)
  - *Bipennate:* Fibers lie at two angles to the force-generating axis. (Example: rectus femoris)
  - *Multipennate:* Fibers lie at multiple angles to the force-generating axis. (Example: deltoid)
- *Parallel (longitudinal):* Fibers are parallel to the force-generating axis. (Example: biceps brachii)
- *Convergent:* Fibers from a broad attachment converge to a narrow attachment, forming a fan shape. (Example: pectoralis major)

TENDER POINTS, TRIGGER POINTS, RELEASE

In examining clients, you will find points on the body that are tender when pressed. Assuming there is no other explanation for the tenderness, such as bruising or other injury, these points are called **tender points.** In the treatment system called *strain-counterstrain,* or *positional release,* developed by the osteopath Lawrence Jones, these points occur in a systematic fashion. They are treated by placing the muscle indicated into a passively shortened position until it relaxes and the tender point dissipates.

A myofascial **trigger point** is a point found in a nodule in a taut band of skeletal muscle tissue that is extremely tender, and that refers or radiates pain in a characteristic pattern. Trigger points are produced by muscle stress, such as overwork, repetitive motion, or sudden excessive stretch. An

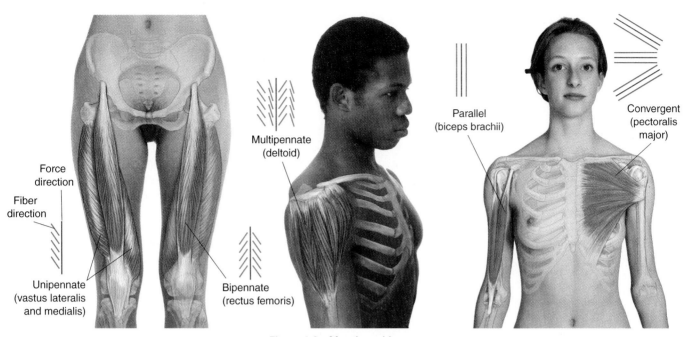

Force direction

Fiber direction

Multipennate (deltoid)

Parallel (biceps brachii)

Convergent (pectoralis major)

Unipennate (vastus lateralis and medialis)

Bipennate (rectus femoris)

Figure 1-3 Muscle architecture

active trigger point is one that is spontaneously producing referred pain in the client; a **latent trigger point** is one that produces pain only when pressure is applied in palpation. A **primary trigger point** is one that is caused by muscle stress; a **satellite trigger point** is one that is produced secondarily by a primary trigger point.

The term **release** is commonly used by massage therapists to refer to the softening and lengthening of soft tissue in response to therapy. A trigger point is said to release when its nodule is felt to soften and it ceases referring pain. A muscle is said to release when it relaxes while a therapeutic maneuver is being performed. Fascia is said to release when the therapist feels it soften and lengthen. The therapist's sense of release in soft tissue is a subjectively experienced phenomenon that is difficult to describe; however, it is difficult to miss when you feel it, and it is a very gratifying feeling for therapist and client alike.

AGONISTS AND ANTAGONISTS

For virtually all skeletal muscle tissue, there is corresponding muscle tissue that pulls in the opposite direction. Although the actual relationships of such corresponding tissues is complex, we generally refer to muscle pairs as **agonists** and **antagonists,** the agonist being the muscle that is carrying out a motion in question and the antagonist

being the muscle that opposes this action. A simple example is biceps brachii (a flexor) and triceps brachii (an extensor), which oppose each other by flexing and extending the arm at the elbow. Not only do these opposing forces produce opposing movements, but the two muscles work in a coordinated way to produce a smooth movement in both directions. When a muscle is contracting to flex a joint by shortening, that is **concentric contraction.** When a muscle functions as the antagonist and contracts to control the movement of a joint while lengthening, that is **eccentric contraction.** The antagonist must overcome its normal resistance to stretch in order for movement to take place. This inhibition of the stretch reflex in antagonists is **reciprocal inhibition.**

We need to be aware of this relationship between muscles because it is reflected in clinical problems. There is a balance in strength between agonists and antagonists under normal circumstances. When muscles are weakened, excessively strengthened, or injured, this balance is upset. When we find a problem of any kind in a muscle, we are very likely to find a problem in its antagonist.

FASCIA

Fascia is a Latin word meaning "band" or "bandage." It is the most pervasive type of tissue in the body: it's everywhere, like ivy on old buildings. It is the infrastructure of the body. Fascia not only gives the body its form, both inside and out, but it also provides the scaffolding for all of the other systems of the body, such as the circulatory, nervous, and lymphatic systems. Fascia might be considered the "skeleton" of soft tissues.

Fascia is a type of **connective tissue,** which takes other such forms as tendons, ligaments, aponeuroses, and scar tissue. It takes different names in different places: around the brain and spinal cord it is the meninges; around bones it is periosteum; around the heart it is pericardium; lining the abdominal cavity it is the peritoneum; and covering the entire body in a layer just under the skin, and enclosing muscles and sections of muscles, it is called fascia.

Fascia serves the following functions:

1. It forms and supports. It gives shape to the body and its component parts and holds them in place.
2. It restricts. By providing firm boundaries, it increases muscle strength. Muscles from which fascia has been removed are significantly weaker.
3. It guides and molds. Damaged bone deprived of periosteum does not heal within appropriate boundaries.
4. It contains and compartmentalizes. Fascia contains and channels body fluids, helping to prevent the spread of infection.
5. It provides infrastructure for branching systems. It supports capillaries and vessels of the circulatory and lymphatic systems, as well as the ubiquitous branching of the nervous system.
6. It gives rise to new connective tissue. Fascia contains connective tissue cells (fibroblasts) which can specialize as needed to thicken connective tissue, help repair tendons and ligaments, and form scar tissue.

Ironically, the healing and restorative functions of fascia can also lead to problems. Enveloping tissues as a spider envelops its prey, fascia can form adhesions between structures that should remain free. It alters the internal structure of muscles with deposits of gristle (fibrosis) that produce pain and limit movement. Such tissue hardens and contracts with time, becoming increasingly refractory to corrective treatment.

One of the most important things to understand about fascia is that *all fascia throughout the body is continuous.*

This fact is the key to the importance it is given by many bodyworkers. Fascia is often compared to a knit sweater, in that a pulled thread anywhere on the sweater will result in a distortion of its shape in places distant from the pull. Many therapists feel that fascial distortions and fascial work have an effect over the whole body, including the internal organs.

The pioneer of fascia-centered bodywork was Ida Rolf. Virtually every therapy focused in any way on fascia is grounded in large measure on her theories and her work. Rolf observed that fascia is made up of collagen fibers in a colloidal ground substance that varies in consistency from gel (the solid or semisolid state of a colloidal solution) to sol (the liquid state of a colloidal solution). When energy (such as pressure or friction) is applied to a gel, it moves toward the sol state. Rolf theorized that applying energy manually to the fascia can turn the ground substance from gel to sol and make the direction and distribution of the collagen fibers more elastic and malleable. Since fascia is continuous throughout the body, the therapist can adjust the "body stocking" of the superficial fascia by releasing restrictions in the deep fascia and breaking up adhesions between fascial layers that restrict free movement of tissues against each other.

Anyone who has worn stockings, pantyhose, tights, or any other tight-fitting garment knows what it is like to have that garment become twisted out of its proper position; it's an unpleasant, nagging sort of feeling. Fascial therapists believe that the fascia, like a body stocking, can become misaligned through habitual body misalignment, and they attempt to loosen, stretch, and realign the superficial fascia manually by means of various techniques.

Superficial Fascia

The superficial fascia is also called the hypodermis, tela subcutanea, subcutis, or stratum subcutaneum. It is located directly under the skin and contains fat, fascicles of muscle tissue, cutaneous blood vessels and nerves, and about half of the fat in the body.

The orientation of the fibers of the connective tissue (collagen) fibers of the dermis follows lines called Langer's lines, or cleavage lines, the direction of which varies from one body area to another (Fig. 1-4). The fibers in a particular region are aligned against the predominate forces expe-

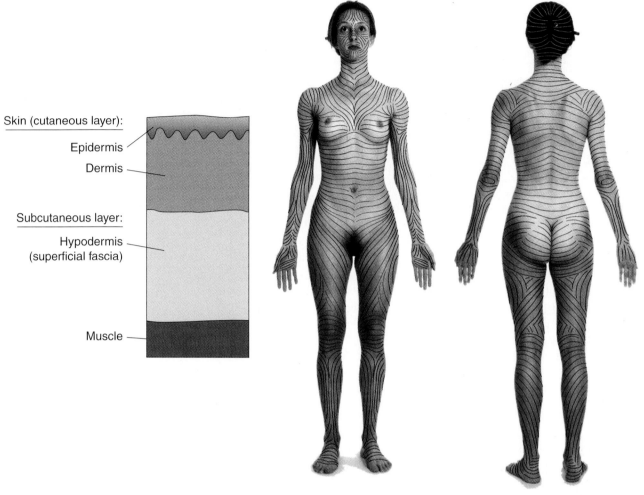

Skin (cutaneous layer):

Epidermis

Dermis

Subcutaneous layer:

Hypodermis
(superficial fascia)

Muscle

Figure 1-4 Langer's lines

rienced by the tissues in that area of the body. Surgeons often follow these lines in making incisions in order to minimize scarring.

Deep Fascia

The deep fascia is all of the fascia that is deep to the superficial fascia, with which it is continuous. For our purposes, deep fascia includes the fascia covering a group of muscles (*investing fascia*), the fascia surrounding the muscles (epimysium), the fascia surrounding the fascicles within the muscle (perimysium), and the fascia surrounding the individual muscle fibers (endomysium) (Fig. 1-1). Each of these layers of deep fascia gives rise to the next deeper layer. Although one of the roles of deep fascia is to restrict the outward (lateral) force of the muscle in contraction to direct and increase contractile

force, excessive restriction or limited elasticity is counterproductive.

Also, as described above, fascial surfaces can develop adhesions that prevent muscles from sliding smoothly against each other in movement. These adhesions must be broken up to restore smooth and pain-free movement.

Types of Fascial Treatment

Extensive treatment of fascia is beyond the scope of this book, but students need to be thoroughly familiar with fascia and its relationship to muscles and remain aware of the importance accorded to fascia by many treatment modalities.

In treating muscles, you are treating fascia: to try to deal with muscle and fascia separately is like trying to deal with a bubble separately from the air inside it. The reason the term *myofascial*

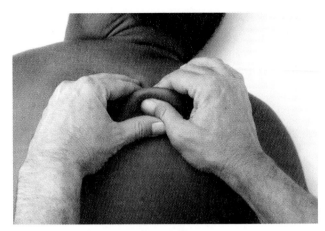

Figure 1-5 Skin rolling

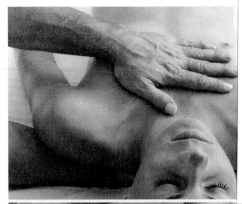

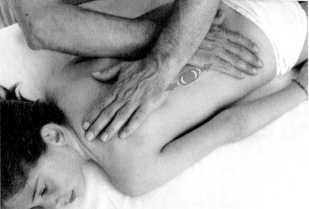

Figure 1-6 Myofascial release

is indispensable is that muscles and fascia are part and parcel of the same package. But just as a particular muscle can be treated in an area where several muscles lie in layers by the intention, depth, and angle of pressure, the fascia can also be singled out by intention and specific techniques.

There are several different approaches to fascial work:

- **Skin rolling** is a technique in which the tissue is picked up from the surface between the thumbs and fingertips. Both hands are usually used in skin rolling. The purposes of this technique are to increase flexibility in the superficial fascia and to treat tender points in the fascial layers (Fig. 1-5).
- **Myofascial release** is a system involving a gentle stretching process, often using two hands to engage and stretch the fascia and move with it according to its inclinations, as sensed by the hands (Fig. 1-6).

Directive fascial approaches (Fig. 1-7) include the following:

- **Bindegewebsmassage** (German, *connective tissue massage*) is a directive technique developed by Elisabeth Dicke.
- **Rolfing™, Hellerwork™,** and **CORE™ Myofascial Therapy** are other directive approaches to the reorientation of the fascia. The latter makes a point of working along Langer's lines, while the former two do not. These descriptions are oversimplifications; therapists interested in learning more about these modalities will need to study them in greater detail.

- **Neuromuscular therapy** is a system of myofascial treatment in which the thumbs are the primary instruments used to engage and release the fascia (Fig. 1-8). There are two chief schools of neuromuscular therapy, the British (Leon Chaitow) and the American (Paul St. John, Judith Walker Delaney).

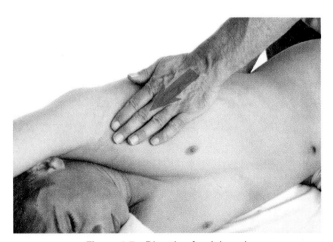

Figure 1-7 Directive fascial work

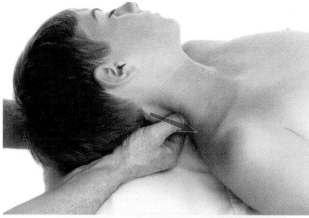

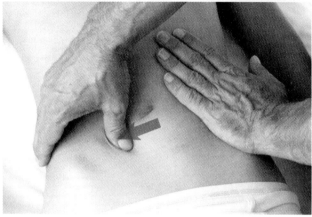

Figure 1-8 Neuromuscular therapy

Treating the Fascia

Fascial work is often a very helpful precursor to specific muscle treatment, as it warms and stimulates the tissue, and gives the muscle more freedom to expand into its fascial sheath. In the ensuing chapters on treatment, we will recommend and describe specific fascial treatments for the torso where we feel it is especially important. However, the principles of fascial treatment are easily transferred to other areas such as the limbs, and its application is helpful over the entire body.

Palpation of the fascia is a skill that can be learned only by experience. Place your hand lightly on any broad surface of skin, and take a few moments to become aware of the skin. Then allow your pressure to increase slightly, and become aware of the superficial fascia underneath the skin. Gently move the skin and fascia back and forth with your hand, becoming familiar with the feeling of moving both layers. Now allow your pressure to increase even more, sinking more deeply into the tissue, and become aware of the fascia as a sheath covering the muscle tissue.

Whenever you do fascial work, take the time to engage the fascia in this way. Once you have familiarized yourself with the sensation of touching the different layers, follow the instructions for fascial work on the torso given in Chapter 4.

BODY MECHANICS

Before addressing specific treatment techniques, we must first consider the demands of the therapist's body and the safest and most effective ways to use it.

Body mechanics is the key not only to safeguarding your own body integrity but also to the performance of effective therapy. It consists entirely of the use of common sense with regard to the placement and movement of weight in relation to gravity. Clients will often ask, "Don't you get tired?" or, "Don't your hands hurt?" If you have mastered good body mechanics, the answer will be no.

Just as massage therapy should take a holistic view of the client, the therapist must think of body mechanics in a holistic way. You do not work only with your thumb, your fingers, your hands, or even your body—you work with your whole self. Your approach to body mechanics, even though there are elements of it that focus on a small area, must take your whole person into consideration, from your emotional attitude to the position of your thumb joints.

Weight and gravity are the foremost mechanical considerations in body mechanics. We take gravity so much for granted that we seldom give it much thought, leaving our relationship to it in the hands of unconscious behavior patterns established early in life as we were learning to walk. But some activities require a conscious awareness of gravity. Dancers, for example, must relearn their relationship to gravity. So should massage therapists, because our work is largely based on the application of pressure, which is best accomplished through the application of our body weight. Therefore, the first principle of body mechanics is:

Use your body weight, rather than muscle force, to apply pressure.

Using your body weight requires less work. Using muscle strength to apply pressure in massage therapy quickly tires the therapist, particularly the local muscles used for the purpose. In addition, the use of weight applies a smoother pressure, lacking in tension, than the use of muscle force. When muscles sustain a contraction over even short periods of time, the process of recruitment and exhaustion at the tissue level results in an uneven pressure, which communicates a sense of tension to the client. To experience this difference, let someone apply pressure to the same part of your body, using the same point of compression (palm, thumb, knuckles, or whatever) with muscle force and then with body weight. Observe the difference in sensation of the pressure.

You do, of course, use your muscles to stabilize your joints. One of the chief functions of muscles in the body is to stabilize joints, and when using your body weight to apply pressure in therapy, this stabilization becomes a key element in the overall process. Therefore,

Keep the joints through which your weight passes relatively straight (but not locked) and avoid hyperextension of your joints (Fig. 1-9).

If you apply weight through locked joints, then the effect is one of total rigidity, like a solid rod. Although the pressure itself should come from the body weight, the joints should retain the "softness" supplied by muscle stabilization rather than being mechanically locked into place.

Hyperextension of joints stresses both the joint itself and the soft tissues that support and stabilize the joint. Use of muscle force in flexing the joint stresses the muscle themselves and communicates tension, as mentioned above. For example, it is known that carpal tunnel syndrome can be caused by repetitive hyperextension of the wrist, but in all

likelihood the actual causal factor is the resulting stress on the soft tissues that control and stabilize wrist and finger movement. To avoid the tissue stress and muscle tension of both flexion and hyperextension,

Let your weight pass through as many joints, in a relatively straight line, as feasible.

The weight that applies the pressure should be as much in line with the joints as possible. The weight that is applied to the client's body is the weight of the therapist's torso, while the point applying pressure is usually some part of the hand or forearm. By lining up the joints between the torso and the point of pressure, you maximize both the stability and the "softness" of the pressure. Since the shoulder joint is the primary joint for transmitting weight from the torso to the arm and hand,

Keep your scapula (glenohumeral joint) rotated downward.

If the glenohumeral joint is rotated upward, the weight of the torso has to be communicated to the arm indirectly by pulling downward at the joint. If it is rotated downward, the torso is above and behind the joint, and communicates the weight directly through the joints.

Support the body part applying the pressure whenever feasible (Figs. 1-10 and 1-11).

Supporting the thumb or fingertips of one hand with the other has two effects. First, it increases po-

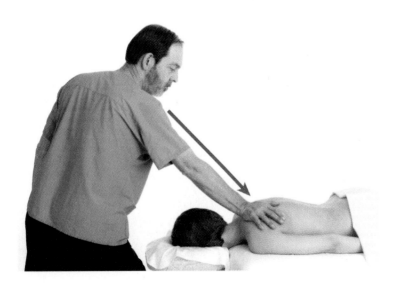

Figure 1-9   Avoid hyperextension of joints

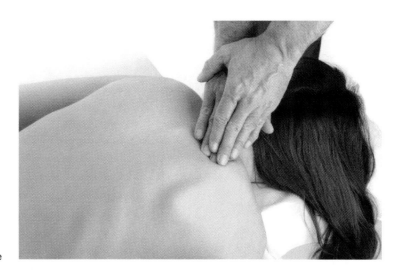

Figure 1-10 Supported pressure

tential pressure, and second, it stabilizes the joints involved to protect the hands from tissue strain.

Whether using muscles for force, stabilization, or movement, use larger, stronger ones rather than smaller, weaker ones.

For example:

Control your center of gravity with your legs; let movement come from your center of gravity and your legs rather than your arms (Fig. 1-12).

The use of the legs to control the placement and movement of one's weight raises an important question: *Should the legs always be placed in bal-* *ance under the center of gravity, or may the center of gravity fall between the legs of the therapist and the body of the client? That is, is it permissible to work off-balance and allow the client's body to support the weight of the torso?* Opinions of qualified therapists vary a great deal on this issue.

It is often helpful to allow the weight of the torso to be supported by the client's body, and it suggests itself intuitively. The biggest danger, of course, lies in the possible loss of balance (Fig. 1-13). This danger is probably greatest when the therapist is still inexperienced and has not yet learned either the subtleties of body mechanics or the qualities of skin (texture, moisture, etc.) that affect the ability to work safely in this way.

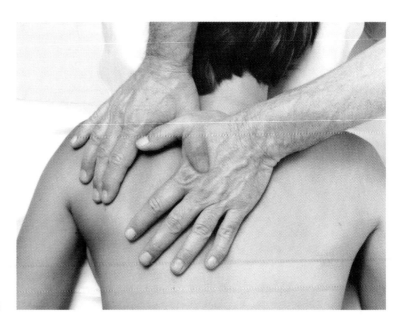

Figure 1-11 Supporting the thumb with the hand

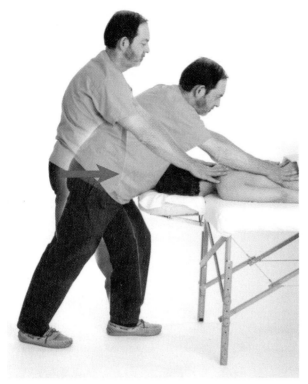

Figure 1-12   Let movement come from your center of gravity and your legs rather than your arms.

Sometimes it is advantageous to work from underneath the client's body, using the client's, rather than the therapist's, weight to apply pressure. This positioning is often an effective way to work, but it must be applied carefully, as its body mechanics is more challenging.

For example, when working from underneath the neck of a supine client, you should be careful not to hyperextend the thumb. When working from underneath on the abdomen or pelvis of a prone client, the same care should be taken with the fingers. Since more muscles are used in these positions to apply force, and smaller muscles are used to stabilize joints, such work should not be done over an extended period. Also, you will need to be even more conscious than usual of feelings of pain or fatigue in your hands.

Sometimes it is advantageous to let your weight generate force through a part of your body other than your shoulder. For example, you can nestle your elbow in your own iliac fossa (just inside your anterior pelvis) and lean into it to transmit force when working on a lateral area on the client's body (Fig. 1-14).

Move into, and out of, pressure slowly.

Slow movement is gentler and less jarring both to the client's tissues (and your own) and to the client's consciousness. Moving slowly into and out of pressure also enables you to monitor the feedback of both your own and the client's body. If your work is not to be purely mechanical, then it is vital that you focus on the tissues you are working with, and take time to exert and release pressure on them. In addition, sensitive tissues (especially the muscles of the lumbar region) are often subject to rebound tenderness. The sudden release of pressure can be painful.

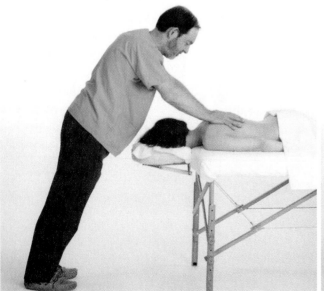
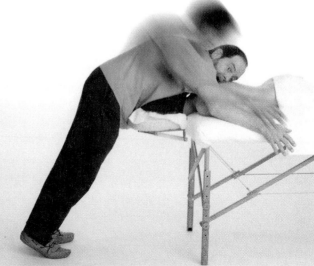

Figure 1-13   Don't lose your balance

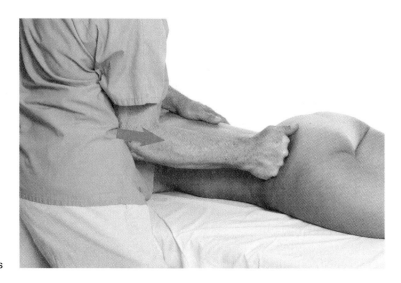

Figure 1-14 Transmitting weight through the pelvis

Finally, pay attention to your body. Get to know your own body, and use the mechanics of your own body.

It is important to get to know your body, its strengths and weaknesses, and its weight distribution. If you've ever watched a baseball game on television, then you've probably heard the announcers comment on the peculiarity of a batter's stance. Every baseball player has to find the batting stance that gives him the greatest control and hitting power. The stance varies from player to player, and your own application of body mechanics in therapy will be somewhat different from anyone else's, although the same general principles apply.

Although it may seem peripheral to body mechanics proper, one final point that needs to mentioned here is the use of the secondary hand.

Use your secondary hand mindfully, not casually.

When one is not performing a two-handed stroke or using one hand to support the other, one hand is used to apply pressure or otherwise manipulate tissue. This hand is called the primary hand. Deciding what to do with the secondary hand is important and should not be made in a casual and unconscious way.

The secondary hand is often referred to by shiatsu practitioners as the "mother hand," which is an apt way of thinking of it. If the hand is not used actively to perform some specific function, it can be used to nurture the client. Even then, be careful and conscious of where the hand is placed. Remember to place each hand carefully and consciously before beginning to work.

VARIETIES OF SOFT-TISSUE MANIPULATION

Remember the third basic premise of clinical massage therapy: *the soft tissues of the body respond to touch.* The touch may be extremely gentle or quite forceful, it may be moving or still, but touch, for reasons not yet understood, elicits a response from the soft tissues. If the touch is artfully applied, then the response can be one of healing.

The classical strokes used in Swedish, or relaxation, massage, are quite effective in inducing a generalized relaxation response from the soft tissues and, thus, in the whole person. But the treatment of specific complaints of myofascial pain and dysfunction require a more specific approach.

Clinical massage therapy requires a thorough knowledge of the anatomy and physiology of the soft tissues and the bones and joints they serve. In addition, knowledge of anatomy and physiology will enable therapists to avoid causing injury or gratuitous pain and to recognize contraindications to the work. Therapists must also be thoroughly familiar with the varieties of approaches to the manipulation of the soft tissues. In the end, however, therapists will range from poor to brilliant according to their mastery of the *art* of clinical massage therapy, which is an indefinable combination of intelligence and intuition. This *art* cannot be forced; it comes with a sense of love and devotion to the work and the desire to do it well, and with time and practice, like learning to speak a foreign language, or sing a song, or to dance or swim or play tennis. It arrives when your therapy becomes more than the sum of its mechanical parts.

The purpose of this book is not to set forth a series of treatments of various muscles in a mechanical fashion, as one might write a manual for small engine repair. Its purpose is to help the student investigate the possibilities for manipulation of each muscle and to explore the responses to such work. Just as each singer must discover, through practice, the optimum control of her own vocal chords, clinical massage therapists must continue to explore touching in a variety of ways, constantly evaluating the results of the touch by feeling and observation and feedback from the client—and not just during the "student" period, but throughout their careers.

The purpose of this section is to introduce you to some of the basic ways in which the soft tissues can be touched and manipulated for therapeutic benefit. The approaches and techniques in this section can be applied to a variety of muscles over the whole body. They will be referred to throughout the book as we deal with each specific muscle or muscle group. These techniques are by no means a comprehensive list of possible approaches to tissue manipulation. They are only the most basic techniques. Therapists will expand their repertoire as they study and gain experience.

The intention of the techniques used in clinical massage therapy is to eliminate pain and/or dysfunction in the tissue by inducing persistently contracted tissue to lengthen. The principal difference between the classic strokes used in Swedish massage and the tissue manipulations used in clinical massage therapy is that the former tend to be broader and more general, the latter to be more concentrated and specific.

The Art of Direct Tissue Manipulation: The "Tissue Dialogue"

The key to the art of tissue manipulation is sensitive palpation. Palpation should always be performed initially with the tips of the fingers or thumbs before compressive treatment is begun. One must palpate for the point of resistance in the tissue, then meet it with pressure. Sometimes the resistance will yield only to firm pressure, sometimes to delicate pressure. *The therapist must gauge the willingness of the tissue to respond and adjust the pressure accordingly.* This mindful sensitivity to the tissue might aptly be called the "tissue dialogue," because the therapist, through palpation, negotiates with the tissue the pressure needed to accomplish release. This "dialogue" is the essence of the art of direct tissue manipulation.

All of these manipulative techniques can be used for both *still compression* and *gliding com-*

pression; in fact, you should find yourself alternating between the two: moving through the tissue, and stopping where the condition of the tissue calls for it.

The Tools of the Therapist's Body

Depending on the area and the purpose, different body parts of the therapist can be used to manipulate tissue:

The Heel of the Hand

The heel of the hand, or thenar and hypothenar eminences, can be used to apply a fairly broad compression. It is especially useful when used on larger muscles, such as leg muscles, gluteals, shoulders, or paraspinal muscles. It is also useful over large bony areas, such as the iliac crest. Set in motion, the heel of the hand compresses a relatively wide swath of tissue (Fig. 1-15).

When using the heel of the hand, avoid hyperextension of your wrist. Feel the tissue as you compress it, and be sensitive to tight, hardened areas. Use this information to determine whether another, more localized, stroke should be applied in certain areas.

The Fist

Another way to apply broad compression is with the closed fist. A particular advantage is the ability to shift between broad compression applied with the full length of the proximal phalanges (the bones of the fingers), and more focused compression with the knuckles (the proximal interphalangeal joints). Again, avoid hyperextension of the wrist. Go slower over hypercontracted areas and negotiate depth of pressure and speed of motion with the tissue.

The Knuckle(s)

The proximal interphalangeal joints, or knuckles, of the index and middle fingers can also be used for compression. Knuckles are helpful as an alternative to fingertips to avoid constant strain to the fingers and thumbs. Because the knuckles present a harder and less sensitive compressive surface than the fingertips, the tissue should first be palpated with the fingers before using a knuckle for compression. In sensitive areas, such as the face, neck, and ribs, fingertips are preferable to knuckles.

The Thumb or Fingertips

Still or gliding compression using the tip of the thumb or finger is ideal for the treatment of small,

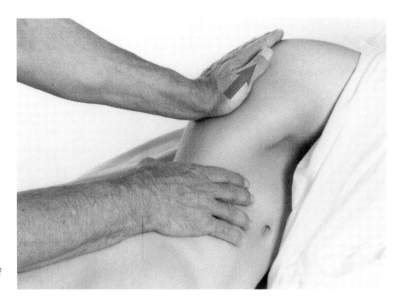

Figure 1-15 Moving compression with the heel of the hand

concentrated areas, such as trigger points or other tender points. It is important to keep body mechanics in mind while applying pressure with the fingers and thumbs, as it can place a tremendous strain on the muscles of the hand and forearm, especially to points deep in the body. It is often wise to support the fingers or thumb with the other hand to help prevent hyperextension of the joints and provide additional pressure. Throughout this book, we will show the use of fingertips and thumbs, sometime supported, sometimes not. In every case, the practitioner may choose whether to support the thumbs or fingertips according to her or his needs.

Remember to line up as many joints in as straight a line as is feasible, and to use your body weight, rather than muscular force, whenever possible. When it is not possible to use your body weight, as in approaching posterior neck muscles in the supine client, you should strive to line up several joints, and pause and alternate hands frequently.

Although they may be used anywhere on the body, the thumbs and fingertips are used almost exclusively in some areas, such as the face, neck, axilla, abdomen, groin, and all internal work, where the touch must be controlled and sensitive (Fig. 1-16).

The Elbow

The elbow, specifically the olecranon process of the ulna (the bony point of the elbow), is an extremely useful tool for compression (Fig. 1-17). Its use has a number of caveats:

1. An extraordinary amount of force can be applied with the elbow; compression should

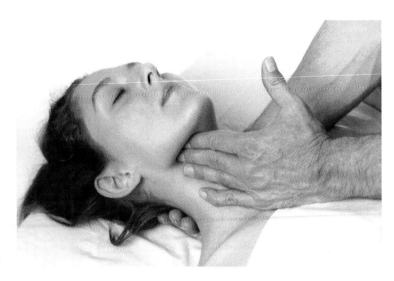

Figure 1-16 Use fingertips in sensitive areas

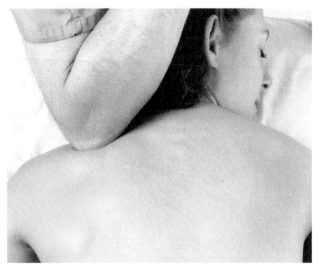

Figure 1-17 Using the elbow for compression

therefore be initiated slowly and applied gradually, with a great deal of attention to the client's responses.

2. The elbow is far less sensitive than the tips of the thumb or fingers. The tissues should be explored first with the fingers, and the elbow used primarily for compression once the need and location have been established.
3. Use of the elbow should be avoided in highly sensitive areas, such as the face, neck, and groin.

The Forearm

The ulnar aspect of the forearm provides a broad surface for deep, gliding compression (Fig. 1-18) of long, straight muscles, such as the erector spinae muscles and many muscles of the leg. Like the elbow, it is comparatively insensi-

tive; palpate the area before treating with the forearm.

Specific Treatment Techniques

Holding

The whole hand, or both hands, may be used to hold an area of the body. Several intentions and effects are possible with this approach:

- *Simple holding* can warm and nurture and communicate intention. Holding a body part in one or both hands involves a physical warming effect and suggests relaxation to the client (Fig. 1-19).
- *Intentional holding* suggests change. The body part is held in one or both hands with a gentle pressure in the direction of a desired change, with the slack being taken up as it occurs.
- *Holding with varying compressions* is a gentle way of applying compression with different parts of the hand. The body part is held in one or both hands and pressure is applied with the fingertips, thumbs, and heads of the phalanges and metacarpals, and possibly even squeezed in places, in varying patterns with varying pressure. These varying applications of pressure may also be combined with intentional holding. This "whole hand work" combines suggestion with an element of confusion that allows muscles to be caught "off-guard" and lengthen.

Compression

Compression consists of pressure exerted perpendicular to the surface of the muscle. Where there

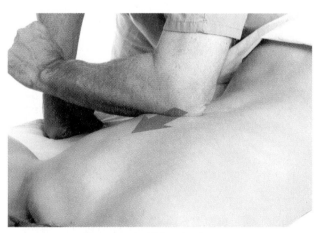

Figure 1-18 Using the forearm

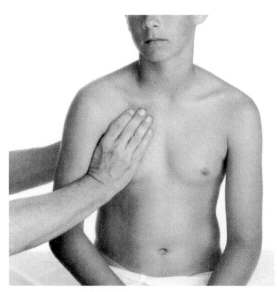

Figure 1-19 Holding

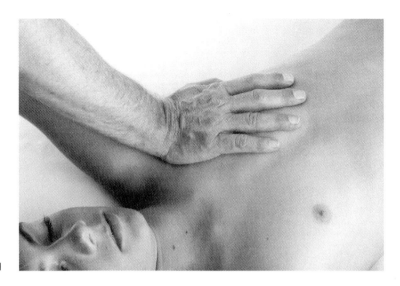

Figure 1-20 Broad compression with the hand

is underlying bone, the muscle tissue is compressed against the bone; otherwise, pressure is exerted against the resistance of the deeper structures of the body. Compression may be firm or light, as appropriate, and may be applied broadly by the entire hand (Fig. 1-20) or on a concentrated point by the thumb, fingertip, or elbow (Fig. 1-21).

Pressure is maintained until release is felt, or until the client reports easing of the pain associated with the point.

Pincer Palpation/Compression

Muscles that present a considerable amount of tissue above the surface of the body can be exam-

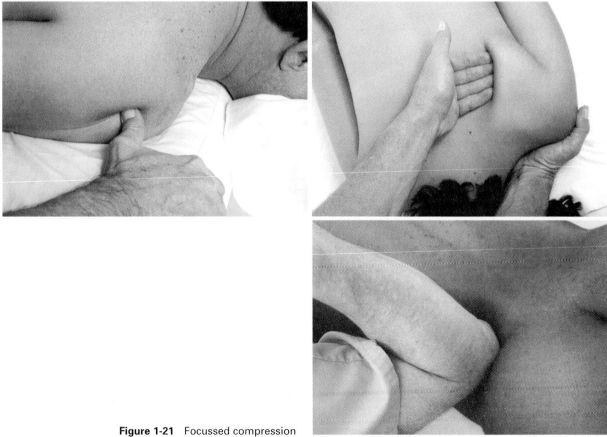

Figure 1-21 Focussed compression

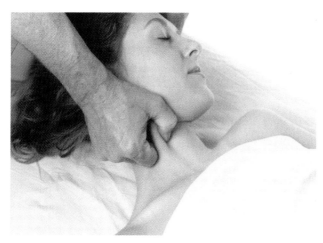

Figure 1-22 Pincer compression of sternocleidomastoid

ined and treated very effectively with pincer palpation and compression. Examples are sternocleidomastoid (Fig. 1-22), pectoralis major, the portion of trapezius that lies on top of the shoulder, and the more proximal aspects of the hip adductors.

To perform this technique, grasp the tissue between the thumb and the tips of the first two or three fingers, or the outside of the bent index finger. Each then provides a firm surface against which the other can palpate and compress. Search the tissues carefully for trigger points or other sensitive points. When you find such a point, hold it until you feel it release, then continue the search.

Stripping or Stripping Massage
This technique involves gliding pressure along a muscle, usually from one attachment to the other in the direction of the muscle fiber (Fig. 1-23).

 Caution

Stripping massage is often called for in areas covered in hair, such as the head, the back of the neck, and the pubic bone. Also, some men have extensive hair on the chest, back, arms, and legs. Painful pulling of body hair is always a danger with stripping massage in these areas. Ask the client to tell you when such pulling occurs. A small amount of lubricant may be helpful. Deep-tissue creams and lotions are generally better for this type of work than oils.

Cross-Fiber Friction
Persistently contracted muscle tissue, lesions in tendons or ligaments, and areas of fibrosis can be effectively treated with friction moving the fingertips, thumb, or elbow back and forth across the muscle perpendicular to the fiber (Fig. 1-24). This technique is most frequently performed on or near the attachment.

Passive Stretching
Although trigger points may be treated directly with any of the above techniques, resolution of them requires passive stretching of the muscle as soon after treatment as possible. The therapist stretches the muscle by moving its attachments away from each other (Fig. 1-25). This technique

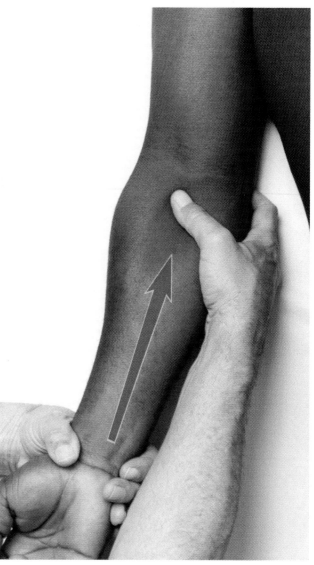

Figure 1-23 Stripping, or stripping massage

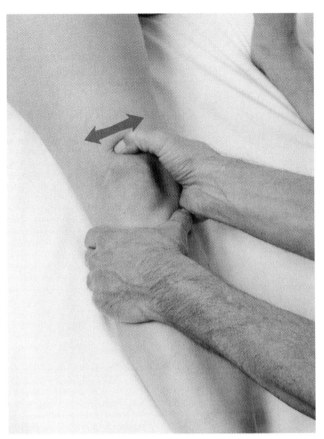

Figure 1-24 Cross-fiber friction

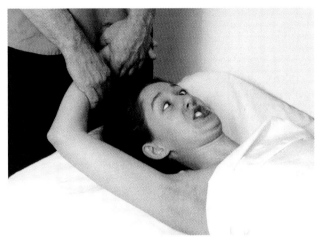

Figure 1-26 Unfortunate passive stretching

requires an intimate knowledge of the anatomy of the joints involved and their range of motion.

Approach stretching with care. Familiarize yourself with the range of motion of each joint, and move into the stretch slowly. It is very easy to place a client in an uncomfortable position (Fig. 1-26).

Most of the manual therapy descriptions in this book are of stripping massage and compression, with a few examples of cross-fiber friction and stretching where such techniques seem particularly appropriate. These descriptions should be taken as examples and starting points, not as an exhaustive repertoire. Each student should experiment with them, as well as with other possibilities not illustrated.

TABLES

Students of massage therapy will certainly be familiar with standard massage tables. The most popular tables are portable, and can be adjusted in height between clients. Therapists generally set the table height according to their own height and the type of work they plan to do. Clinical massage therapy, however, makes special demands. The optimum table height may vary according to the type of work being done and the position of the client. You may use several different treatment approaches in a session, and place the client in several different positions. To accommodate this flexibility in treatment, the ideal solution is an adjustable electric table. There is a wide variety of such tables available, either mechanical or pneumatic, at a wide variety of prices. These tables are considerably more expensive than a standard portable table, but the investment is well worthwhile, since it enhances both the quality of the work that can be done and the comfort and health of the therapist.

In addition, many therapists find an arched table to be a helpful addition to the treatment room. Such tables include the BodyBridge™ (Fig. 1-27A) or the Khalsa Bodywork Table™ (Fig. 1-27B).

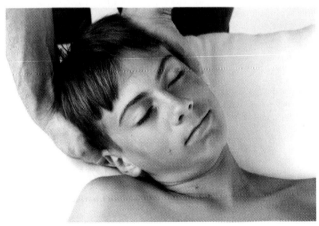

Figure 1-25 Passive stretching

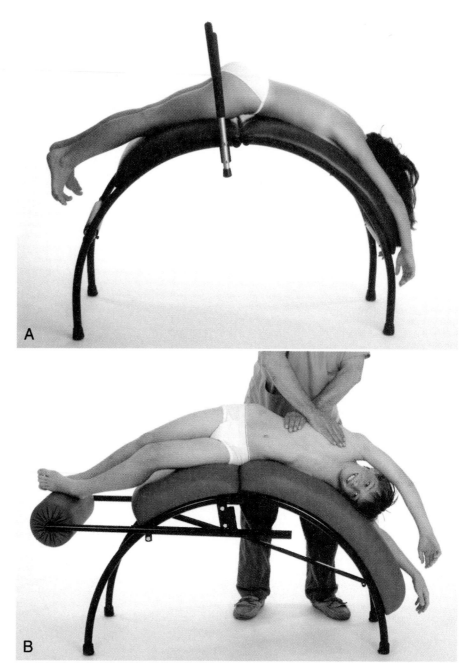

Figure 1-27 Arched tables: Body-Bridge (A) and Khalsa Bodywork Table (B)

DRAPING

Most examination and treatment in massage therapy and bodywork require some exposure of the body. Therefore, we need to consider ways of respecting the client's feelings of privacy and modesty, while still accomplishing the therapeutic goal. *Draping* is the term commonly used for the covering of the parts of the client's body that are not being examined or treated. The term originated in the art world, where it referred to the drapery of the subject of a painting or sculpture. In the last century it came to be used in photography as well, and from that field was adopted by the medical profession.

The codes of ethics and standards of practice of various organizations vary somewhat, but all require consideration of the client's feelings of privacy and modesty. The National Certification Board for Therapeutic Massage and Bodywork states in its Code of Ethics that the certificant shall "provide draping and treatment in a way that ensures the safety, comfort, and privacy of the client," and in its Standards of Practice that the certificant shall "use appropriate draping to protect the client's physical and emotional privacy." Although these requirements are unequivocal about the need to consider the client's sense of privacy and modesty, they are not specific in describing precisely what draping is to be used. Therapists, therefore, have the responsibility to determine the best ways to meet these requirements in their own clinical settings with regard to each individual client.

In addition to requirements of professional organizations, therapists must also consider the laws of the jurisdictions in which they practice. In states where massage therapy is licensed, there will normally be a board that issues guidelines for the conduct of practitioners. These guidelines often contain more or less specific provisions regarding draping of clients. Some guidelines, for example, specifically permit the uncovering of buttocks or female breasts with the consent of the client, while others may specifically prohibit such exposure. In states that do not have licensure, laws may exist either at the state or local level that restrict their conduct in some way. Therapists must, therefore, take the responsibility for investigating the laws and guidelines that govern their practices.

Early in the chapter we saw that clinical massage therapy is the result of the coalescence of traditional massage, osteopathic and other techniques, and the bodywork heritage of Wilhelm Reich and Ida Rolf. In traditional massage, the client normally lies prone or supine on a table, with private areas of the body covered by a towel or a sheet. Each area is uncovered by the therapist

as necessary for treatment. In the bodywork tradition, the emphasis is on the structure of the body as a whole. For that reason, clients are first observed while standing, usually in underwear. Most schools of massage therapy teach conservative, traditional draping techniques, and require that these techniques be used when practicing massage therapy in the school setting. As therapists move beyond basic Swedish massage, however, they are likely to need more flexibility in methods of draping to perform the variety of techniques for examination and treatment available to them.

Therefore, depending on the approach, the therapist, the client, and applicable regulations, the client may wear underwear or not, be covered by a sheet or towel, wear an examination gown, or any combination of these choices. With the understanding that both therapists and clients vary widely in their needs, we will present a variety of illustrations of suggested draping for the examination and treatment of each area of the body. Throughout the chapters on treatment, our technique for illustrating internal structures dictates that adult models be shown with only minimal draping and child models in underwear, but we will refer back to the appropriate draping illustrations for the benefit of the student.

We show the basic techniques of draping clients with sheets in supine and prone positions. In conjunction with the technique for draping female breasts for abdominal massage, we show a way of arranging the drape for treating the chest muscles. We also show techniques for draping clients in a sidelying position. This position is well suited for performing certain techniques. It is also appropriate for the general treatment of pregnant women, and we provide illustrations for that specific situation.

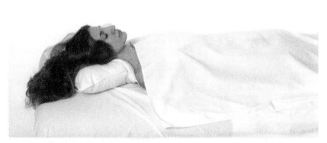

1: Head and neck

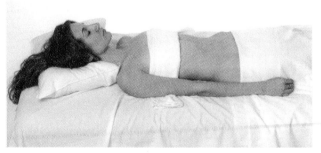

2: Abdomen

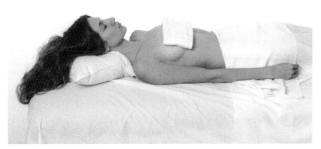

3: Chest muscles

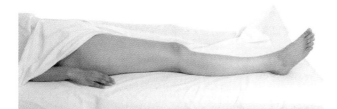

4: Anterior leg

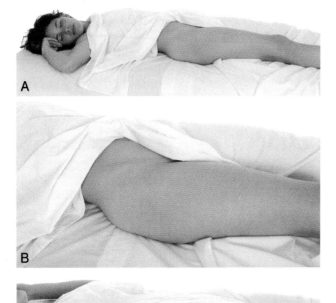

A

B

C

5: Groin and lower abdomen (A and B, sheet; C, examination gown)

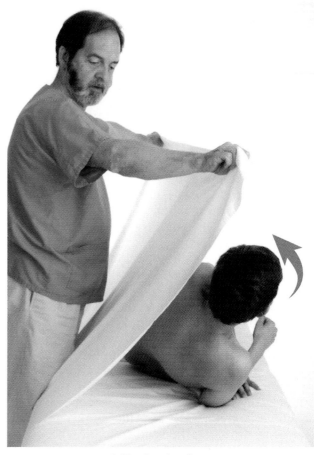

6: Turning the client

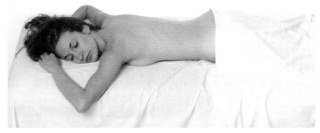

7: Back

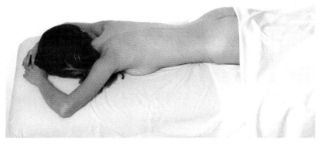

8: Between buttocks

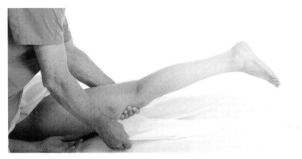

9: Positioning the sheet under the leg

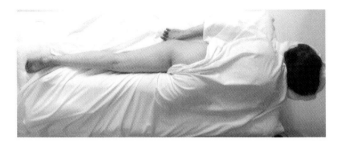

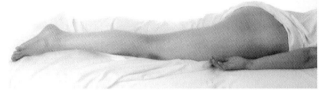

10: Posterior leg and buttock

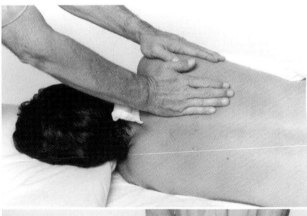

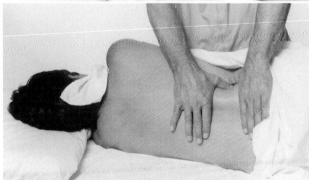

11: Sidelying: shoulder and back (pregnant client)

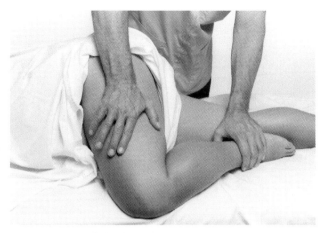

12: Sidelying: thigh (pregnant client)

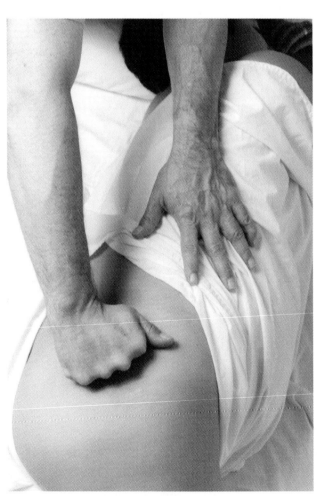

13: Sidelying: buttock (pregnant client)

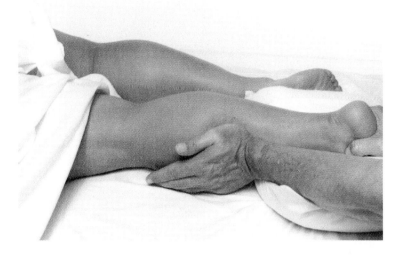

14: Sidelying: lower leg (pregnant client)

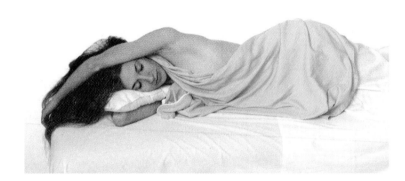

15: Sidelying: shoulder and chest (examination gown)

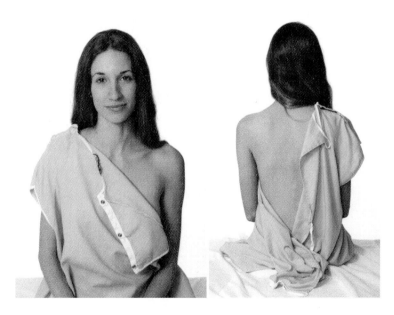

16: Sitting: shoulder and chest (examination gown)

Some therapists may find it helpful to use an examination gown in some situations, either instead of or in addition to a sheet, towel, or underwear. The most versatile such gown for massage therapy unfastens across each shoulder. The use of these gowns is illustrated as an option for treatment of some areas.

CHAPTER SUMMARY

1. Massage therapy is experiencing a renaissance as more and more people discover its effectiveness not only for promoting relaxation and relief from stress, but also for resolving pain and dysfunction. Clinical massage therapy and bodywork are the result of the coalescence of several historical currents, including the work of such pioneers as Wilhelm Reich, Ida Rolf, Janet Travell, David Simons, Leon Chaitow, and many others.

2. A basic understanding of the microanatomy and physiology of muscles and fascia and their relationship to the nervous system helps the massage therapist comprehend the issues involved in myofascial pain and dysfunction, and the treatment and resolution of such problems in the clinical setting. As therapists work from the outside in, they must learn the art of fascial palpation by experience, and prepare areas of the body for more specific work by first stretching and releasing the fascia from the superficial to the deeper levels.

3. One of the keys to successful bodywork is the awareness and care for the therapist's own body. It is important, therefore, for the therapist to learn good body mechanics, both for effective therapy and for the therapist's safety.

4. Various parts of the therapist's arm and hand, including fist, thumb, fingertips, knuckles, forearm, and elbow, are used as tools in the treatment of the soft tissues. There are many different ways of applying these tools, the most basic being compression, stripping massage, cross-fiber friction, and passive stretching.

5. Although a standard portable table is usually sufficient for the practice of Swedish massage, the demands of clinical massage therapy make an adjustable electric table preferable. Many bodyworkers also use a specialized table, such as an arched table, in their practices.

6. The therapist must consider the privacy and comfort of the client when unclothed. Local regulations, requirements of professional organizations, the specific professional setting in which the therapist works, and the personal comfort of both the practitioner and the client need to be taken into consideration in making decisions about draping the client.

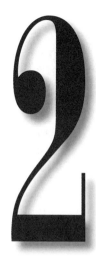

"One must always think of everything."
— *Eugene Ionesco,* The Bald Soprano

Approaching Assessment

The purpose of any system of clinical assessment is to describe pathology or dysfunction in a way that suggests effective treatment. The term *clinical* massage therapy is more accurate than *medical* massage therapy because clinical massage therapists view the body from a different perspective than that of the physician. We do not treat conditions according to medical diagnostic criteria, but according to clinical massage therapy assessment criteria.

For example, a physician might diagnose a patient as having tendinitis. This diagnosis implies an inflammation of a tendon, indicating a prescription for anti-inflammatory medication, rest, and application of ice. The same person might be assessed by a clinical massage therapist as having persistently contracted muscle tissue with referred pain from trigger point activity, indicating deep tissue therapy and trigger point compression. The physician and the clinical massage therapist are addressing the same complaint in the same patient from two different perspectives. Neither is wrong, and each perspective may inform the other. Therefore, it is important for the clinical massage therapist to develop a familiarity with medical diagnostic terms and concepts, and learn to consider them when assessing the client.

The first priority in relaxation (Swedish) massage is the client's comfort. Within appropriate limits, the wishes and personal preferences of the client take precedence, and the objective is to give the client a pleasant and relaxing experience. The first priority in clinical practice, however, is to offer effective treatment, with all procedures subject to the informed consent of the client. The first step in treating clients effectively is to correctly identify the areas that need treatment. For this reason, a systematic and intelligent approach to examination and assessment is essential in clinical massage therapy.

Good assessment requires that we look for the following (after Leon Chaitow, DO):

■ Patterns of misuse
■ Postural imbalances
■ Shortened postural muscles
■ Weakened muscles
■ Problems in specific muscles and other soft tissues, such as trigger points, tender points, and areas of persistent shortening
■ Restrictions in joints
■ Dysfunctional patterns in coordination, balance, gait, respiration

The epigraph to this chapter, "One must always think of everything," may seem daunting at first, but it emphasizes the comprehensive nature of effective examination in clinical massage therapy. The body is a system of interdependent elements, and all of those elements must be considered when determining how to solve problems of pain and dysfunction.

The primary methods used to gather information about a client's problem include taking the client's history (both written and oral), observing the client informally, measuring the client's body, formally observing or measuring certain activities, and manually examining the tissues. It is important to remember that examination and assessment do not end in the initial session; it is an ongoing process. This constant reexamination and reassessment is a particular feature of clinical massage therapy, since the hands-on nature of the work involves sensory feedback that regularly informs the direction of treatment.

CLIENT HISTORY

Designing a Form for Client Information

Practitioners usually need to gather certain client information for business purposes, such as the client's name, address, phone number, and so on. This information is most easily acquired by having clients fill out a form at the initial visit. It can also be helpful to use the same form to gather information about the client's circumstances and history. The form can serve as a starting point for the gathering of more information in the history interview.

In designing a form, think about what information is best obtained in writing and what information requires a more personal, in-depth exploration. Personal data, family information, occupation, and names of primary health care practitioners (or current specialists) are best acquired on a form. These items are fairly easy to decide on.

It is more difficult to decide, however, what to ask about health history on a form. On the one hand, it's best not to leave all health history to the interview, because it's too easy to digress and overlook important issues. On the other hand, an overly lengthy and complicated history questionnaire may seem tedious and irrelevant. The object is to compose a form that both is succinct and accounts for most possibilities.

In addition to the form itself, clients may be given a drawing of the human form on which they can mark the areas where they are feeling pain or have felt pain recently. On the following sample form, this information is sought both in words on the form itself (Fig. 2-1) and on the accompanying figures (Fig. 2-2). This duplication serves as a double-check to make sure all the possibilities are covered.

Remember that clients have their own points of view. They may consider the information to be irrelevant that we see as important, and not think to mention it. It is our job to collect all the data that we may need for our purposes, while clarifying the relevance of this data to the client.

Conducting the Interview

Although the primary purpose of the history interview is to gather information and establish rapport, it is also a good time to begin educating your

INFORMATION FORM

Name: _____   Height _____   Weight _____

Address:

_____

Home phone: _____   Work phone: _____   Cell phone: _____   E-mail: _____

Date of birth: _____   Sex: M   F   Living status: Coupled   Uncoupled

How did you hear of The Pain and Posture Clinic? _____

Name, sexes and ages of children in the home:

History of injuries, illnesses and/or surgeries:

Regular physical activities/sports:

Circle any of the following that you have or have had within the past year:

PAIN: Headaches   Back   Chest   Abdomen   Hip   Leg

       Shoulder   Neck   Arm   Pelvis   Groin

       Buttock

DISORDERS: Digestion   Cramps   Seizures   Asthma   Fibromyalgia/CFS

           Scoliosis   Depression   Anxiety

Other:

_____

Present medications:

_____

Family or general physician:

_____

Specialist:

_____

Figure 2-1   Intake form

client. For example, clients with possible work-related problems may need to consider ergonomics, repetitive motions, or other problems, such as holding the telephone with their shoulders or working at a poorly set up computer station. Some people undertake exercise programs without proper advice. The initial interview provides an opportunity to introduce these issues.

During the interview you may find yourself "thinking out loud"—that is, sharing your

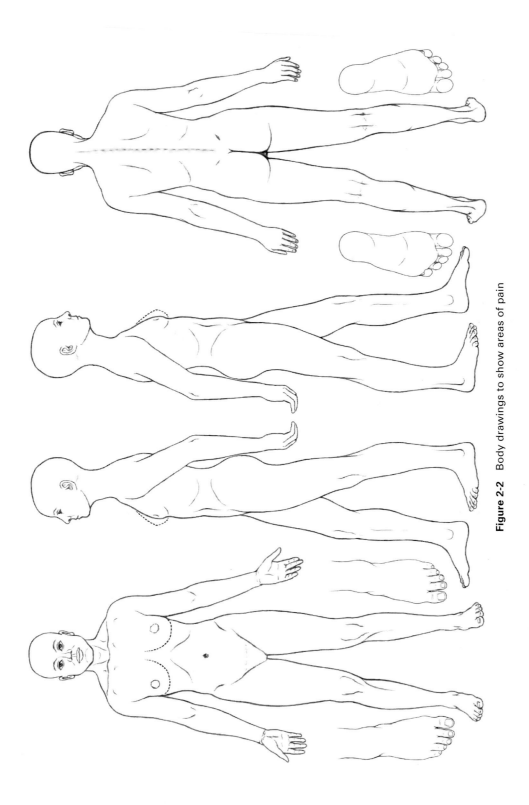

Figure 2-2 Body drawings to show areas of pain

thoughts with the client as the interview progresses. Including the clients as you process their information may encourage them to think about their muscular system in a new way. It also builds a team approach to therapy.

Like other aspects of the assessment process, the interview has a dual purpose—both holistic and reductionistic. On the one hand, you are seeking to build a broad picture of the client and the circumstances of his or her life to determine what may be causing problems and what kinds of solutions may be most effective. On the other hand, you must remain alert to clues to the cause of the specific complaint. In some cases, the injury may have occurred at a specific time when performing a precise movement (e.g., "I lunged after the ball and felt a sharp pain in my groin.") Most of the time, however, the onset and origin of the presenting problem will be much more vague, and will require some detective work on your part. The key to the solution will often lie hidden in the information gathered in the interview.

Ideally, taking a history should be a warm, human encounter, rather than a mechanical process in which the therapist sits with pen poised, reading questions and taking down answers. You should develop the ability to hold a relaxed, conversational interview while also keeping a mental checklist of important areas to cover. In the beginning of your practice, you may want to have a written checklist to consult. This checklist will vary somewhat, of course, from one client and one problem to the next, but the overall territory will remain the same. Above all, do not assume that the client will volunteer important information. Remember that what is important to you may seem trivial to the client. Be thorough.

Your checklist should include the following items:

Presenting Problem:
- What brought you here?
- Where do you hurt?
- What doesn't work right?
- How long has it been this way? When did it start?
- If the pain is the result of a specific injury, exactly how did the injury occur? What physical position were you in when the injury occurred? What was the course of the rest of the day, and of the next couple of days? Describe the pain, swelling, limitation of motion, and treatment (including self-treatment) that occurred over the course of the rest of the day, as well as the days following the injury.
- Have you ever had this problem before? When, and under what circumstances? When was the first time?
- When is the pain worse? When is it better?
- What makes the pain worse? What makes it better? In what physical position does it feel worst and best?
- Whom else have you consulted? What did they say and do?

Health History:
- How is your general health?
- Have you had any recent illnesses, injuries, surgeries?
- Have you ever had any major illnesses, injuries, surgeries?
- Do you have a history of heart problems or neurological problems?
- Is there any history in your family of brain or neurological disorders, such as stroke?
- Are you under a doctor's care for any condition? If yes, what condition? Are you taking any medications?
- Who are your regular caregivers? Do you see a chiropractor, osteopath, naturopath, or any other sort of physician? Any other kind of health professional?

Athletic History:
- Do you play any sports? Work out? Have you ever?
- As a child or teenager, did you take dance? Were you a cheerleader? What were your activities?

Personal/Family/Social History:
- Are you married? Single? Any children?
- Describe any recent stressors in your home environment.
- What do you do for recreation?
- What are your primary sources of stress?

Occupational History:
- What is your occupation? What does it involve—i.e., what do you do all day? How much do you sit, stand, move about? Is there any heavy lifting? Repetitive motion? Does any work activity cause pain?
- How often do you take breaks, and for how long? What do you do during breaks?

■ What types of work have you done in the past?

■ Have you ever had any work-related injuries?

Feel free to add to this checklist; your own knowledge and imagination will find questions to ask and leads to pursue that lie beyond these boundaries. You should certainly follow up on any questions in your mind.

WHOLE-BODY ASSESSMENT

Most of our clientele is accustomed to thinking in terms of traditional medical approaches. If they present with a specific injury, then they expect the examination and treatment to focus on the injury and its immediately surrounding area. In many cases this expectation may be appropriate: it is certainly possible to suffer an isolated injury at a precise site that can be specifically treated. In most cases, however, a broader approach is needed. Most myofascial pain or dysfunction results from alignment problems of long duration, and most local injuries, if left untreated, will eventually affect other parts of the body. For this reason, it is usually appropriate and desirable to evaluate the alignment of the body as a whole before initiating treatment.

Some clients will refuse such an evaluation and insist on strictly local treatment. The need for informed consent requires that therapists share their assessment of the problem with the client and propose a course of examination and treatment, including possible alternatives. One of the alternatives is, of course, palliative treatment. As long as therapists are honest with clients about what they believe is wrong and what they believe to be the ideal course of action, it is appropriate to work with such clients to alleviate their symptoms on a short-term basis. For such clients, the therapist may perform a more abbreviated interview, confined largely to the circumstances that seem relevant to the chief complaint, then skip directly to examination of the area of the presenting problem.

For those clients, however, who agree to pursue a whole-body approach, an examination of body alignment can be crucial to forming the clinical picture. The extent of such an examination can vary according to the skills and judgment of the therapist and the specific situation. A description of the basic requirements for an assessment is presented in the following sections.

Informal Observation

In this first step in the whole-body assessment, the therapist observes the client carefully, beginning with the first encounter in the waiting area. How does the client sit? Stand? Walk? Sit down again in the treatment room? The clinical massage therapist should cultivate this observational habit, which can easily be practiced in any public place.

Formal Alignment Examination

A thorough, formal examination of body alignment, or posture, should be carried out with the client wearing as little clothing as possible, since it involves not only global observation but fairly precise scrutiny of surface landmarks and their movements. A complete examination is most commonly carried out with clients wearing underwear, but individual therapists can establish their own protocols.

Photographs

Many therapists take photographs of clients as part of a complete alignment examination. Advantages of this practice include:

■ The client is able to see what the therapist sees.

■ The therapist has access to the photographs in the absence of the client for treatment planning purposes.

■ If the therapist has a computer, then photographs can be scanned in (or taken initially with a digital camera), and lines or grids can be drawn to help analyze deviations. Copies can be printed for the client.

■ Photographs taken before and after treatment can provide documentation of changes.

Note: Photographs should be taken either with a digital camera or a Polaroid camera, since sending film out to be processed compromises client privacy and confidentiality.

Whether being photographed or observed without photography, clients should be asked to stand in a way that feels reasonably straight, but relaxed and normal, with the hands at the sides. Clients whose hair falls below the shoulders should be asked to push it back for a front view and forward for a back view.

The client should first be photographed full front, full back, left side, and right side. Then the client may be asked to cross the wrists and stretch the arms overhead as high as possible. This stance

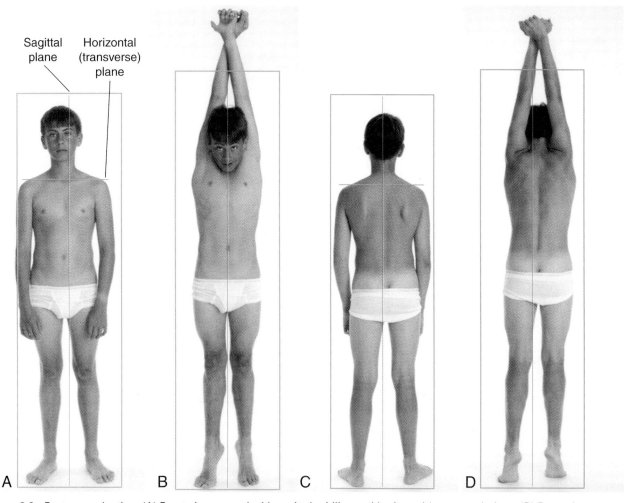

Figure 2-3 Posture evaluation: (A) Front view normal with sagittal midline and horizontal (transverse) plane. (B) Front view stretched with sagittal midline. (C) Back view normal with sagittal midline and horizontal (transverse) plane. (D) Back view stretched with sagittal midline

shows the corrections or exaggerations that take place in a stretched position. Crossing the wrists guides the arms directly overhead, and their position in relation to the midline shows which side is more flexible and which is more constricted. Once the photographs are taken, the normal and stretched views can be placed side-by-side for comparison (Figs. 2-3 and 2-4). If the client has **scoliosis,** it is helpful also to take a close-up of the back, from head to coccyx, and to photograph the client bending over with arms hanging straight down to document rotation of the ribcage (Fig. 2-5). It is useful to routinely examine children and early teens in this way for scoliosis. The presence of a **rib hump** (Fig. 2-6) is evidence of the vertebral rotation of **idiopathic scoliosis,** and the parent should be encouraged to consult the child's physician.

Some clients may prefer not to be photographed, or some therapists may choose not to use this technique. In these cases, the therapist can still observe the client in all of the above positions.

Some additional positions and movements that are helpful for observation, but need not be photographed, include bending to each side from the waist, and bending backward with the arms stretched overhead.

The goal of asking the client to assume these various positions and stances is to observe the dynamic structure of the body. Even when the client is in a normal resting position, we are actually observing muscles at work. Just as a bird's leg muscles are always working, even in sleep, to keep it on the perch, our muscles must always respond to gravity. The ideal posture of a person standing at rest demands minimal muscle activity to maintain

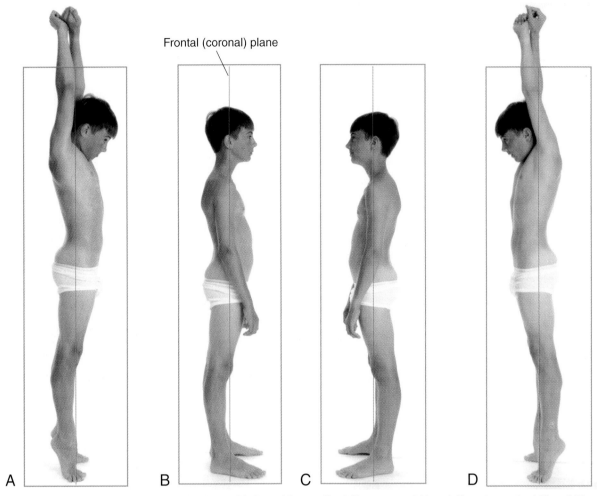

Frontal (coronal) plane

A   B   C   D

Figure 2-4   Posture evaluation: side views with frontal (coronal) midline—normal (A and C) and stretched (B and D)

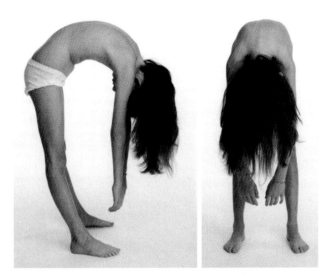

Figure 2-5   Scoliosis screening: side and front views

an upright posture. The ideal functioning of the body of a person in motion uses minimal muscle activity to accomplish any task, and will use larger and stronger rather than smaller and weaker muscles whenever possible.

The Body at Rest
When we observe a client standing at rest, we view the body in relation to certain planes. Although we work with these planes as lines, it is important to remember that they are planes, or we will be deceived.

Looking at the client from the front, the sagittal plane (Fig. 2-3A and B) is a midline that begins at a point midway between the feet (since that is the resting point for the weight) and passes through the pubic symphysis, the navel, the xiphoid process, the manubrium, the center of the chin,

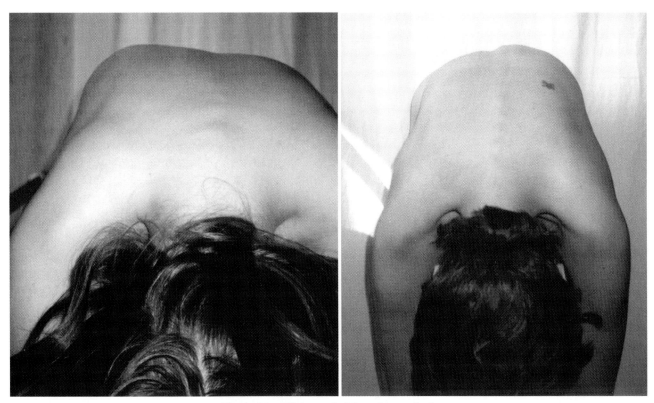

Figure 2-6 Rib hump in idiopathic scoliosis

and the nose. Note any deviation from that line. Also observe the kneecaps and feet. Do they point forward, or do either of them deviate inwardly or outwardly?

Viewing the client from behind, the sagittal plane (Fig. 2-3C and D) is a line that again begins midway between the feet and passes through the gluteal cleft and the coccyx, straight up through the spinal column, and through the middle of the head.

Comparing these two views can teach you how to think in planes rather than lines—in other words, how to see a client in a three-dimensional, rather than two-dimensional, view. Often the upper body of the client appears to lean to one side when viewed from the front, but lean to the opposite side when viewed from behind. This illusion is created by seeing lines rather than planes. In reality, the client's upper body is slightly rotated, placing the landmarks on the torso to one side of the midline in front and to the other side in back.

Viewing the client from each side, the frontal plane (Fig. 2-4) is a line passing just in front of the ankle through the knee, the greater trochanter, the glenohumeral joint of the shoulder, and the ear. Again, note any deviation from this line.

Therapists who do not take photographs or use a computer may find a plumb line helpful in making these observations. A long string weighted at one end (a two- or three-ounce fishing sinker works well) can be suspended in a place where the client can stand behind it to be observed. The plumb line gives the therapist a visual reference point for observing alignment deviations (Fig. 2-7).

In addition to the sagittal and frontal planes, the horizontal plane (Fig. 2-3A and C) should be considered in relation to the shoulders and hips:

- Are the shoulders level?
- Are the shoulders rotated medially and pulled forward in a slump?
- Is the pelvis tilted to one side or the other?
- Is the pelvis tipped forward?

You can make these same observations with the client's arms stretched overhead, with the wrists crossed in order to see if the shoulders yield evenly on both sides. Notice various body landmarks in a stretch: do the deviations you may have already observed correct themselves, worsen, or reverse themselves? The breasts or nipples move with the tissue overlying the ribcage, and the po-

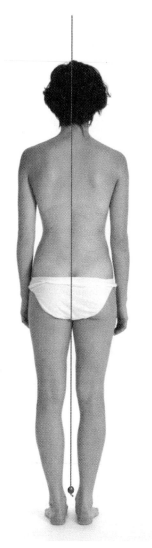

Figure 2-7   Using a plumb line

sition of the breasts is normally visible even if covered: how do they change in relation to each other in a stretch?

You may want to make notes of all your observations, particularly if you do not take photographs. *And remember that no individual view is sufficient to yield significant information.* Each view is merely one piece of a three-dimensional puzzle. Merely viewing the body at rest is insufficient to give a full assessment of the client's body. There are still more pieces of the puzzle to consider.

The Body in Motion

The first step in assessing the body in motion is to observe the client's gait (Fig. 2-8) from the back, front, and side. Do the legs swing straight forward, or do they deviate from that course, even slightly, along the way? Notice individual aspects of the legs: is there a medial pulling motion on the

inner thigh? Do the kneecaps always point forward? Do the feet point straight ahead throughout the swing of the leg? Viewed from behind, does the pelvis tilt from side to side, or swivel with the gait?

Ask the client to bend over backward with arms stretched overhead (Fig. 2-9). Does the body form a graceful arch? What happens to the lumbar curve? Does the head go backward with the rest of the body or does it remain upright? Is the client able to stay balanced in this position?

Ask the client to bend the torso to the left and the right, with the arms resting at the sides (Fig. 2-10). Notice any differences in flexibility between the two sides.

Sitting behind the standing client, place your hands on the ilium with your thumbs pressing into the dimples at the posterior superior iliac spines (PSIS). Ask the client to bend forward, and follow the PSISs with your thumbs (Fig. 2-11). Do they remain even, or does one move upward ahead of the other? In other words, does the sacrum rotate during forward bending?

Make notes of all deviations during movement, just as you did for the body at rest. These findings contribute to the solution of the puzzle.

Measurements

For many therapists, the observations described above will suffice for an analysis of the overall alignment of the body. Others, however, may

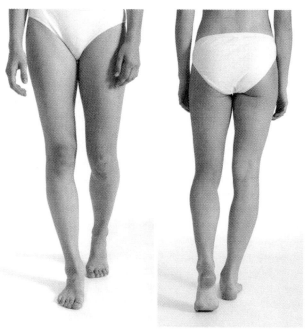

Figure 2-8   Gait assessment

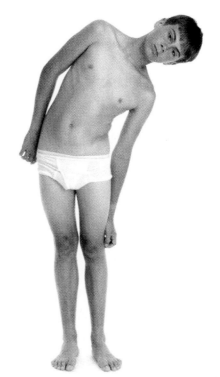

Figure 2-10 Assessment of client in side bend

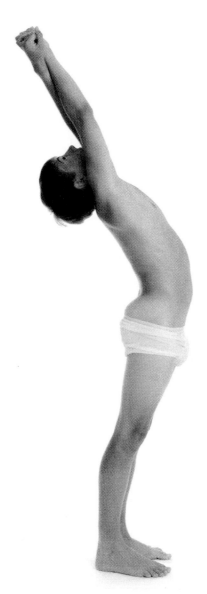

Figure 2-9 Assessment of client in backward bend

want to take specific measurements, either to document change for the client's records or medical reports, or for formal or informal clinical research. Such measurements are easy to take, depending on the measurement tools used.

Range of Motion

A complete examination includes measuring the range of motion (ROM) of the hips and shoulders. These measurements are normally taken with a goniometer, a widely available and fairly inexpensive instrument for measuring the angles of joints. These measurements should be made with the client lying supine (Fig. 2-12).

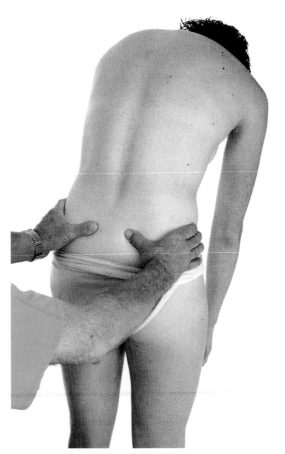

Figure 2-11 Examination of PSIS movement

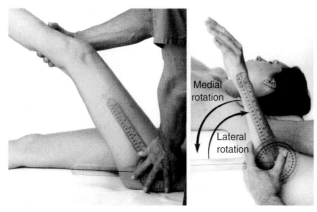

Figure 2-12   Measuring range of motion: hip flexion, shoulder rotation

To determine the ROM of the hip, stand at the side of the client at the hip and raise the client's leg by holding it by the calf, fully extended, until the knee attempts to bend slightly to accommodate the stretch of the hamstrings. Measure the angle of the joint in relation to the horizontal plane.

To determine the ROM of the shoulder, the shoulder should be abducted 90° and the elbow flexed 90°, so that the fingers point to the ceiling. Stand beside the client at the level of the shoulders. Place your hand nearest the head of the client on the shoulder with your fingers lying over the superior border of the scapula. Rotate the forearm toward the table (medial rotation of the shoulder) until it lies flat, or until movement is felt in the scapula. If the forearm does not lie flat without movement of the scapula, the angle should be measured and noted. Then rotate the arm upward (lateral rotation of the shoulder) until it lies flat or movement is felt in the scapula, and again measure and note the angle. Feeling for movement in the scapula is necessary to determine actual *glenohumeral* rotation, rather than rotation that may be accommodated by movement of the scapula.

Body Alignment
The most useful device for measuring body alignment is the inclinometer, which is the equivalent of the carpenter's spirit level adapted for bodywork purposes. The inclinometer indicates the relationship of a given line, such as the line of the hips or shoulders, to the horizontal plane.

One of the most useful devices on the market for this purpose is the PALM (PALpation Meter), made by Performance Attainment Associates (Saint Paul, MN). The PALM is a combination inclinometer, caliper, and special slide rule (Fig. 2-13). The caliper tips are held with the fingers against any two points on the client's body (Figs. 2-14 and 2-15). The gauges show the distance between the two points and the angle of deviation of the line between them from the horizontal. Using these two figures, the slide rule device calculates the exact height difference in inches or centimeters between the two points. This system allows the relationship of any two points on the body to be determined with a high degree of specificity.

In reality, the angle is the most important piece of information for the therapist, since the height differential will vary according to the size of the client even at the same angle. A larger client who has the same angle of deviation as a smaller client will have a greater height differential, since the points being measured are farther apart. The height differential is of use primarily to give the client an idea of the amount of deviation. The primary advantage of the PALM lies in the ability of the therapist to use the fingertips as the caliper tips, hence the name, "PALpation Meter." The measurements made with the PALM can be recorded on a form for the client's record (Fig. 2-16).

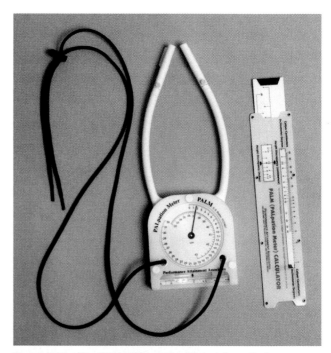

Figure 2-13   The PALM (PALpation Meter) from Performance Attainment Associates (Saint Paul, MN)

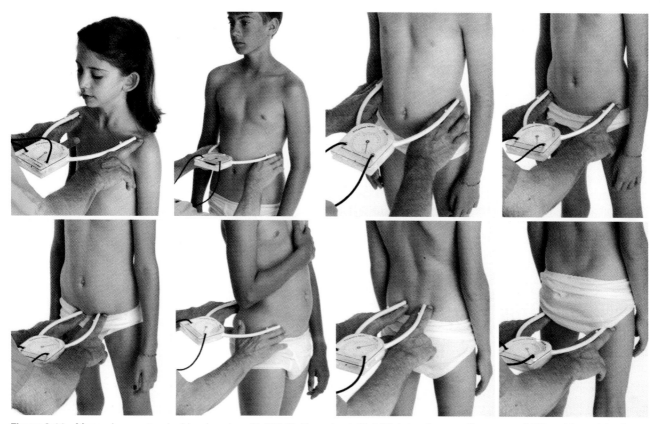

Figure 2-14 Measuring anatomical landmarks with PALM: (from top left) AC joints, rib cage, iliac crests, ASIS, pubis, pelvic tilt, PSIS, gluteal folds

Testing Areas Specific to the Complaint

By carefully noting and analyzing the type and location of discomfort produced by the following combination of tests, the therapist can gain valuable information about the likely nature of the dysfunction. Therefore, the next step in assessment is to test the area or areas specific to the complaint. First, determine the position that best suits this purpose. Usually, the client stands to have the hip joint tested, sits to have the shoulder

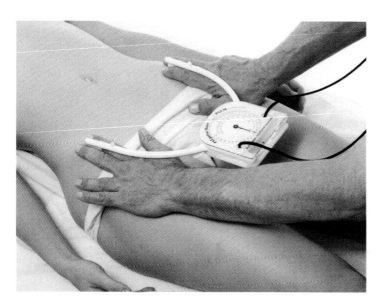

Figure 2-15 Measuring anterior iliac crest height differential supine with PALM

joint tested, and sits and stands for testing of the knees. More of the area may be accessible when the client is standing or sitting than when the client is lying down, and in these positions you can easily palpate the tissue while the client moves the joint.

Joints should be tested both actively and passively. The client moves the joint through its full ROM, reporting any pain, discomfort, or barriers to movement. In passive testing, the therapist *carefully* moves the joint through the same range, with the client instructed to relax the limb and give control to the therapist. The client should be asked to describe any differences in feeling between active and passive movement.

Then, in whatever position is suitable, the therapist tests active movement of the joint against resistance. The client is instructed to move the limb in a particular direction while the therapist resists the motion and report any feelings associated with that effort.

There are far too many specific tests for soft-tissue disorders in particular areas of the body to be included in this book. However, Appendix D, Suggested Readings, lists some excellent references to help you with assessments.

POSTURAL ALIGNMENT EXAMINATION

Name of patient: _____   Date: _____

Age: _____ Sex: F M   Height: _____ Weight: _____ Scoliosis: idiopathic   postural   none

Measurement: 1st   2nd   3rd   4th   5th   Final

AC joints	DISTANCE _____	ANGLE _____	Low R L	HEIGHT DISC. _____
Iliac crests	DISTANCE _____	ANGLE _____	Low R L	HEIGHT DISC. _____
ASIS	DISTANCE _____	ANGLE _____	Low R L	HEIGHT DISC. _____
PUBIS	DISTANCE _____	ANGLE _____	Low R L	HEIGHT DISC. _____

Inferior angle of scapulae	DISTANCE _____	ANGLE _____	Low R L	HEIGHT DISC. _____
PSIS	DISTANCE _____	ANGLE _____	Low R L	HEIGHT DISC. _____
ASIS/PSIS angle	RIGHT _____ LEFT _____			

AS APPLICABLE

Leg lengths   RIGHT FEMUR _____   LEFT FEMUR _____

                RIGHT TIBIA _____   LEFT TIBIA _____

Glenohumeral ROM: L _____   R _____   Hip ROM: L _____   R _____

Figure 2-16 Form for recording measurements

The Breathing Examination

An essential element in assessment is examining the client's breathing technique. Many, if not most, older children and adults have developed the habit of "paradoxical breathing," i.e., expanding and raising the upper rib cage while keeping the abdomen and lower rib cage constricted.

Paradoxical breathing is detrimental to muscle health and posture for a number of reasons. Inappropriate use of neck and shoulder muscles in breathing causes chronic tightness in those areas, which can result in forward positioning of the head and the development of trigger points or nerve entrapment. Tight chest muscles pull the shoulders forward and rotate the arms internally. Inflexibility in the muscles of the chest and abdomen can pull the anterior rib cage forward and down, exaggerating a thoracic kyphosis. Finally, good diaphragmatic breathing techniques use the full capacity of the lungs, optimize the exchange of blood gases, and enhance relaxation. Therefore, if your examination indicates that the client breathes paradoxically, it will be important to incorporate training in diaphragmatic breathing technique. The complete procedure for assessing and teaching breathing will be found later in the text.

The Manual (Palpatory) Examination

This part of the examination begins with the client sitting or standing, according to the circumstances. Throughout the examination, the client will sit, stand, or lie successively supine and prone on the table in whichever order the therapist finds most useful and efficient. It is often best to perform the palpatory examination of the area of complaint before or during the specific testing described above. If the client chooses to be examined and treated only for relief of the specific complaint, then you should limit your palpatory examination to those areas likely to be contributing to it. In any case, finding and treating the immediate source of pain or dysfunction is one of your primary objectives.

You may find it useful to refer to Appendix C (Index of Pain Referral Zones by Location) in choosing the range of muscles to examine to determine the source of the client's pain. Thereafter, each muscle description in Part II presents a list of "Other Muscles to Examine." Do not stop with a single positive finding; a trigger point that reproduces the client's pain may not be the sole source of the problem. Thorough exploration of the muscles in a particular body region will increase the accuracy, efficiency, and effectiveness of your treatment.

Broadly speaking, the palpatory examination has two parts: (1) general assessment of the tissues in each area, and (2) precise palpation for taut bands in the muscles, and tender or trigger points. Both parts are continuous and contiguous with therapy: as you treat, you examine. In the initial evaluation, the information you gain through palpation is an essential adjunct to the information you obtain through observations and measurements.

The palpatory examination begins again with observation: look at the area you are about to examine. Notice its color, especially in comparison with other areas of the body. Is it pale or pasty? Does it have the angry redness of inflammation? Or does it appear gently flushed (as healthy tissue should be), without radical contrast to other areas?

Begin with a broad, gentle, general touch. Lay your hand on the area you are examining and just let it rest there for a moment. Feel the temperature of the area. Is it cold? Cool? Hot? Warm? Does it feel damp or sticky, or is it unpleasantly dry? Healthy skin should have a subtly moist feeling to it, without dryness, dampness, or stickiness. Allow your hand to press a bit deeper, and move the skin around over the underlying layers. Does it seem stuck, or does it seem loose? Or does it feel firm but mobile, as if connected to the layers underneath but not adhered to them? Draw your finger across the skin, noting whether there is "drag" in the tissue that impedes your motion. Such palpable phenomena at the levels of the epidermis, dermis, and superficial fascia often reflect underlying tissue dysfunction.

Note any marked differences in an area. Differences in temperature and moisture can be signs of sympathetic nervous system activity in response to problems in the underlying tissue. Fascial tightness and tissue congestion are usually signs of a myofascial problem. Remember also the classic signs of local inflammation: heat, redness, pain, and swelling. This combination is a contraindication for local massage work.

At this point you can move deeper still, and begin to use your fingers and thumbs in whatever sort of palpation suits the shape of the tissue. You are feeling the muscle tissue, and you want to learn whether it is flabby or firm or hard or contracted. Move your hands, palpating different parts of the muscle to feel for taut bands and knots in the tissue. Ask the client to let you know what areas are tender, ticklish, numb, or feel in any way "strange." Also be aware of the client's nonverbal responses: clients will not always verbally communicate to you about everything they feel. Be alert to wincing or face-making or intakes of breath that indicate that the client is feeling something significant.

You can certainly palpate at this point for trigger points or other sensitive points, but you should also be careful not to press too deeply into trigger points. Arousing them before you are prepared to treat them will only cause needless pain for the client.

Obviously it is impossible to do a focal examination for tender points or trigger points over the entire body in a reasonable amount of time. However, a general assessment of the principal muscles of posture and movement is possible. As you gain experience, you will know the most likely spots to explore more carefully for sensitivity. Also, your awareness of the client's complaint and history will guide your choices about areas to examine more closely.

One rule to remember when examining muscular tissue is to *always examine the antagonists.* If there is a problem in a particular muscle, there is a problem in its antagonists. This rule is one more reason why a thorough knowledge of anatomy and kinesiology is needed in clinical massage therapy.

The information that you gain from the palpatory examination should be recorded for easy reference. One way to keep this information organized is to design a form like the one suggested earlier for clients, with four body views, on which you can make notations according to your own style.

SUMMATION AND DETECTIVE WORK

You now have the following sets of data to work with:

- The chief complaint
- The history
- Informal and formal observations of body alignment and movement
- ROM assessment
- Palpatory examination

Table 2-1 shows some questions to ask in your mind, with sources of information about each.

As you think in problem-solving terms, the first question you should consider is,

What is the likelihood that the cause and treatment of this problem lie outside my scope of practice?

This issue is extremely important, both for the client's health and your own legal protection. Al-

TABLE 2-1

QUESTION	SOURCE OF INFORMATION
What muscles may refer pain to the area of complaint?	Charts, your knowledge of referral zones
What muscles seem shortened or tight? Where are tender points or trigger points?	ROM assessment, palpatory examination, body alignment
What are the antagonists of the muscles in the area of complaint?	Presenting complaint, your knowledge of anatomy and kinesiology
If there was a specific injury, then what muscles were stretched and what muscles were shortened?	Presenting complaint, your knowledge of anatomy and kinesiology
What muscles are regularly challenged by this client?	Occupational and athletic history, alignment examination
What was the client doing around the time the problem started?	Personal, occupational, and athletic history
What activities in the client's past could have injured these muscles?	Personal, occupational, and athletic history
Could this problem be related to a compensation for some other injury?	Health history, observation of movement
To what degree might stress in the client's life be activating a dormant tissue problem?	Personal, athletic, and occupational history

ways keep in mind that your assessment may be wrong.

Although clinical massage therapists should become highly adept at examination and assessment of the musculoskeletal system and work towards mastery of the process, this system is only one aspect of the whole person. Thus, our scope of examination and treatment is necessarily limited. It is always safest to assume that, since we are working within a limited range, our knowledge and awareness may be incomplete. We should never discourage clients from seeking the opinions of other professionals, including their physician. In fact, we should encourage it.

In some cases, the therapist should defer treatment of a client until a physician has evaluated and cleared the client for massage therapy. Such clients include those with internal pain (chest, abdomen, or pelvis), or any client with suspected musculoskeletal injuries such as a dislocated or broken bone or torn muscles, tendons, or ligaments.

Otherwise, the therapist may continue with treatment. When the problem is likely to be myofascial in origin, and direct manipulation of the tissue clearly represents no danger to the client, it is normally safe to proceed. However, the therapist should continue to consider the possibility that other factors may be involved, and be prepared to refer the client at the slightest suspicion that another form of treatment might be called for.

SYNTHESIZING YOUR FINDINGS

Correctly assessing a client's problem and developing a treatment plan depends on recognizing that problems in the body do not occur in isolation. *A problem anywhere in the musculoskeletal system compromises to some degree the integrity of the entire system.* Therefore, you must think simultaneously at both the local and whole-body levels. The longer you are in practice, the more seamless this process will become, because all the pieces of the puzzle will fit themselves into place as you gather them.

When thinking through muscular problems, keep these two frameworks in mind:

- Think of muscles in terms of groups that work together (myotatic units) and consider agonist/antagonist relationships.

- Think of joints as well as muscles, since the primary function of muscles is to move or stabilize joints.

At this point, all of the information you have gathered needs to be synthesized in a view of the whole person. Here is a useful order for considering and synthesizing this information:

- In your observation of the whole body, what are the differences in the front and back sides? How do these differences mesh? Add the two side views to let your mind build a hologram of the body. Do you see deviations in a single plane, or is there a spiral effect to the deviations that would indicate twisting?
- Consider any measurements you have taken. Do the measurements support the three-dimensional picture you have built? For example, if the measurements show that the right anterior superior iliac spine (ASIS) is lower than the left in front, but the right PSIS is higher than the left in back, does your picture indicate a spiral effect or twisting of the torso?
- How does the pain and/or dysfunction reported by the client fit into the picture? Does the pain or restriction occur in an area where muscles appear to be chronically shortened or lengthened? Could the pain be causing compensatory posture or movement?
- Consider your palpatory examination. Where are tender spots, and how do these areas compare with areas of pain reported by the client? Compared with your holographic picture of the client, are they in areas where muscles are chronically shortened or lengthened?
- Did you encounter trigger points that reproduce the client's pain?
- Now add the history. What does the client do now, either at work or in recreation, that might affect the problem areas? What about past activities, injuries, surgeries?
- Finally, what recent stressors might be causing an already existing problem to surface?

COMMUNICATING WITH CLIENTS

When the examination is completed, it's time to share your thinking with the client. Since most people are naturally curious, it's a good practice to share your observations with the client throughout the examination. It's annoying to have someone who is examining you say nothing but, "Hmmm." But now you can let the client know how the information is coming together for you, what your working assessment is, and what sort of work you propose to do. For example:

"I think that when you sprained your ankle last year, you favored your right leg for a while. That got your left hip muscles working overtime, and shortened the muscles supporting your pelvis on the right. Since you're young and in good shape, you didn't feel the effects at first, but your new job pressures have made you tense and lowered your pain threshold, so now those muscles are finally making themselves felt. I'd like to work on your left hip to give you some immediate relief from the pain in your leg, but I think we also need to work on your low back and abdominal muscles, since they're pulling your pelvis out of balance."

Clients may sometimes question why the examination and proposed treatment wanders so far afield from the specific area of their complaint. For this reason, it is important to educate them about the nature of myofascial pain. This education need not be highly technical. Metaphors are often useful in explaining what seems to be going on. For example, one might describe the relationship of agonists and antagonists as being like two people in bed fighting over the covers, or characterize the gradual spreading of muscle cell involvement in an injured area as a revolution or a labor dispute.

This educational process is another good reason for documentation such as photographs and recorded measurements. These concrete bits of information support your assessment.

The most important aspect of communication with the client is to establish a relationship in which the client becomes an active and informed participant in the overall process. You are the authority, that's why the client consulted you; however, it is your job to help clients become more knowledgeable and take greater responsibility for their own health and well-being.

APPLYING YOUR SYNTHESIS TO TREATMENT

Your first responsibility is to give the client relief from the presenting complaint as quickly as is feasible. Therefore, in most cases, begin treatment

eliminating trigger points, tender points, and tightness in the area where the pain is and those areas that appear to be causing it or contributing to it. In Chapters 3 through 10, the pain referral zone is listed for each muscle, as well as a list of other muscles to examine that may refer pain to similar areas.

In the case of multiple trigger points, there will be a **primary trigger point** accompanied by **satellite trigger points.** The only way to distinguish them is to treat them and observe the results. Resolving a primary trigger point will eliminate referred pain, while resolving satellite trigger points will not.

Once the presenting problem has been treated and alleviated, it is appropriate to address the issues of postural alignment and other mitigating factors that are responsible for the client's pain. A detailed discussion of postural analysis is beyond the scope of this book; however, most of the postural misalignments that result in myofascial pain are a matter of common sense, good judgment, and a thorough knowledge of musculoskeletal anatomy. Clinical experience and additional study and training will round out your skills in this area.

The general order of treatment should proceed:

- From the areas specific to the complaint to the overall body alignment
- From superficial to deep
- From general to specific
- From bottom to top

COMMUNICATING WITH OTHER HEALTH PROFESSIONALS

Communicating effectively with other health professionals is important for three reasons:

- It is potentially helpful in the care of specific clients.
- It affects your image as a health professional, and helps create the degree of respect you will be accorded in the present and future.
- It affects the image of the bodywork profession as a whole, and will ultimately determine the degree of acceptance we all achieve.

The first requirement in effective professional communication is to master your terminology. On the one hand, do not go out of your way to use the most technical language you can, because it will simply be seen as an attempt to impress. On the other hand, you should know anatomical terms and be able to spell and pronounce them properly, or it will be assumed that you don't know what you're talking about. Keep a medical dictionary handy and use it regularly. If you use a computer, get a medical spell-check program.

Some good policies to follow regularly:

■ Ask clients to tell their other health care providers to feel free to contact you.
■ With the client's consent, write letters to other health care providers to inform them about your assessment and treatment of the client and the results.
■ If another health care provider refers a client to you, then write a letter of thanks that includes your report, with your client's consent.

You will find your own style, but two sample reports are included here as examples.

SAMPLE 1

Name:	Amanda P. Fundlethwaite
Chief Complaint:	Pain in neck and left shoulder, radiating into left arm to hand.
Treatment Dates:	Jan. 23; Feb. 1, 7, 10, 17, 28; March 6, 17

I saw the above-named patient on the indicated dates for complaints of pain resulting from an automobile accident in which her car collided with another car while her left arm was resting on the car's windowsill.

I treated her for severe trigger point activity in the scalene muscles, particularly the middle scalene and scalenus minimus, and related spasms and trigger point activity in pectoralis minor, rhomboids, levator scapulae, and rotator cuff muscles. Techniques employed consisted primarily of trigger point compression and deep tissue therapy.

Some temporary relief was achieved, but her problem is complicated by two factors: (1) treatment did not begin until 8 months after her accident, and (2) the constant weight of the ribcage on the scalenes continues to irritate the muscles.

Ms. Fundlethwaite informs me that she has been told by her physicians that she has nerve damage. I can't comment directly on that, but I do believe that improvement can be achieved with additional work on the muscles themselves. This treatment would necessarily be long-term because of the time that has passed since the injury.

SAMPLE 2

Patient:	Esther Megillah
Date of Birth:	8/24/85
Complaints:	Frequent headaches (at least 3X per week), back pain
Measurements:	■ Left shoulder (AC joint) 1" lower than right ■ Left shoulder blade (inferior angle of scapula) .4" lower than right ■ Left iliac crest .4" lower than right ■ Left ASIS .3" lower than right ■ Left PSIS .2" lower than right ■ Left gluteal fold .4" lower than right ■ Pelvic tilt: 16° left, 19° right
Photographs:	Photographs show significant rotation of torso from hips counterclockwise (from above). Tightness in chest muscles is indicated by difficulty in raising arms fully overhead and in pulling forward of shoulders, particularly on the right. Lumbar lordosis indicates excessive pelvic tilt, which is confirmed in measurements.
Manual Examination:	Excessive tenderness found in chest, back, abdomen, buttocks, and legs.
Conclusions:	Measurements indicate landmarks on left side to be consistently .3° to 1° lower than on right side. Photographs confirm this and indicate rotation of torso and pelvic tilt. Manual examination confirms muscular constriction in legs, abdomen, buttocks, back, and chest.
Recommendations:	Alignment therapy (neuromuscular and connective tissue therapy) is recommended to correct the above imbalances and mis-

alignments and could eliminate or alleviate headaches and back pain. This procedure is also likely to increase her flexibility for gymnastics and other activities.

SPECIAL POPULATIONS

Pregnant Women

Pregnant women can certainly benefit from massage therapy, since the added weight and imbalance in their bodies can cause considerable soft-tissue pain, especially in the low back, hips, and legs. Certain precautions must be taken, however, and special requirements need to be considered.

A pregnant woman may not be able to lie on her stomach, and may be uncomfortable lying on her back for any significant period of time. Depending on the area being treated, she may be in a seated position or she may lie on her side. The use of pillows may enable her to lie on her stomach. She should be allowed to arrange these herself, as she can determine her needs better than the therapist. Commercial systems are also available, such as the Body Cushion (Polymer Dynamics, Inc., Allentown, PA), which can be arranged to allow a pregnant woman to lie prone. Any problems can usually be solved in collaboration with the client.

There are certain points on the body that many acupressure practitioners believe induce labor.

Although there is little in the literature to support this assumption, you may find it preferable to avoid these points (Fig. 2-17). In addition, the following guidelines have been established by the American College of Obstetrics and Gynecology. A woman in any of these categories should obtain a release from her primary care provider before receiving massage.

- The pregnancy is high risk, i.e., the mother has used fertility methods to get pregnant or has had difficulty getting pregnant naturally.
- She has miscarried in the first trimester of previous pregnancies.
- She has a cardiac disorder (heart or pulmonary problems).
- She has a history of problems in pregnancy.
- There is a multiple pregnancy (twins, triplets, etc.).
- The mother is under age 20 or over 35.
- The mother has asthma.
- The mother has been exposed to illegal drugs.

The Elderly

The work described in this book is appropriate for the treatment of older clients, with the following specific cautions:

- Be sure to take a thorough medical history, and be aware of any problems such as stroke, heart disease, blood clots, surgeries, medications, etc.
- Osteoporosis occurs frequently in older adults. Ask about this condition in the client's history.

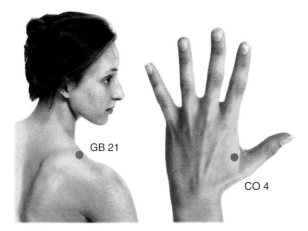

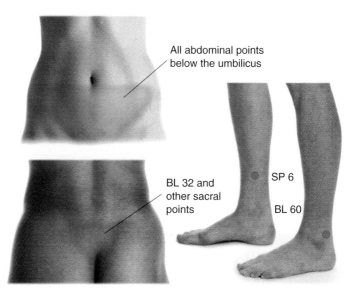

Figure 2-17 Acupressure points to be avoided on pregnant women

Avoid intense pressure on any bones, particularly the ribs, in therapy.

■ Avoid treatment directly over implanted devices, such as pacemakers.

■ Older people tend to have thinner skin that is more apt to tear. Exercise caution in pulling the skin during treatment.

Children and Adolescents

Adolescent clients may be treated essentially as adults. This work is also appropriate for children, with certain cautions and considerations:

■ Most children have not developed a perspective that allows them to deal well with pain in treatment. They therefore have a lower pain tolerance than adolescents or adults.

■ However, the soft tissues of children tend to be more responsive and resilient, so that the work usually does not need to be as deep or intense as may be required in adult clients.

■ Children tend to be more ticklish than adults, and palpation that elicits pain in adult clients will often elicit ticklishness in children. You will need to learn to distinguish between superficial ticklishness (evoked by light touch) and deep ticklishness (evoked by deep touch). The latter should be seen as equivalent to a pain response in an adult.

Posturally-oriented bodywork can be done very effectively with school-age children, depending on their cooperativeness. An ideal time for this work is from the ages of 8 or 9 through puberty. The child is old enough to understand and participate in the work, and it will provide some preventive advantage as the child progresses through the adolescent growth spurt. It may also help the growing child in dealing with body issues at that sensitive age.

CONCLUSION

Effective examination and assessment are the keys to good clinical work. Intelligent assessment of the problem is essential to gaining the trust of the client and working with confidence. In the beginning, the process may seem artificial and mechanical, but as you gain experience and self-assurance, it will develop a natural flow. You will

master it by touching many bodies, again and again and again, and by using your eyes, hands, and brain to put together coherent concepts of the whole, individual human being. Soon, the dialogue between you and your clients, both physical and verbal, will become as natural to you as breathing.

CHAPTER SUMMARY

1. The priority of clinical massage therapy is effective treatment. Effective treatment requires effective assessment.

2. The client's history is taken, both on a brief form and in an interview, including
   ■ Presenting problem
   ■ Health history
   ■ Athletic history
   ■ Personal history
   ■ Occupational history

3. The client is examined in these areas:
   ■ Observation
   ■ Alignment examination
   ■ Photos, if desired
   ■ The body in motion
   ■ Measurements
   ■ ROM
   ■ Testing of affected muscles
   ■ Breathing examination
   ■ Palpatory examination of the area of complaint
   ■ Palpatory examination of the rest of the body

4. The information must then be summarized, and a synthesis and working hypothesis made.

5. Your thoughts, reasoning, and recommendations must be communicated effectively to the client.

6. You must be able to communicate with other health professionals who may be involved in the client's treatment.

7. Some special considerations may apply to particular kinds of clients:
   ■ Pregnant women
   ■ The elderly
   ■ Children and adolescents

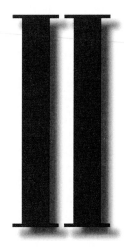

Approaching Treatment

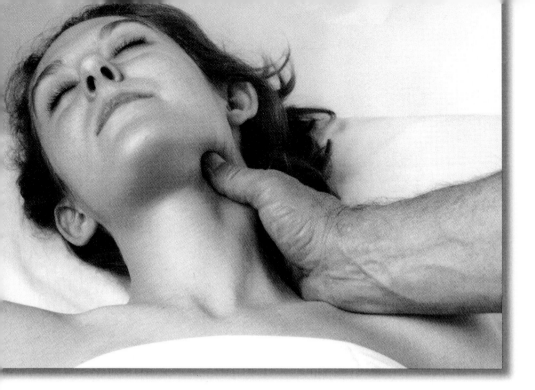

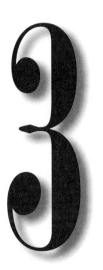

The Head, Face, and Neck

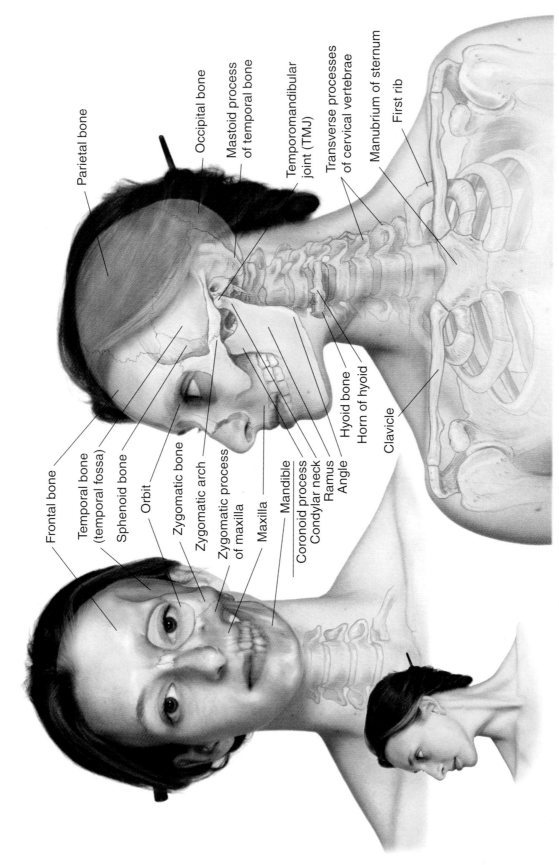

Parietal bone

Occipital bone

Mastoid process of temporal bone

Temporomandibular joint (TMJ)

Transverse processes of cervical vertebrae

Manubrium of sternum

First rib

Frontal bone

Temporal bone (temporal fossa)

Sphenoid bone

Orbit

Zygomatic bone

Zygomatic arch

Zygomatic process of maxilla

Maxilla

Mandible

Coronoid process

Condylar neck

Ramus

Angle

Hyoid bone

Horn of hyoid

Clavicle

Plate 3-1 Skeletal features of the anterior and lateral head and neck

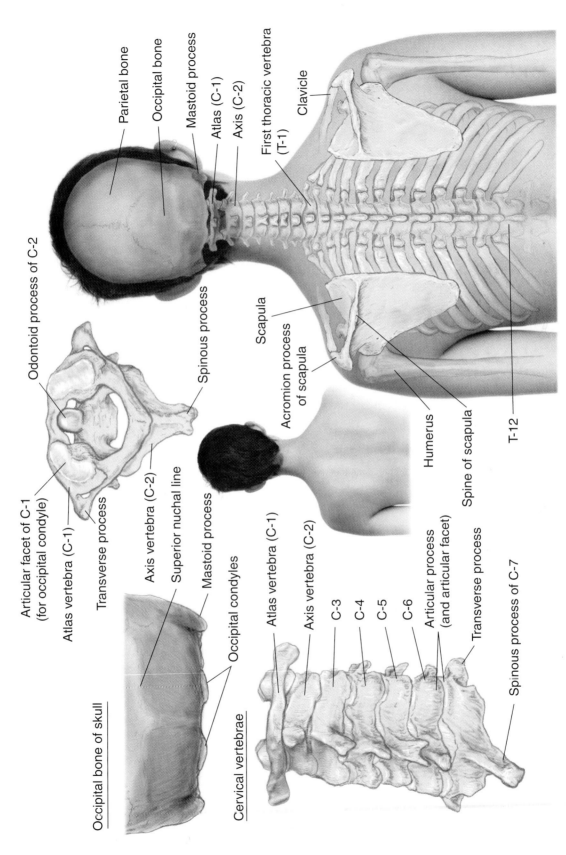

Plate 3-2 Skeletal features of the posterior head and neck

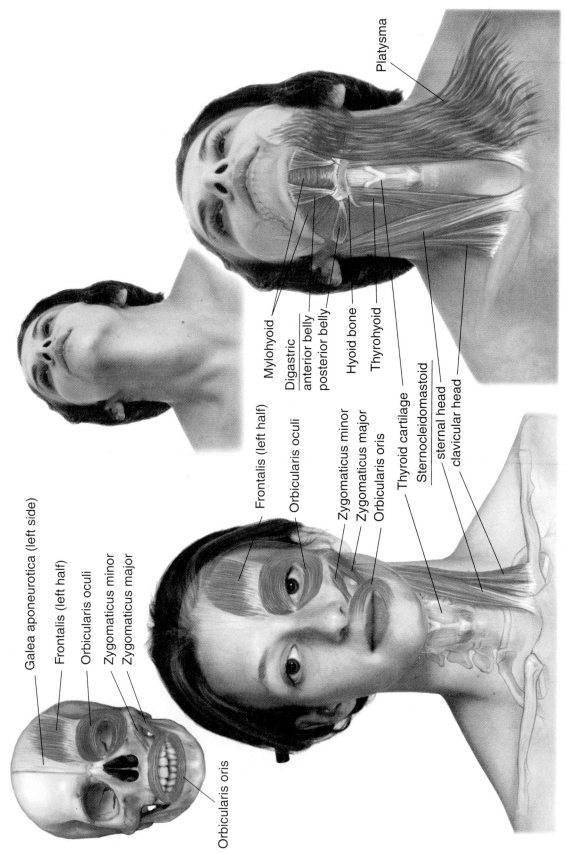

Galea aponeurotica (left side)
Frontalis (left half)
Orbicularis oculi
Zygomaticus minor
Zygomaticus major

Orbicularis oris

Frontalis (left half)
Orbicularis oculi

Zygomaticus minor
Zygomaticus major
Orbicularis oris

Thyroid cartilage
Sternocleidomastoid
sternal head
clavicular head

Mylohyoid
Digastric
anterior belly
posterior belly
Hyoid bone
Thyrohyoid

Platysma

Plate 3-3 Muscles of the anterior head and neck

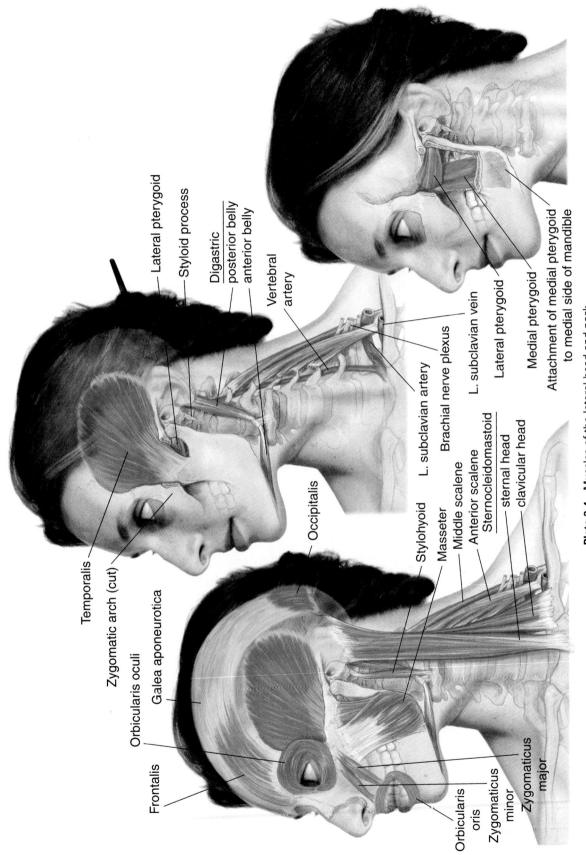

Lateral pterygoid

Styloid process

Digastric
posterior belly
anterior belly

Vertebral
artery

Temporalis

Zygomatic arch (cut)

Orbicularis oculi

Galea aponeurotica

Frontalis

Occipitalis

L. subclavian artery

Brachial nerve plexus

L. subclavian vein

Lateral pterygoid

Medial pterygoid

Attachment of medial pterygoid
to medial side of mandible

Stylohyoid

Masseter

Middle scalene

Anterior scalene

Sternocleidomastoid
sternal head
clavicular head

Orbicularis
oris

Zygomaticus
minor

Zygomaticus
major

Plate 3-4 Muscles of the lateral head and neck

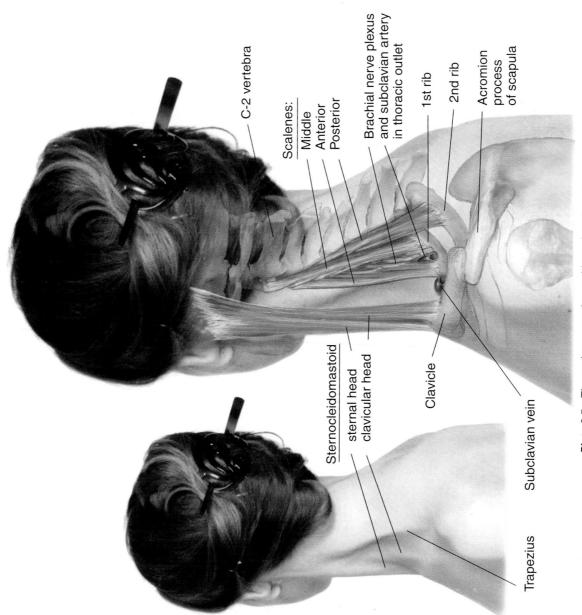

C-2 vertebra

Scalenes:
Middle
Anterior
Posterior

Brachial nerve plexus
and subclavian artery
in thoracic outlet

1st rib

2nd rib

Acromion
process
of scapula

Sternocleidomastoid
sternal head
clavicular head

Clavicle

Subclavian vein

Trapezius

Plate 3-5 The scalene muscles and lateral neck anatomy

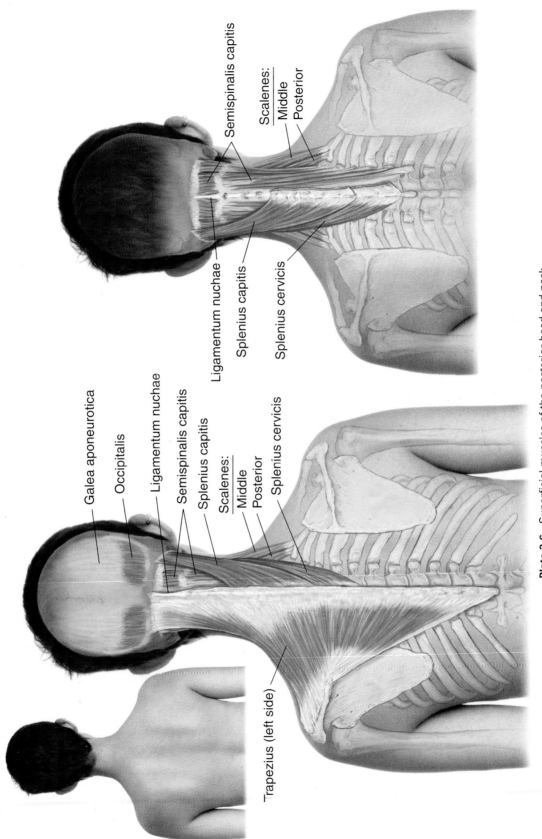

Semispinalis capitis

Scalenes:
Middle
Posterior

Ligamentum nuchae

Splenius capitis

Splenius cervicis

Galea aponeurotica

Occipitalis

Ligamentum nuchae

Semispinalis capitis

Splenius capitis

Scalenes:
Middle
Posterior

Splenius cervicis

Trapezius (left side)

Plate 3-6 Superficial muscles of the posterior head and neck

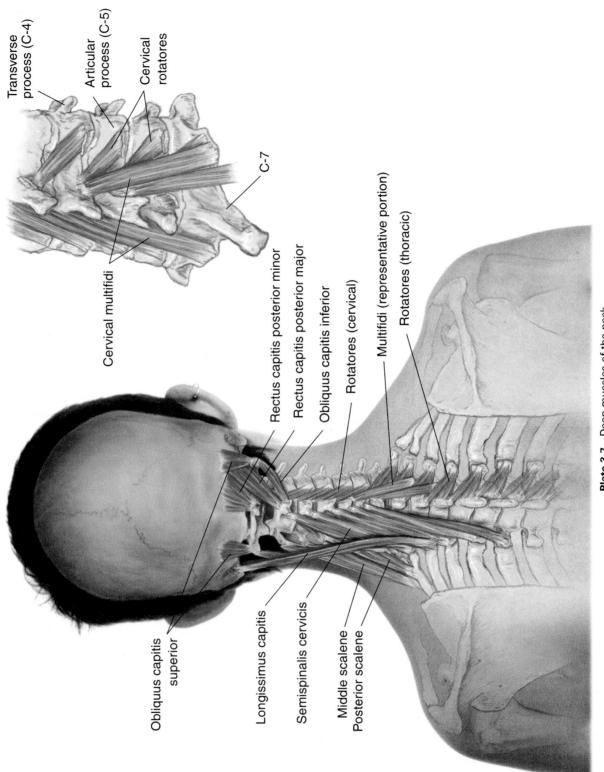

Transverse process (C-4)

Articular process (C-5)

Cervical rotatores

C-7

Cervical multifidi

Rectus capitis posterior minor

Rectus capitis posterior major

Obliquus capitis inferior

Rotatores (cervical)

Multifidi (representative portion)

Rotatores (thoracic)

Obliquus capitis superior

Longissimus capitis

Semispinalis cervicis

Middle scalene

Posterior scalene

Plate 3-7   Deep muscles of the neck

Chapter 3 The Head, Face, and Neck **61**

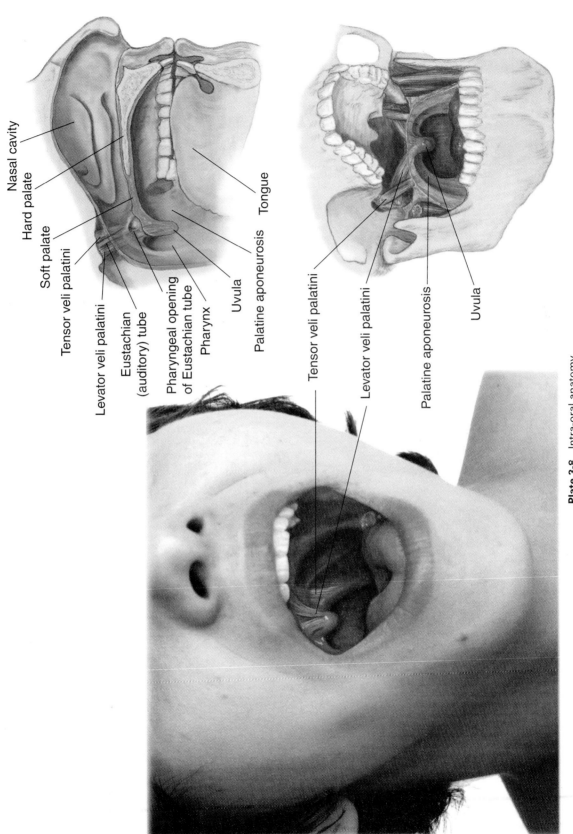

Nasal cavity

Hard palate

Soft palate

Tensor veli palatini

Levator veli palatini

Eustachian (auditory) tube

Pharyngeal opening of Eustachian tube

Pharynx

Uvula

Palatine aponeurosis

Tongue

Tensor veli palatini

Levator veli palatini

Palatine aponeurosis

Uvula

Plate 3-8   Intra-oral anatomy

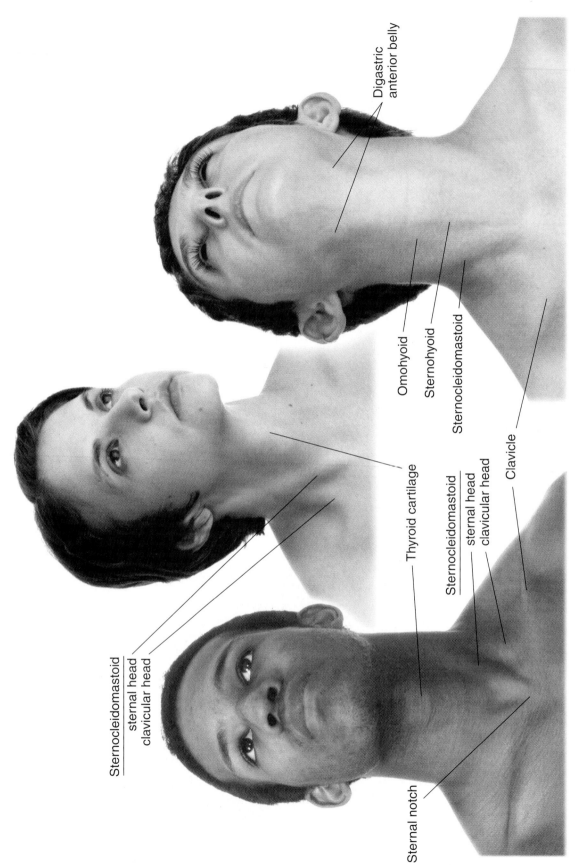

Plate 3-9 Surface anatomy of the anterior neck

Digastric
anterior belly

Omohyoid

Sternohyoid

Sternocleidomastoid

Clavicle

Thyroid cartilage

Sternocleidomastoid
sternal head
clavicular head

Sternocleidomastoid
sternal head
clavicular head

Sternal notch

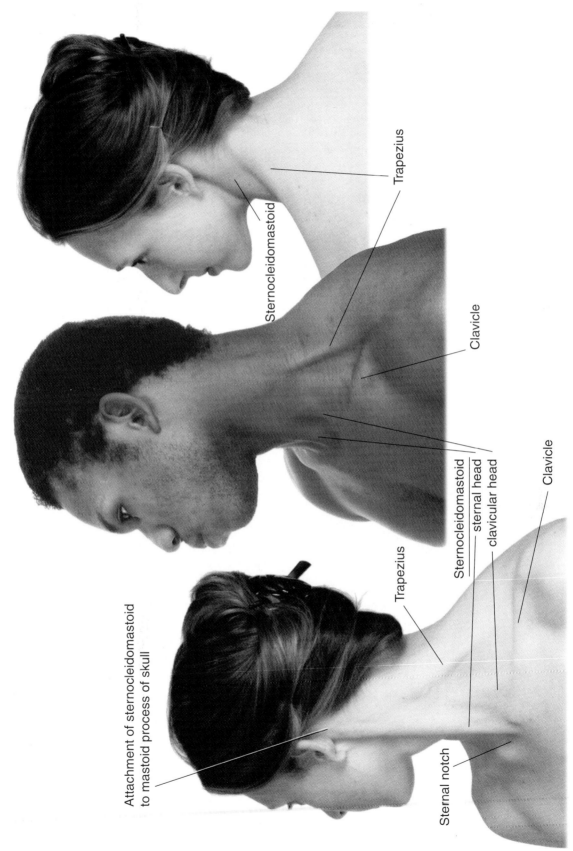

Trapezius

Sternocleidomastoid

Clavicle

Trapezius

Sternocleidomastoid
sternal head
clavicular head

Clavicle

Attachment of sternocleidomastoid
to mastoid process of skull

Sternal notch

Plate 3-10   Surface anatomy of the lateral and posterior neck

OVERVIEW OF THE REGION

The head is the capital of the body. It's the headquarters. It's worth noting that:

- The head houses the brain, the control center of the body and, according to some, the seat of consciousness.
- It's the home of the face. The face tells others who we are and what we are feeling (Fig. 3-1).
- It's the point from which the voice issues. The voice is how we transmit information about ourselves to the rest of the world.
- It is the exclusive residence of four of the five traditional senses. The head houses the organs of vision, hearing, taste, and smell. In addition, the head contains the primary organs of balance.
- Finally, it contains the entrance to the respiratory and digestive systems. The two functions that are essential to the sustenance of life, breathing and eating, begin here.

The neck serves two essential functions:

- It connects the head and its functions to the rest of the body.
- It supports and moves the head.

Clinical observation confirms that many headaches originate in trigger points in the neck muscles. Such headaches can be reduced in frequency and intensity, if not completely eliminated, by resolution of these trigger points. Many people carry their heads with the ears well forward of the sagittal midline (Fig. 3-2). This misalignment often results in the development of myofascial trigger points in the posterior neck[1]. According to David G. Simons, MD, "The head-forward posture activates posterior neck MTrPs [myofascial trigger points] by overloading them causing chronic contraction without relaxation periods" (Simons, David G., MD, private communication, September 23, 2001). Note, however, that treatment of the posterior cervical trigger points alone will seldom solve the pain problem. Overall correction of the

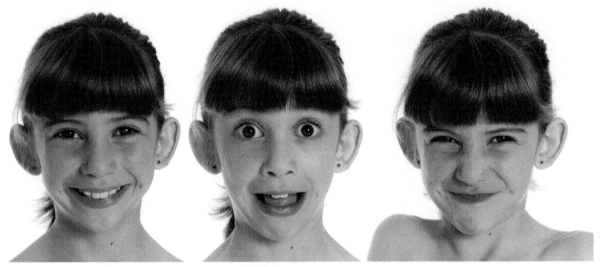

Figure 3-1 Muscles produce facial expressions

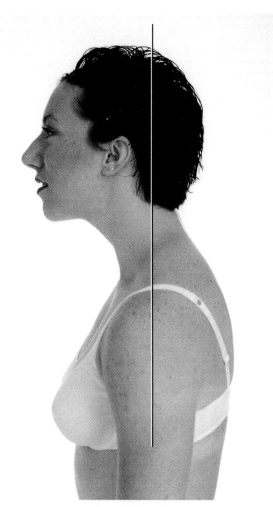

Figure 3-2 Posture with ear forward of sagittal midline

causes of postural misalignment is required to achieve long-term relief (see Chapter 4, Pectoralis Major).

The skull consists of 22 cranial bones, only one of which, the **mandible,** is generally considered movable. The cranial bones are joined by sutures and are regarded by most anatomists as being fused. Craniosacral therapists believe that the cranial bones are capable of small but significant movement, and their treatment approach attempts to influence the movement and positioning of these bones. The arguments for and against craniosacral theory are beyond the scope of this book.

The skull itself rests on the first cervical vertebra or **atlas;** the **occipital condyles** of the skull rest on two kidney-shaped facets on the superior surface of the atlas. The atlas is a bony ring with essentially no body or spine. In turn, the atlas rests on the second cervical vertebra, or **axis,** which has a toothlike projection, the **odontoid process,** projecting up into the ring of the atlas (see Plate 3-2). Turning the head consists of rotation around the odontoid process.

The head is quite heavy. For this reason, and because of the importance of the mobility of the head for using the senses (particularly vision), the neck muscles are numerous, and many are thick and strong. They are all susceptible to pain and dysfunction.

The muscles of the head, face, and neck can be classified as follows:

- Scalp muscles, primarily occipitalis and frontalis (or occipitofrontalis, if viewed as one muscle), and the more dorsal aspects of temporalis. These muscles move the scalp and forehead.
- Face muscles, involved primarily in controlling facial expressions.
- Jaw muscles, which open and close the jaw by moving the mandible.
- Neck muscles, which support and balance the head on the spinal column and move it in all directions.

NOTE: Some of the treatment techniques described in this chapter require work inside the mouth. Two principles should be observed:

- Working inside any body orifice may have emotional implications for the client. Always obtain permission first and discuss any hesitations the client may have.
- Examination gloves should always be worn when working inside any body orifice.

Frontalis

fron-TAL-is

Etymology   Latin, pertaining to the front

Overview

Frontalis (Fig. 3-3) is sometimes regarded as one belly of the muscle occipitofrontalis, since it is connected directly to the occipitalis by the galea aponeurotica, a tendinous sheet of connective tissue that lies over the skull from front to back. Tightness in either the frontalis or occipitalis muscles, or bellies, therefore produces an overall sense of tightness in the scalp. Note that frontalis connects partially to orbicularis oculi (see Plate 3-5); both muscles are commonly involved in headaches.

Attachments

- Superiorly, to the galea aponeurotica
- Inferiorly, to the skin over the eyebrow, partially to the orbicularis oculi, and to the root of the nose

Actions

- Raises the eyebrow and wrinkles the forehead
- Working with occipitalis, helps shift the scalp posteriorly, raising the skin of the forehead and causing the hair to stand up, as in horror

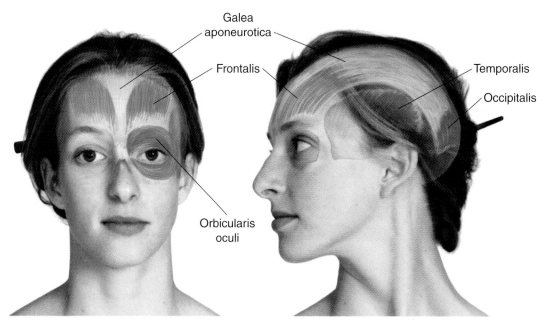

Galea aponeurotica
Frontalis
Temporalis
Occipitalis
Orbicularis oculi

Figure 3-3   Anatomy of frontalis (occipitofrontalis), and galea aponeurotica

Referral Area

Local, with pain radiating over the forehead

Other Muscles to Examine

- Occipitalis
- Orbicularis oculi
- Temporalis
- Sternocleidomastoid
- Zygomaticus major
- Scalenes
- Posterior neck muscles

Manual Therapy

CROSS-FIBER STROKING
- The client lies supine.
- With the fingers spread over the sides of the client's head, place the thumbs at the center of the forehead just over the eyebrows.
- Pressing firmly into the tissue, slowly spread the thumbs apart (Fig. 3-4) until they have covered the forehead to the lateral ridges of the frontal bone.
- Shifting your hands superiorly, repeat this process as far as the hairline.

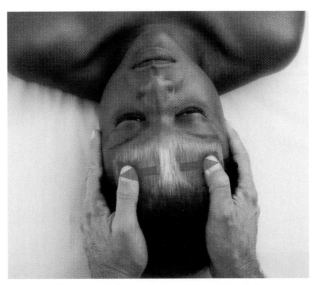

Figure 3-4   Cross-fiber stroking of frontalis

STRIPPING
- The client lies supine.
- Place the tip or flat of the thumb on the forehead at the hairline just next to the center line of the forehead.
- Pressing firmly into the tissue, slide the thumb inferiorly to the medial end of the eyebrow
- Shifting your hand laterally, repeat this process as far as the lateral end of the eyebrow.

Occipitalis

ock-sip-it-TAL-is

Etymology   Latin *occiput*, back of the head

Overview

Occipitalis (Fig. 3-5) is sometimes regarded as the posterior belly of the muscle occipitofrontalis, since it is connected directly to the frontalis by the galea aponeurotica, a tendinous sheet of connective tissue that lies over the skull from front to back. Tightness in either the frontalis or occipitalis muscles or bellies, therefore, produces an overall sense of tightness in the scalp.

Attachments

- Superiorly, to the galea aponeurotica
- Inferiorly, to the superior nuchal line of the occipital bone

Actions

- Anchors and retracts the galea aponeurotica, thus pulling the scalp posteriorly. See frontalis for further discussion (page 66).

Referral Area

Radiates pain locally to the back and top of the head and can refer pain to the ipsilateral eye.

Other Muscles to Examine

- Frontalis
- Temporalis
- Orbicularis oculi
- All lateral and posterior neck muscles

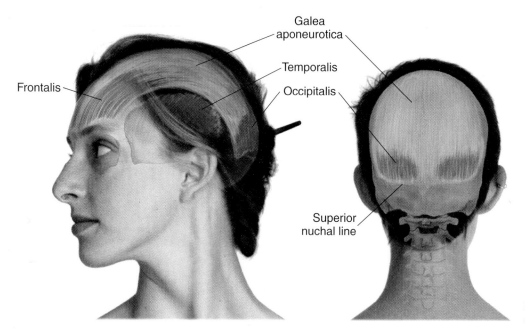

Galea aponeurotica

Temporalis

Frontalis

Occipitalis

Superior nuchal line

Figure 3-5   Anatomy of occipitalis

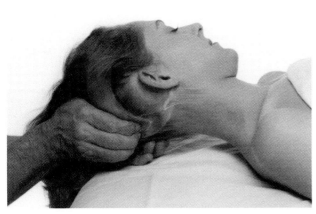

Figure 3-6 Stripping occipitalis with the fingertips

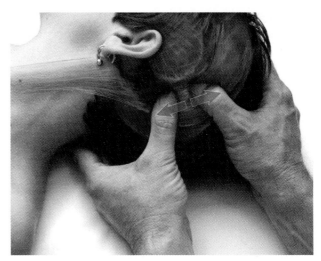

Figure 3-7 Stripping of occipitalis with thumbs

Manual Therapy

STRIPPING (1)
- The client lies supine.
- Place the hands under the head, the fingers curled upward so that the fingertips touch the base of the skull.
- Pressing superiorly and using the weight of the client's head to generate pressure, draw the hands very slowly toward yourself, so that the fingertips treat the entire occipitalis belly (Fig. 3-6).
- Pause where the client reports tender points.

STRIPPING (2)
- The client lies either supine or prone with the head turned away from the therapist.

- Holding the head with one hand, place the other thumb at the center line of the occiput, on a line with the upper part of occipitalis.
- Pressing firmly into the tissue, draw the thumb laterally across occipitalis.
- Placing the thumb in a position closer to the neck, repeat the procedure until you have covered the entire muscle belly.

STRIPPING (3)
- The client lies either supine or prone with the head turned away from the therapist.
- Hold the client's head in both your hands, so that the thumbs rest on the upper part of occipitalis at its center.
- Pressing firmly into the tissue, spread the thumbs apart as far as the outer aspects of the muscle belly (Fig. 3-7).
- Shifting the thumbs to a position nearer the neck, repeat the procedure until the whole muscle belly has been treated.

Orbicularis Oculi

or-bic-yu-LAR-is OCK-yu-lee

Etymology   Latin: *orbiculus,* a small disk + *oculi,* of the eye

Overview

Orbicularis oculi (Fig. 3-8) encircles the eye and provides for voluntary closure of the eyelid. Its trigger points can be activated by frowning and squinting and by trigger points in sternocleidomastoid.

Attachments

- Medially, to the medial palpebral ligament, frontal, and maxillary bones, and to the tissue of the eyelid
- Superiorly and medially, to the orbit

Actions

- Intentional blinking and strong closure of the eyelid.
- Squinting

Referral Area

Superior to the eye and down the side of the nose

Manual Therapy

COMPRESSION
- Using the thumb, seek a common tender or trigger point near the lateral end of the eyebrow.
- Compress and hold for release (Fig. 3-9).

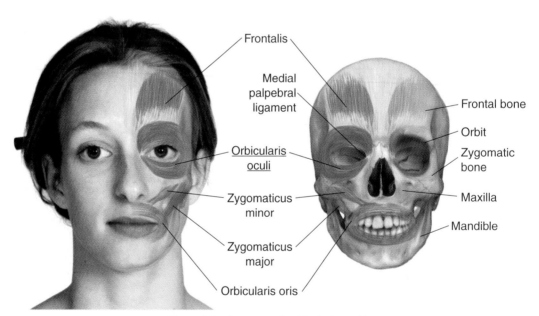

Figure 3-8   Anatomy of orbicularis oculi

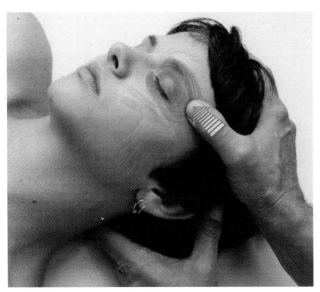

Figure 3-9 Trigger point compression of orbicularis oculi

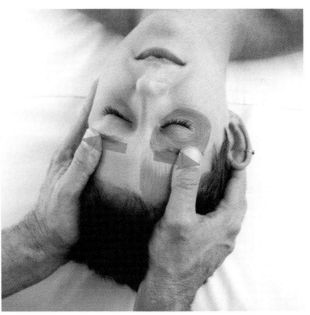

Figure 3-10 Stripping orbicularis oculi superior to the orbit

STRIPPING
- Place the tip of a thumb or finger on the medial end of the eyebrow.
- Pressing firmly into the tissue, slide the thumb or finger outward to the lateral end of the eyebrow (Fig. 3-10).
- Repeat once just superior to the eyebrow, and again just inferior to it, pressing superiorly against the orbit (Fig. 3-11).

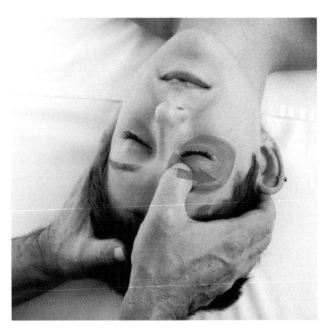

Figure 3-11 Stripping orbicularis oculi pressing upward against the orbit

Zygomaticus Major and Minor

zye-go-MAT-ik-us

Etymology   Greek *zygon,* yoke or joining

Overview

Zygomaticus major and **minor** (Fig. 3-12) are the principal smiling muscles; their trigger points arise from trigger point activity in the chewing muscles (masseter and the pterygoids) (see Plates 3-3 and 3-4). It is best examined by pincer palpation with the index finger in the mouth and the thumb outside the mouth, or vice versa.

Attachments

- Superiorly, to the zygomatic bone
- Inferiorly, to the tissues at the corners of the mouth, blending with fibers of orbicularis oris

Actions

Pull the corners of the mouth up and back, as in smiling

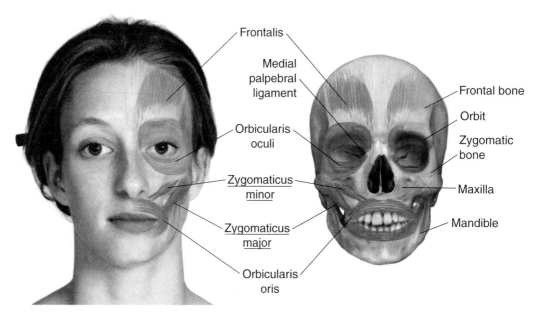

Figure 3-12   Anatomy of zygomaticus

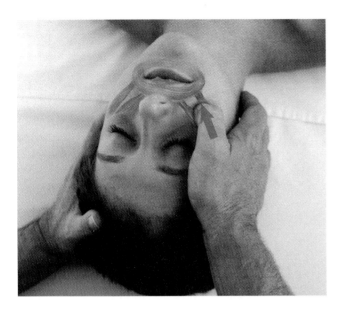

Figure 3-13 Stripping of zygomaticus

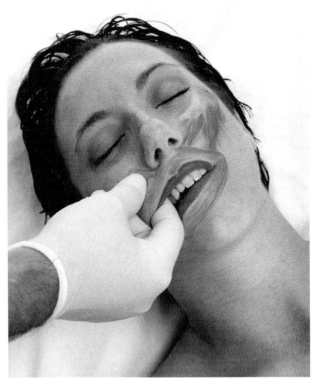

Figure 3-14 Intraoral pincer compression of zygomaticus

Referral Area

Up the cheek and along the side of the nose, past the medial corner of the eye and the eyebrow, and over the medial aspect of the forehead

Other Muscles to Examine

- Masseter
- Pterygoids
- Orbicularis oculi

Manual Therapy

STRIPPING
- The client lies supine.
- Place the edge of the thumb against the zygomatic bone (cheekbone).

- Pressing firmly into the tissue, slide the thumb slowly inferiorly to the corner of the mouth (Fig. 3-13).

COMPRESSION
- The client lies supine.
- Place the index finger inside the mouth in the pouch of the cheek.
- Place the tip of the thumb on the outside of the cheek.
- Using pincer palpation, explore the length of the muscle for trigger points or tender points. Compress and hold each point until it releases (Fig. 3-14).

Temporalis

TEM-per-AL-is

Etymology   Latin, relating to the temple

Overview

Temporalis (Fig. 3-15) is a large, scallop-shaped muscle covering the side of the head in front of, superior to, and behind the ear. It is a muscle of the temporomandibular joint (TMJ). It should be examined and treated in all clients complaining of headaches or TMJ problems. Therapists usually pay a lot of attention to the anterior and middle portions, but the posterior section of the muscle should be addressed as well.

Attachments

- Superiorly, to the bone and fascia in the temporal fossa superior to the zygomatic arch

- Inferiorly, to the coronoid process of the mandible and the anterior edge of the ramus of the mandible

Actions

- Closes the jaw
- Moves the jaw posteriorly and laterally
- Maintains the resting position of the mandible

Referral Areas

To all or part of temporal region, eyebrow region, cheek, and incisor and molar teeth.

Other Muscles to Examine

- Masseter
- Pterygoids
- All facial muscles
- All anterior, lateral, and posterior neck muscles

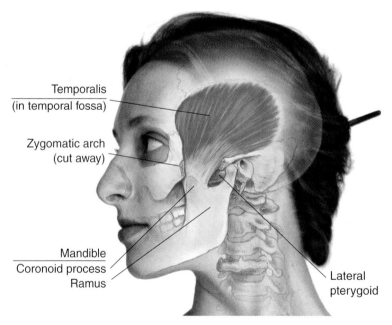

Temporalis
(in temporal fossa)

Zygomatic arch
(cut away)

Mandible
Coronoid process
Ramus

Lateral
pterygoid

Figure 3-15   Anatomy of temporalis

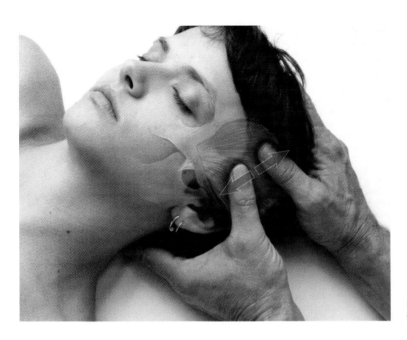

Figure 3-16 Cross-fiber stroking of temporalis with thumbs

Manual Therapy

STRIPPING
- The client lies supine.
- Place fingertips at top of anterior part of muscle (superior and lateral to eyebrow).
- Pressing firmly medially, glide the fingertips inferiorly toward zygomatic arch.
- Place fingertips at the top of the muscle more posteriorly on head. (Note that the muscle is shaped like a scallop, so that it begins higher on the head toward its center, then lower toward the back of the head.) Repeat movement toward zygomatic arch, pressing firmly.
- Continue until the entire muscle is covered.

STROKING ACROSS THE FIBER (1)
- The client lies supine.
- Place fingertips on sides of client's forehead at the anterior edge of temporal fossa (superior to lateral end of eyebrows).
- Pressing firmly, glide the fingertips across the muscle to its posterior edge behind the ear.
- Moving downward, repeat the procedure to cover the entire muscle.

STROKING ACROSS THE FIBER (2)
- The client lies supine.
- Hold the client's head in your spread hands, with your thumbs resting together on the anterior aspect of temporalis.
- Pressing firmly into the muscle with the edges of your thumbs, glide your thumbs apart, so that each thumb slides an inch or two (Fig. 3-16). Move the hands posteriorly, repeating the procedure, until the entire temporalis muscle is covered.

Masseter

MASS-e-ter

Etymology   Greek, masticator

Overview

Masseter (Fig. 3-17) is the most prominent chewing muscle. It should be treated first in TMJ problems, since it is in an easily accessible position.

Attachments

- Superiorly, to zygomatic process of the maxilla and to the zygomatic arch

- Inferiorly, superficial layer of muscle to external surface of the mandible at its angle and to the inferior half of its ramus; deep layer of muscle to superior half of the ramus, possibly extending to the angle of the mandible

Action

Raises mandible in conjunction with temporalis and pterygoids

Referral Area

- To upper and lower jaw, side of face, ear, and superior to eyebrow.
- May also cause tinnitus (ringing in the ears).

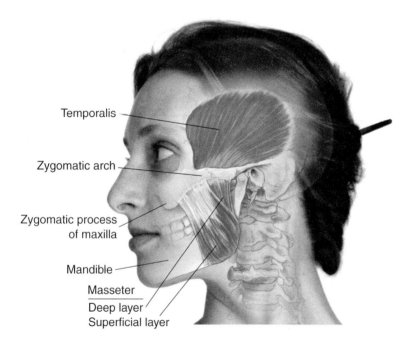

Temporalis

Zygomatic arch

Zygomatic process of maxilla

Mandible

Masseter
Deep layer
Superficial layer

Figure 3-17   Anatomy of masseter

Other Muscles to Examine

- Temporalis
- Pterygoids
- All facial muscles
- All muscles of anterior, lateral, and posterior neck

Manual Therapy

STRIPPING

- The client lies supine.
- Place the thumb or fingertips at the upper aspect of the muscle, just anterior to the opening of the ear canal.
- Pressing firmly inward, glide the thumb (Fig. 3-18A) or fingertips (Fig. 3-18B) downward along the length of the muscle to the mandible.
- Pause at barriers or tender spots until release is felt.
- Make as many passes as necessary, starting nearest the ear and working forward, to cover the entire muscle (usually one or two passes will suffice).
- When a great deal of tenderness is present, repeat the above process, beginning lightly and pressing in more deeply each time.

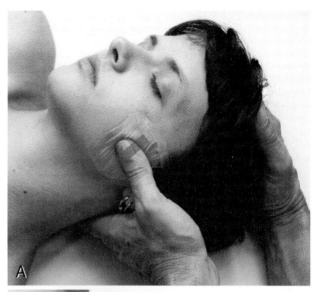

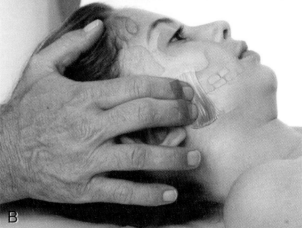

Figure 3-18 External stripping of masseter (A) with the thumb, (B) with the fingertips

Pterygoids

TER-ri-goids

Etymology Greek *pteryx*, wing + *eidos*, resemblance; "winglike"

Overview

The **pterygoids** (Fig. 3-19) are jaw (temporomandibular joint, or TMJ) muscles that radiate in a winglike pattern, hence their name. They are a complex set of muscles, with different parts of the muscles participating in all jaw movements, and stabilization of the TMJ. A small part of the lateral pterygoid can be accessed from outside the mouth, while the medial pterygoids must be examined and treated intraorally. Examination and treatment of the pterygoid muscles can be somewhat awkward and uncomfortable, but they are often key factors in pain in the jaw, face, and ear. They are also major players in TMJ syndrome.

NOTE: The head is anatomically complex, and the attachments of the pterygoids are particularly challenging to illustrate. For this reason, and because these attachments are not necessarily relevant to the massage therapist, not all of them can be seen in the anatomy plates. The student interested in more detail should consult an anatomy atlas.

Medial or Internal Pterygoid

Attachments

- Superiorly, to the inner surface of the lateral pterygoid plate and the lateral surface of the palatine bone, and to the maxilla
- Inferiorly to the lower border of the ramus of the mandible, close to the angle of the mandible, and to the medial surface of the ramus of the mandible near the angle.

Actions

- Participates in raising the mandible
- Protracts the mandible
- Acting alternately, moves the mandible from side to side in grinding motion

Referral Area

- Jaw in front of ear
- Side of jaw (both outside and inside mouth)

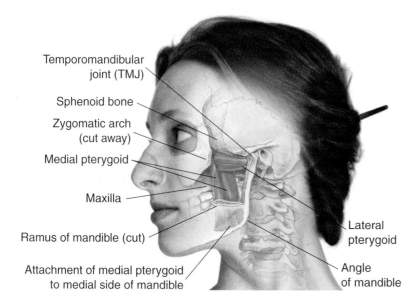

Temporomandibular joint (TMJ)
Sphenoid bone
Zygomatic arch (cut away)
Medial pterygoid
Maxilla
Ramus of mandible (cut)
Attachment of medial pterygoid to medial side of mandible
Lateral pterygoid
Angle of mandible

Figure 3-19 Anatomy of pterygoids

Lateral or External Pterygoid

This muscle has two divisions: superior and inferior. Note that the two divisions of the lateral pterygoid are antagonists.

Attachments

Superior attachments:

- Superiorly, to infratemporal crest and inferior lateral surface of greater wing of sphenoid bone
- Inferiorly, to lateral surface of lateral pterygoid plate

Inferior attachments:

- Superiorly, backward, and somewhat downward toward the TMJ, to the ligament of the joint capsule, the articular disc, and the lateral pterygoid plate of the sphenoid
- Inferiorly, diagonally upward to condylar neck and ramus of the mandible just inferior to the joint, to the neck of the mandible, articular disc, and capsule of the temporomandibular joint

Actions

- The two divisions of this muscle are involved in raising and lowering the mandible, as well as moving the mandible posteriorly, anteriorly, and laterally.

- Depresses and protracts the mandible
- Acting alternately, produces side-to-side grinding

Referral Area

- TMJ region
- Face around cheekbone

Other Muscles to Examine

- Masseter
- Temporalis
- All facial muscles
- Anterior, posterior, and lateral neck muscles

Manual Therapy

All of the following are performed with the client supine.

EXTERNAL COMPRESSION (1)
- Use the thumb to find the space just anterior to the TMJ.
- Compress upward, downward, and forward, seeking tender points (Fig. 3-20). Hold each tender point until it releases.

EXTERNAL COMPRESSION (2)
- Place the thumb or two fingertips just under the angle of the mandible.
- Press superiorly and into the medial surface of the mandible, moving slowly and gently, seeking tender points.
- Compress any tender points against the medial surface of the mandible (Fig. 3-21).

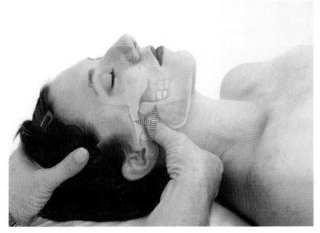

Figure 3-20 Compression of pterygoids (1)

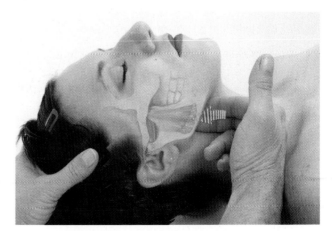

Figure 3-21 Compression of pterygoids (2)

Levator Veli Palatini, Tensor Veli Palatini, and the Palatine Aponeurosis

le-VAY-ter VEL-lee pa-LAT-in-ee

TEN-ser VEL-lee pa-LAT-in-ee

PAL-a-tine ap-o-new-RO-sis

Etymology Levator veli palatini: Latin *levator*, raiser + *velum*, veil or sail + *palatini*, of the palate; "raiser of the veil of the palate"

Tensor veli palatini: Latin *tensor*, tightener + *velum*, veil or sail + *palatini*, of the palate; "tightener of the veil of the palate"

Aponeurosis: Greek, the end of a muscle, where it becomes tendon, from *apo*, from + *neuron*, sinew

Overview

Levator and **tensor palatini** (Fig. 3-22) both attach to the Eustachian (auditory) tube at one end and the palatine aponeurosis at the other. Although further research is needed, they may be involved in the cause of chronic ear infections, as they play a role in keeping the Eustachian tube open.

Attachments

Levator:

- Superiorly, to cartilage of auditory tube and petrous part of temporal bone
- Inferiorly, to palatine aponeurosis

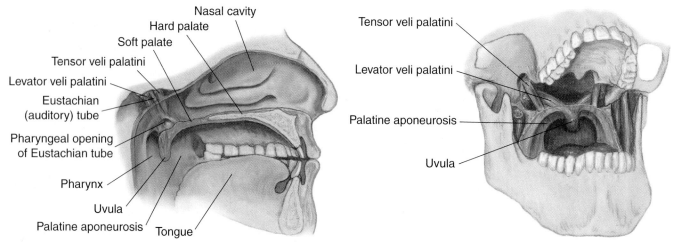

Figure 3-22 Anatomy of tensor and levator veli palatini

Tensor:

- Superiorly, to cartilage of auditory tube, medial pterygoid plate, and spine of sphenoid bone
- Inferiorly, to palatine aponeurosis

Actions

As their names imply, the levator raises the soft palate, and the tensor tenses the soft palate. Both muscles also open the auditory tube to equalize air pressure between the middle ear and the pharynx.

Referral Area

Because these muscles can be accessed only via the palatine aponeurosis, we have no knowledge of trigger points or referral zones for them; however, they are highly suspect in the presence of ear pain and infection.

Other Muscles to Examine

- Temporalis
- Masseter
- Pterygoids
- All anterior, lateral, and posterior neck muscles

Manual Therapy for the Jaw Muscles: Intraoral Work

All of the following are performed with the client supine. Have the client open the mouth as wide as is comfortable.

MANUAL THERAPY FOR THE PALATINE APONEUROSIS (LEVATOR VELI PALATINI, TENSOR VELI PALATINI)

- Place the gloved fingertip on the roof of the mouth just medial to the upper molars.
- Pressing firmly (but gently) superiorly, glide the fingertip back toward the pharynx.
- Maintaining pressure, carefully glide the fingertip along the soft palate toward the center (medially) (Fig. 3-23).

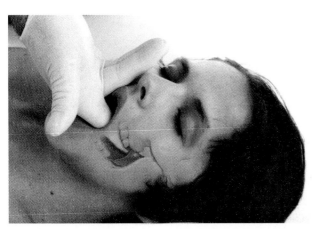
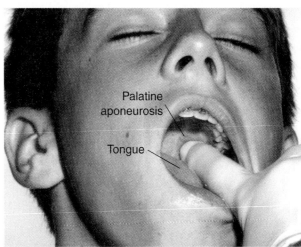

Palatine aponeurosis

Tongue

Figure 3-23 Release of palatine aponeurosis (1)

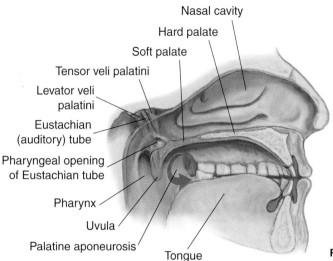

Nasal cavity
Hard palate
Soft palate
Tensor veli palatini
Levator veli palatini
Eustachian (auditory) tube
Pharyngeal opening of Eustachian tube
Pharynx
Uvula
Palatine aponeurosis
Tongue

Figure 3-24 Release of palatine aponeurosis (2)

MANUAL THERAPY FOR THE INNER ASPECT

■ Beginning just posterior to the last upper molar on the medial side, press the tissue against the bone firmly, gliding in a deep (posterior) direction. The movement should form a "U" shape (Fig. 3-24) as it passes over the inner aspect of the maxilla and mandible just posterior to the teeth, first inferiorly, then anteriorly just posterior to the last upper molar.

MANUAL THERAPY BETWEEN THE MAXILLA AND MANDIBLE

■ Place the fingertip at the deepest point (the bend) of the "U" movement just made; that is, on the medial aspect of the mandible.
■ Pressing the tissue firmly against the bone, move the finger laterally between the teeth (Fig. 3-25).

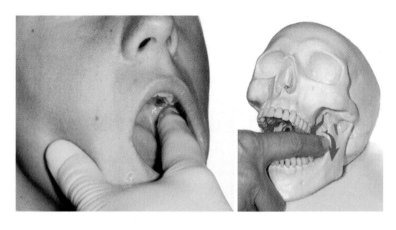

Figure 3-25 Stroking between the maxilla and mandible

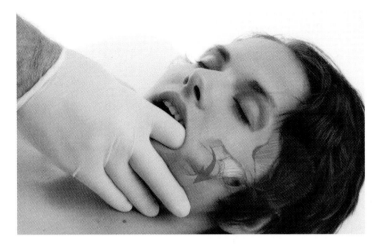

Figure 3-26   Intraoral stroke over the coronoid process

MANUAL THERAPY OF OUTER ASPECT
- Beginning just posterior to the last upper molar on the lateral side, press the tissue against the bone firmly, moving in a deep (posterior) direction. The movement should form a "U" shape as it passes over the coronoid process and inside (deep to) the masseter, first inferiorly, then anteriorly to just posterior to the last lower molar (Fig. 3-26).
- Repeat the above movement pressing outward to work the masseter from inside. You can also work the front border of the masseter with the fingertip (Fig. 3-27).

 Caution
- If you are worried about being bitten, use a finger of the non-treating hand to press the cheek between the client's teeth.
- To suppress the gag reflex while working medially, have the client curl the tongue backward into the pharynx.

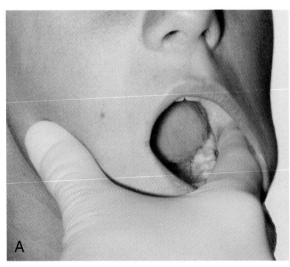
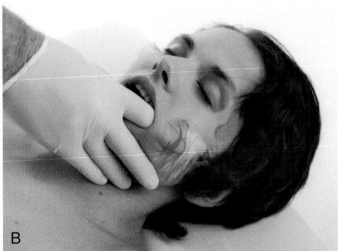

Figure 3-27   Intraoral compression of masseter: (A) intraoral view, (B) lateral view

Platysma

pla-TIZ-ma

Etymology Greek, a flatplate

Overview

Platysma (Fig. 3-28) is a thin, flat, subcutaneous muscle. It lies parallel to sternocleidomastoid, and its trigger points tend to occur in conjunction with that muscle.

Attachments

- Superiorly, to the corner of the mouth and the other facial muscles in that region, and to the lower aspect of the mandible
- Inferiorly, to the superficial fascia of the upper anterior chest

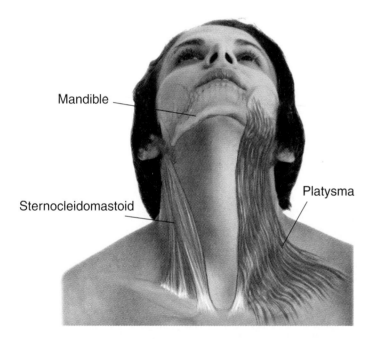

Mandible

Sternocleidomastoid

Platysma

Figure 3-28 Anatomy of platysma

Actions

- Pulls the corner of the mouth downward and the skin of the chest upward.
- Tenses the skin of the neck (as in horror)

Referral Area

Over the anterior neck in the area of the sternocleidomastoid; may also be a hot, prickly sensation to the upper chest

Other Muscles to Examine

Sternocleidomastoid

Manual Therapy

STRIPPING

- Place the fingertips on the chest 2 or 3 inches below the clavicle, just medial to the anterior deltoid.
- Pressing firmly into the tissue, glide the fingertips superiorly over the clavicle and up the neck, then over the mandible and halfway up the cheek.
- Shift the fingertips medially to the next uncovered area and repeat the procedure (Fig. 3-29), ending the stroke at the mouth.
- Repeat the procedure across the chest, with the last stroke beginning at the sternum.
- The same procedure may be performed from superior to inferior using the edge of the thumb.

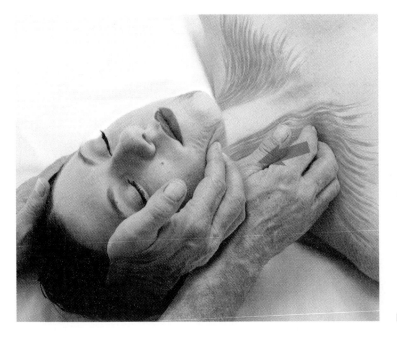

Figure 3-29 Stripping platysma with fingertips

Muscles Attached to the Hyoid Bone

Etymology Greek, *hyoeides,* shaped like the letter upsilon (u- or v-shaped)

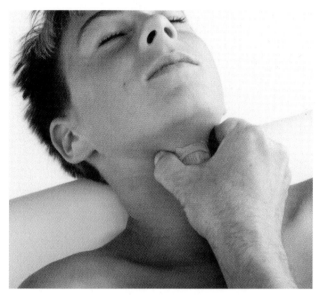

Figure 3-30 Locating the hyoid bone by palpation

Overview

The **hyoid bone** lies just superior to the thyroid cartilage at the level of the body of the third cervical vertebra. It is the first resistant structure below the chin. To find it, place your thumb and index finger on either side of the anterior neck below the chin about 3 or 4 inches apart. Squeeze gently. If you don't feel resistance, shift your fingers a little farther down and squeeze again. Repeat until you feel a resistant structure (Fig. 3-30). It may also help to ask the client to swallow, which will cause a palpable movement of the hyoid bone.

Many muscles attach to the hyoid bone (Fig. 3-31). Those superior to the hyoid bone are called **suprahyoid** muscles; those inferior, **infrahyoid** muscles. They fan out from the hyoid bone both above and below. It is not necessary in basic clinical massage therapy, and therefore this book, to distinguish them all; they can be worked as a group above and below. The principal muscle involved in pain referral and clinical treatment is the digastric muscle, which is discussed separately on page 88. Geniohyoid and sternothyroid are not illustrated because they lie deep to mylohyoid and sternohyoid; their anatomical details are not essential to the purposes of this book.

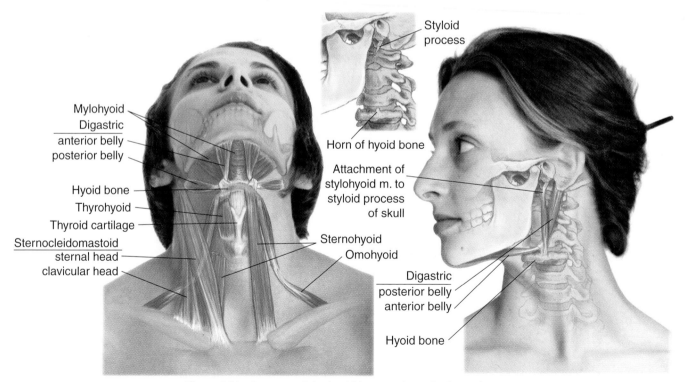

Figure 3-31 Anatomy of the hyoid bone and attached muscles

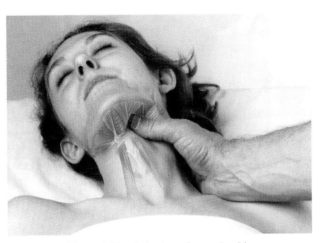

Figure 3-32 Stripping of suprahyoids

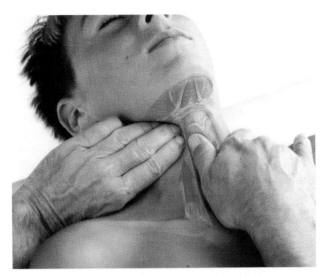

Figure 3-33 Stripping of infrahyoids

Suprahyoid muscles:

- Digastric (indirectly attached to the hyoid bone)
- Stylohyoid
- Mylohyoid
- Geniohyoid (not illustrated)

Infrahyoid muscles:

- Sternohyoid
- Thyrohyoid
- Omohyoid
- Sternothyroid (not illustrated)

Manual Therapy of the Suprahyoid Muscles

STRIPPING

- Locate the hyoid bone with your thumb and index finger.
- Place your thumb just superior to the hyoid bone medial to its horn (end) (Fig. 3-32).
- Pressing gently into the tissue, glide the tip of your thumb slowly superiorly to the inner surface of the mandible at the center.
- Starting again superior to the hyoid bone, place your thumb slightly lateral to the previous starting point.
- Slide the thumb slowly superiorly to the inner surface of the mandible, parallel to the first pass.

- Repeat the process, letting the path of your thumb fan out from the hyoid bone until it ends at the styloid process between the angle of the mandible and the mastoid process, just inferior to the ear.

Caution

Do not exert excessive pressure on the styloid process; it can be broken.

Manual Therapy of the Infrahyoid Muscles

STRIPPING

- With the side of one thumb or finger, gently press the thyroid cartilage laterally away from you.
- Place the thumb or fingertips of the other hand just superior to the manubrium next to the trachea.
- Pressing gently, glide the thumb or fingertips slowly up to the hyoid bone (Fig. 3-33). Place the tip of the thumb just over the clavicle slightly lateral to the sternal notch and repeat the above procedure.
- Repeat this procedure until you have covered a fan-shaped area extending to the clavicular attachment of sternocleidomastoid.

Digastric

die-GAS-trick

Etymology Greek *di*, two + *gaster*, belly

Overview

One of a group of muscles that attach to the hyoid bone, **digastric** (Fig. 3-34) is close to and difficult to distinguish from the **stylohyoid.** Digastric takes its name from its two bellies: one is between the mastoid process and the hyoid bone, the other between the hyoid bone and the mandible.

Attachments

- Inferiorly, both bellies attach to the hyoid bone.
- Superiorly, the posterior belly attaches to the mastoid process deep to longissimus capitis, splenius capitis, and sternocleidomastoid; the anterior belly attaches to the inferior edge of the mandible near the center.

Actions

- Lowers the mandible (opening the jaw)
- Raises the hyoid bone
- Retracts the mandible
- Participates in swallowing and coughing
- Steadies the hyoid in coughing, swallowing, and sneezing

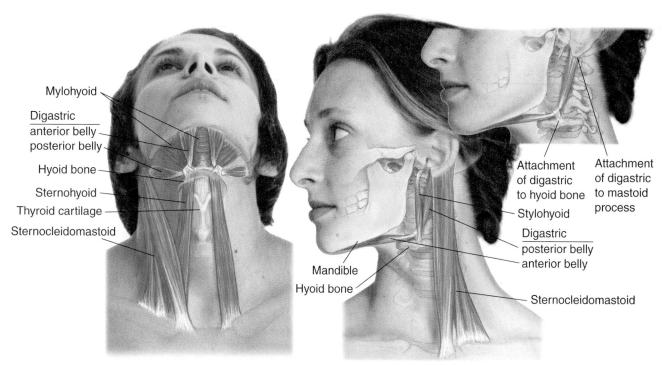

Figure 3-34 Anatomy of digastric and stylohyoid

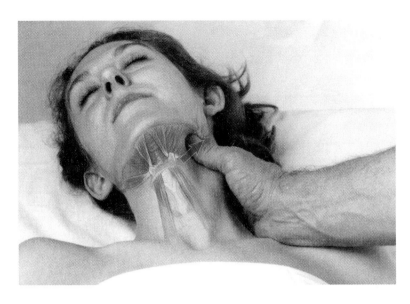

Figure 3-35   Stripping of posterior belly of digastric

Referral Area

Posterior belly: inferior to, over, and behind the angle of the mandible; over the mastoid process; into the occipital region
Anterior belly: to the four lower incisors and directly inferior to them

Other Muscles to Examine

- Other muscles of the anterior and lateral neck
- Occipitalis

Manual Therapy

STRIPPING

- Gently locate the hyoid bone using the tips of your thumb and index finger.
- Place the tip of the thumb or a finger just superior to one side of the hyoid bone.
- Pressing gently, follow the posterior belly to the mastoid process (Fig. 3-35).
- Starting at the same position, follow the anterior belly to a point just to one side of the center of the underside of the mandible.
- Pause where tenderness is found and wait for release.
- Repeat on the opposite side.

Sternocleidomastoid

STERN-o-KLIDE-o-MASS-toid

Etymology   Greek: *sternon*, chest + *kleis*, clavicle + *mastos*, breast + *eidos*, resemblance

Overview

Sternocleidomastoid (usually abbreviated **SCM**) (Fig. 3-36) is a two-headed muscle with major responsibilities for stabilizing, turning, and flexing the head and neck. It is also a common site for many trigger points that cause a wide variety of headaches. Sternocleidomastoid should be examined carefully in all clients complaining of headaches. Its two heads are the **sternal,** which is more anterior, medial, and superficial; and the **clavicular,** which is more posterior, lateral, and deep. Note that the sternocleidomastoid also maintains posture by helping to compensate for tilting of the shoulder girdle.

Attachments

- Superiorly to the lateral surface of the mastoid process and the lateral half of the superior nuchal line of the occipital bone

Inferiorly:

- Sternal head: to the anterior surface of the manubrium

- Clavicular head: to the medial third of the anterior surface of the clavicle

Actions

Bilateral:

- Stabilizes the head and neck
- Resists neck hyperextension and backward movement of the head (whiplash)
- Flexes the neck
- Participates to some degree in swallowing and breathing

Unilateral:

- Rotates face to the opposite side
- Tilts face upward
- With trapezius, bends the head and neck to the side

Referral Area

- Sternal head: into the occipital region, in an arc over the eye, the top of the head, the cheek, and areas on and inferior to the chin
- Clavicular head: into the ear, behind the ear, and into the frontal region bilaterally

Other Muscles to Examine

All other muscles of the anterior, lateral, and posterior neck

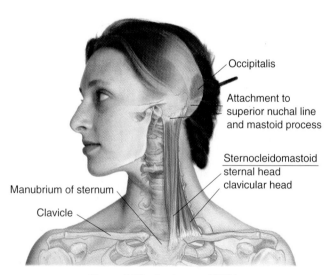

Figure 3-36 Anatomy of SCM

Occipitalis

Attachment to superior nuchal line and mastoid process

Sternocleidomastoid
sternal head
clavicular head

Manubrium of sternum

Clavicle

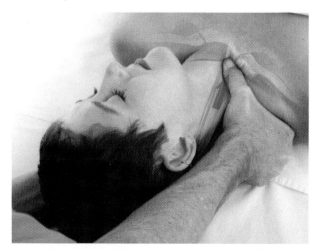

Figure 3-37 Stripping of sternal head of SCM

Manual Therapy

STRIPPING

- The client is supine. Hold the client's head in one hand and turn it slightly to the side opposite to the muscle you intend to work on.
- Place the thumb or fingertips of the other hand on the attachment of the muscle at the mastoid process.
- Pressing firmly into the tissue, slide the thumb or fingertips slowly down the sternal head all the way to the attachment at the manubrium, pausing at tender spots until they release (Fig. 3-37).

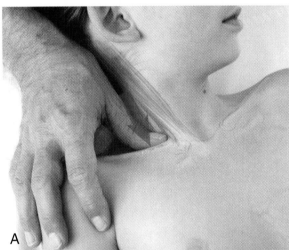

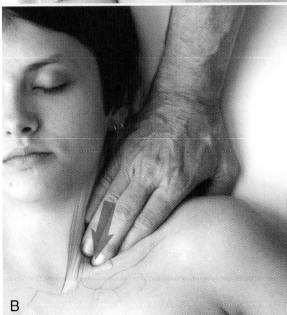

Figure 3-38 Stripping of clavicular head of SCM with thumb (A) and fingertips (B)

- Beginning at the superior attachment again, repeat the process on the clavicular head, all the way to the attachment on the clavicle (Fig. 3-38).
- Repeat the above process on the other side.

PINCER COMPRESSION

- Hold the client's head in one hand, firmly supporting the back of the head and base of the skull.
- Lift the head a few inches to induce sternocleidomastoid to stand out; turn the head slightly away from the side on which you intend to work.
- Starting as close as possible to the mastoid attachment, grasp the sternal head between your thumb and either the side of your index finger or the tips of your index and middle fingers (Fig. 3-39).
- Compress firmly but gently, asking the client for feedback about tenderness and/or pain referral. If there is tightness or tenderness, hold until release.
- Shift your fingers down slightly, repeating until you get as close to the manubrium as possible.
- Turn the client's head a little farther from the side you are working on, and repeat the above process with the clavicular head. Note that this head is more difficult to grasp, as it lies deeper than the sternal head.
- Repeat the entire process on the other side.

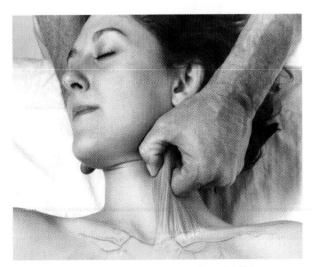

Figure 3-39 Pincer compression of SCM

Scaleni (Scalenes)

ska-LEN-ee

Etymology   Greek, *skalenos,* uneven

Overview

The **scalenes** (Fig. 3-40) are known for their propensity to refer pain. Although they have the fairly simple function of tilting the head to either side, we also tend to use them to hold up the ribcage, and as inappropriate accessory muscles in paradoxical breathing (see Chapter 4, Muscles of Breathing). As a result, we subject the scalenes to substantial tension. Few people escape problems with these muscles.

The term **thoracic outlet** is used to refer to the entire area defined by scalenes and the first rib, or to the passage between the anterior and middle scalenes. On their way to the arm, the axillary (subclavian) artery and brachial plexus pass between these two muscles, then between the first rib and the clavicle. They can become entrapped at some point in this area by tightness in the anterior and middle scalenes. It is sometimes difficult to distinguish pain referred by the scalenes from pain resulting from entrapment of the brachial plexus.

NOTE: Scalenus minimus is not found in everyone, and often occurs on only one side. Although it can have a trigger point, it is difficult to isolate manually, and may be treated as an aspect of the anterior scalene.

Attachments

Anterior scalene (scalenus anterior):

- Superiorly, to the front of the transverse processes of C3 through C6
- Inferiorly, to the inner upper edge of the first rib

Middle scalene (scalenus medius):

- Superiorly, to the back of the transverse processes of C2 through C7
- Inferiorly, to the outer upper edge of the first rib

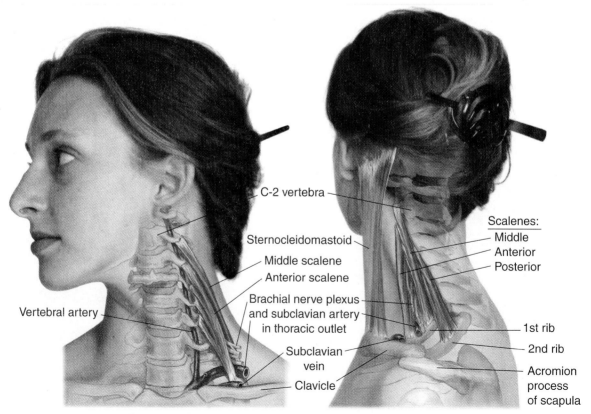

Figure 3-40 Anatomy of the scalenes and the thoracic outlet

Posterior scalene (scalenus posterior):

- Superiorly, to the back of the transverse processes of C5 or C6 and C7
- Inferiorly, to the lateral surface of the second rib, and sometimes also the third

Scalenus minimus (found in most, but not all, people):

- Superiorly, to the front of the transverse process of C7
- Inferiorly, to the top of the pleural dome and the inner edge of the first rib

Actions

- Primary lateral flexors of the cervical spine
- Anterior scalenes: bilaterally, assist in flexion of the neck
- Posterior scalenes: stabilizers of the neck, participate in inspiration, also tend to be involved in raising the ribcage in lifting and carrying

Referral Area

- Over the shoulder and down the medial side of the shoulderblade
- Over the upper anterior chest
- Down the front of the upper arm

- Down the radial half of the forearm and into the thumb and fingers, especially the index finger
- Scalenus minimus: dorsum of the forearm and hand

Other Muscles to Examine

All muscles of the rotator cuff, anterior chest, and arm

Manual Therapy
STRIPPING (1)
- The client lies supine.
- Stand at the client's head. Hold the head underneath with one hand.
- Place the fingers of the other hand under the client's neck, and with the thumb find the upper part of the anterior scalene (Fig. 3-41).
- Pressing firmly into the tissue, slide the thumb slowly along the muscle as far as you can reach, into the space behind the clavicle.
- Repeat the process, this time finding the middle scalene.
- Repeat the process, this time finding the posterior scalene and following it as far as you can into the space just anterior to the edge of trapezius (Fig. 3-42).
- Repeat the entire process on the other side.

As an alternative to the above procedure, you can use the fingertips rather than the thumb (Fig. 3-43).

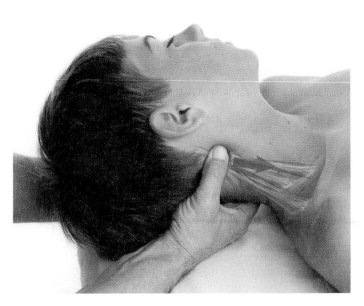

Figure 3-41 Stripping of anterior scalene

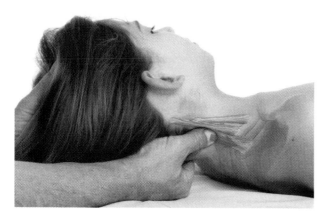

Figure 3-42 Stripping of posterior scalene with thumb

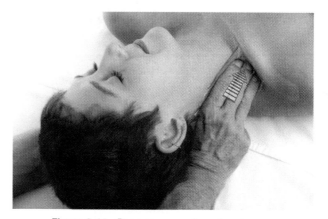

Figure 3-44 Deep compression of scalenes

DEEP COMPRESSION
- The client lies supine.
- Stand or sit at the client's head. Place the fingertips on the scalenes at the base of the neck. Press deeply into the tissues in a diagonal direction toward the chest on the opposite side of the client. Hold until the muscles release (Fig. 3-44).

COMPRESSION
- The client lies prone.
- Stand beside the client facing the client's head. Place your hand at the base of the client's neck, with the heel of the hand resting over trapezius and levator scapulae.
- Curl the fingers over trapezius so that they grasp the scalenes at the base of the neck.

- Squeeze, at first gently, then with increasing firmness, as you feel the scalenes release.

STRIPPING (2)
- The client lies prone.
- Stand at the client's head facing the client.
- Holding the head steady with one hand, find the superior portion of the middle scalene with the other thumb.
- Pressing firmly into the tissue just anterior to the edge of trapezius (Fig. 3-45), slide the thumb along the anterior scalene as far as it will go.
- Repeat for posterior scalene.
- The previous procedure may also be performed using the knuckles (Fig. 3-46).

STRIPPING (3)
- The client is seated.
- Stand behind seated client.
- Place the thumb on the middle scalene at its superior attachment (Fig. 3-47).
- Pressing deeply into the tissue, glide the thumb along the muscle to its inferior attachment.
- Repeat above procedure for anterior and posterior scalenes.

POSTERIOR NECK MUSCLES

Overview

Because of the large number of overlapping muscles in the posterior neck, it is difficult to isolate them and their tender points manually. When you

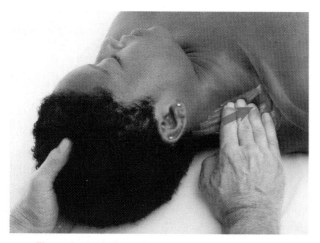

Figure 3-43 Stripping of scalenes with fingertips

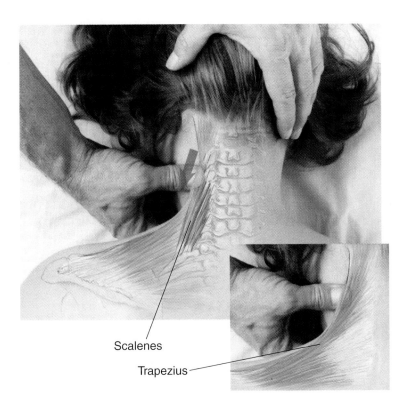

Scalenes

Trapezius

Figure 3-45 Stripping of scalenes with client prone: thumb is on the scalenes. Inset shows thumb under the edge of trapezius.

find a tender point by pressing deeply a little inferior to the skull, for example, is the tender point located in trapezius, splenius capitis, or semispinalis capitis? Often you can only make an educated guess, usually based on the referral area.

Fortunately, for the purposes of this book, it is not necessary to isolate the location of a trigger point in a particular muscle of the posterior neck

with absolute precision. Because all of these muscles are frequently in a state of strain due of reading, desk work, or poor posture, and because they are all commonly responsible for headaches, they should be treated together. It is important, however, to become familiar with their individual attachments and actions, since more advanced approaches require precise isolation.

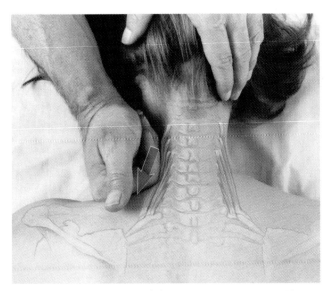

Figure 3-46 Stripping of the scalenes with the knuckles

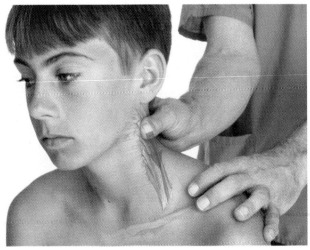

Figure 3-47 Stripping of scalenes with client seated

Trapezius

tra-PEEZ-ee-us

Etymology Greek, *trapezium,* a table, from *tetra,* four + *pous,* foot

Overview

Trapezius (Fig. 3-48) covers a vast territory and performs a wide variety of functions. Although it is an important posterior neck muscle, it is also a shoulder and back muscle. Problems in trapezius may cause a great deal of pain and discomfort. It is the muscle most commonly addressed in informal backrubs between friends, because it is so ac-cessible and because manual therapy of trapezius gives tremendous relief. For most people, it is the chief repository of day-to-day tension.

Trapezius lies superficial to all other muscles of the posterior neck, shoulders, and upper back; therefore, examination and treatment of the other muscles of this region inherently involve examination and treatment of trapezius. It is important to be aware of its attachments, actions, and referral patterns because of the major role it plays in upper body pain and dysfunction.

In general, examination and treatment of the cervical portion of trapezius is accomplished through examination and treatment of the other muscles of the posterior neck. The same is true for the portions of middle trapezius over and around the scapula.

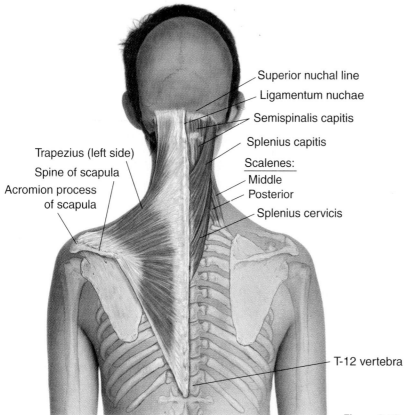

Figure 3-48 Anatomy of trapezius

Attachments

Upper trapezius:

- Superiorly and medially, to the superior nuchal line, the ligamentum nuchae, and the spinous processes of C1 through C5
- Inferiorly and laterally, to the outer third of the clavicle

Middle trapezius:

- Medially, to the spinous processes and ligaments of C6 through T3
- Laterally, to the acromion and upper aspect of the spine of the scapula

Lower trapezius:

- Medially, to the spinous processes and ligaments of T4 through T12
- Laterally, to the medial end of the spine of the scapula, next to the lower attachment of levator scapulae

Actions

- Elevates the scapula (with levator scapulae)
- Rotates the scapula upward (moves the glenoid fossa upward)

- Retracts the scapula (pulling toward the spinal column)
- Depresses the scapula
- Extends the head and neck (bilateral action)
- Turns the head and neck (unilateral action)

Referral Area

- Trigger points in the part of upper trapezius overlying the shoulder refer pain up the neck to the mastoid process and over the ear to the temporal region; also to the angle of the mandible.
- Trigger points in middle and lower trapezius refer pain into the posterior neck at the base of the skull, across the posterior shoulders, and between the shoulder blades.
- Trigger points in middle trapezius, particularly toward the lateral end near the acromion, refer pain to the outer surface of the arm proximal and inferior to the elbow.

Other Muscles to Examine

All muscles of the posterior and lateral neck, the upper back, and around the scapula.

Manual Therapy

STRIPPING

- The client lies prone.
- Stand at the client's head and place one hand flat on the client's shoulder at the base of the neck, the fingers pointing inferiorly.
- Using your body weight and pressing firmly into the tissue, slide the hand inferiorly between the vertebral column and the scapula all the way to the end of the thoracic spine, transmitting your weight primarily to the client through the heel of your hand (Fig. 3-49).

- Place the same or opposite hand—whichever is most comfortable for you—at the same starting point.
- Using the same weight and motion, and shifting the position of your feet so that your weight is behind the movement of your hand, slide your hand diagonally along the back just inside the medial edge of the scapula, past the inferior angle of the scapula.
- Place the heel of your opposite hand just lateral to the lower cervical vertebrae.
- Pressing firmly, slide your hand over the upper aspect of the scapula continuing to the acromion (Fig. 3-50).
- Repeat this procedure on the other side.

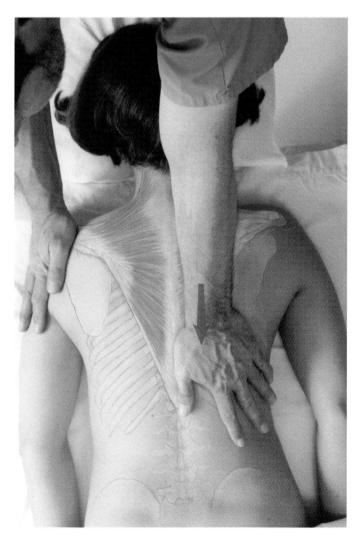

Figure 3-49 Deep stripping of trapezius

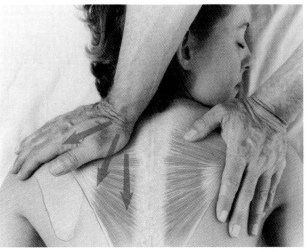

Figure 3-50   Deep stripping of superolateral trapezius

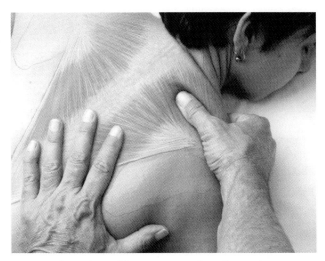

Figure 3-51   Pincer compression of trapezius

PETRISSAGE
- Stand at the side of the prone client at the elbow, facing the client's head.
- Place both hands on the client's near shoulder on the upper trapezius.
- Squeeze and pull the tissue, first with one hand, then with the other, beginning gently and allowing your grasp to become firmer as the tissue relaxes.
- To finish, grasp the muscle with one hand and shake it several times.
- Move to the other side of the client and repeat the procedure.

PINCER COMPRESSION
- Stand at the side of the prone client at the elbow, facing the client's head.
- Place the hand that is closest to the client's head on the client's upper trapezius.
- Grasp it firmly between your fingers and thumb, and hold it. Begin with a gentle grasp, assessing the tissue, and allow your grasp to become firmer as the tissue releases (Fig. 3-51).
- Alternate holding the tissue with a back and forth movement of your thumb and fingers.

Semispinalis Capitis and Cervicis, Longissimus Capitis

SEM-ee-spin-AL-iss CAP-it-iss, SERV-iss-iss, long-GISS-im-us

Etymology   Latin *semi,* half + *spinalis,* of the spine + *capitis,* of the head
semi, half + *spinalis,* of the spine + *cervicis,* of the neck
longissimus, longest + *capitis,* of the head

Overview

Semispinalis capitis and **cervicis** and **longissimus capitis** (Fig. 3-52) are involved in support of the head when carried or tilted forward. As a result, they are commonly overused and in a state of strain and are among the chief culprits in headache pain.

Attachments

- Inferiorly, to the transverse processes of T1 through T6 (semispinalis capitis also to C3 through C6)
- Superiorly, semispinalis cervicis to the spinous processes of C2 through C5; semispinalis capitis to the base of the occiput; longissimus capitis just lateral to semispinalis capitis.

Actions

Semispinalis capitis and longissimus capitis:

- Extends head, flexes the neck laterally to the same side (side bending)
- Supports the head when tilted forward

Semispinalis cervicis:

- Extends the neck
- Flexes the neck laterally
- Rotates the head to opposite side.

Referral Area

- Semispinalis and longissimus capitis: a band across the side of the head, especially in the anterior part of the temporal region
- Semispinalis cervicis: back of the head (the classic tension headache)

Other Muscles to Examine

- All other posterior, lateral, and anterior neck and head muscles
- Levator scapulae

Occipital bone (occiput)

Ligamentum nuchae

Semispinalis capitis

Splenius capitis

Middle scalene
Posterior scalene

Splenius cervicis

Figure 3-52   Anatomy of posterior neck muscles

Splenius Capitis, Splenius Cervicis

SPLEN-ee-us CAP-it-iss, SER-viss-is

Etymology Latin *splenius*, bandage (from Greek, *splenion*, bandage) + *capitis*, of the head
splenius, bandage (from Greek, *splenion*, bandage) + *cervicis*, of the neck

Overview

Splenius capitis and splenius cervicis (Fig. 3-53) are head-turners and neck extenders, and are involved in much headache pain.

Attachments

Inferiorly, to the spinous processes of C3 through T6
Superiorly:

- Splenius cervicis attaches to the back of the transverse processes of the first two or three cervical vertebrae.
- Splenius capitis attaches to the mastoid process and a small part of the occipital bone next to it.

Actions

These muscles extend the neck and turn the head to the same side.

Referral Area

Splenius capitis: to the top of the head
Splenius cervicis:

- To the eye
- Over the temporal region and the ear to the occipital region
- To the angle of the neck

Other Muscles to Examine

- All posterior neck muscles
- Levator scapulae
- Trapezius
- Sternocleidomastoid

Occipital bone (occiput)

Ligamentum nuchae

Semispinalis capitis

Splenius capitis

Splenius cervicis

Middle scalene
Posterior scalene

Figure 3-53 Anatomy of splenius capitis and splenius cervicis

Multifidi and Rotatores

mul-TIFF-id-ee, ro-ta-TORE-ace

Etymology Latin, *multus,* much + *findus,* divided
Latin, *rotatores,* rotators

Overview

Multifidi and **rotatores** (Fig. 3-54) are small, deep intervertebral muscles that occur over the entire length of the spine. They function less as movers than as restrainers; they keep the individual vertebrae from bending or rotating too far out of position when the spine is bent by larger muscles.

The rotatores in the cervical region are poorly defined and not present in everyone. Multifidi cross two to four vertebral joints, rotatores only one or two (Fig. 3-55).

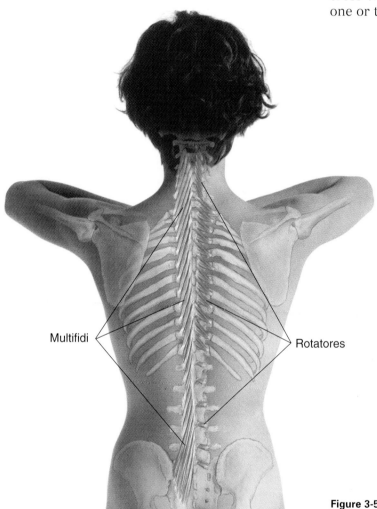

Multifidi

Rotatores

Figure 3-54 Attachment patterns of multifidi and rotatores of entire spine

Attachments

- Superiorly, C2 through C5
- Inferiorly, C4 through C7

Actions

Although technically considered extensors, lateral flexors, and rotators of the spine, these functions are actually carried out primarily by larger muscles. These small muscles seem to be chiefly involved in small positional adjustments of individual vertebrae.

Referral Area

- To an area just inferior to the base of the skull and another just medial to the root of the spine of the scapula
- To a band between those areas extending slightly over the shoulder

Other Muscles to Examine

- Other posterior neck muscles
- Levator scapulae
- Serratus posterior superior

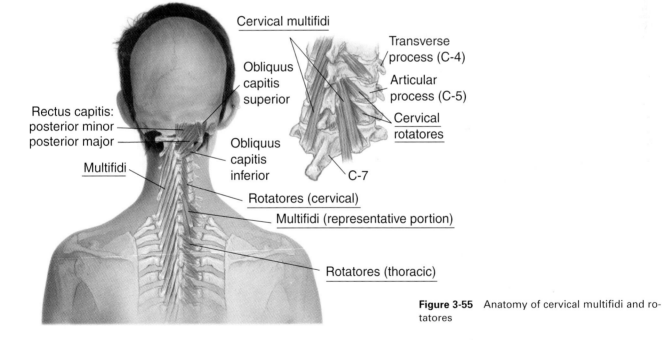

Figure 3-55   Anatomy of cervical multifidi and rotatores

Suboccipital Muscles

Obliquus capitis superior, obliquus capitis inferior rectus capitis posterior major, rectus capitis posterior minor

Etymology   Latin *sub*, under + *occiput*, back of head
Latin *obliquus*, oblique + *capitis*, of the head + *superior*, higher
Latin *obliquus*, oblique + *capitis*, of the head + *inferior*, lower
Latin *rectus*, straight + *capitis*, of the head + *posterior*, toward the back + *major*, larger
Latin *rectus*, straight + *capitis*, of the head + *posterior*, toward the back + *minor*, smaller

Overview

The triangle formed by the suboccipital muscles (Fig. 3-56) (except rectus capitis posterior minor) is called the **suboccipital triangle**; it surrounds the vertebral artery. The suboccipital triangle muscles, which are often involved with other posterior neck muscles in general headache pain, are treated along with these other muscles. Their trigger points are virtually impossible to differentiate from those of the overlying muscles. They are best treated with compression and stretching.

 Attachments

Obliquus capitis inferior connects the first two cervical vertebrae; the remaining muscles connect the first two cervical vertebrae with the occipital bone.

 Actions

- Extends and rotates the head
- Tilts the head to the same side

 Referral Area

- Over the back of the head
- In a band over the side of the head to the eye

 Other Muscles to Examine

- All other posterior neck muscles
- Sternocleidomastoid

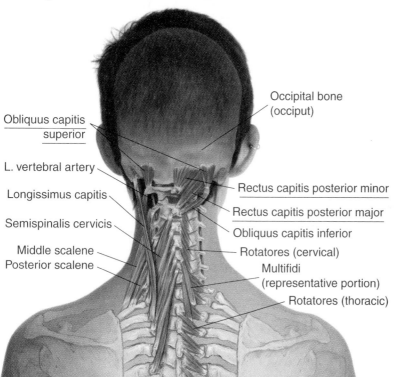

Obliquus capitis superior

L. vertebral artery

Longissimus capitis

Semispinalis cervicis

Middle scalene
Posterior scalene

Occipital bone (occiput)

Rectus capitis posterior minor
Rectus capitis posterior major
Obliquus capitis inferior
Rotatores (cervical)
Multifidi (representative portion)
Rotatores (thoracic)

Figure 3-56 Anatomy of suboccipital muscles

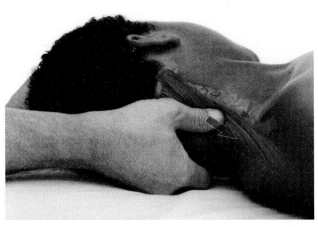

Figure 3-57   Stripping of posterior neck muscles with thumb

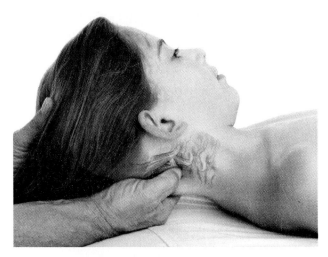

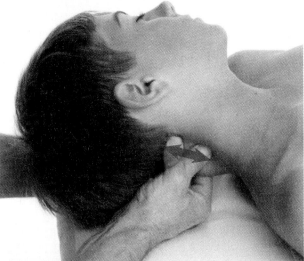

Figure 3-58   Bi-directional stripping of posterior neck muscles with thumb

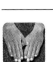

Manual Therapy for All Posterior Neck Muscles

STRIPPING AND COMPRESSION

- The client lies supine.
- Seated beside the client's head and using the hand nearest the client's head to support it from underneath, place the other hand under the client's neck with the fingers on the far side and the thumb on the near side.
- Press the thumb into the posterior muscles of the neck at the base of the skull just lateral to the spinous processes of the upper cervical vertebrae.
- Pressing firmly into the tissue, glide the thumb toward the torso, pausing at tight or tender spots and waiting for them to release (Fig. 3-57). Take the thumb as far as it will comfortably go along the base of the neck.
- Slide the thumb back along the same path to the base of the skull, again stopping at tender or tight spots to release them (Fig. 3-58).

- Shift the thumb laterally toward yourself and repeat the process until you have covered the posterior neck as far as the posterior aspect of the scalenes.

■ At the base of the skull, press the thumb upward and deep into the sub-occipital muscles.

■ Hold for release (Fig. 3-59).

MOVING COMPRESSION WITH FINGERTIPS

■ The client lies supine.

■ Seated centrally at the client's head, push both hands flat under the client's shoulders on both sides until your fingertips rest on either side of the thoracic spine.

■ Curl your fingers so that their tips press into the muscles on either side of the spine.

■ Slowly draw your hands toward yourself, gliding your curled fingertips along the muscles on either side of the spine until your fingers reach the base of the skull (Fig. 3-60).

CROSS-FIBER STROKING

■ The client lies supine.

■ Standing at the client's head and facing the client, place one hand under the client's neck at the base of the occiput and curl the fingertips into the lateral aspect of the posterior neck muscles (Fig. 3-61).

■ Pressing firmly up into the tissue, continue to curl the fingers, drawing the tips toward yourself until they reach the spine.

■ Move the hand downward toward the base of the neck and repeat.

■ Repeat on the other side.

CROSS-FIBER STROKING WITH THE THUMB

■ The client lies prone.

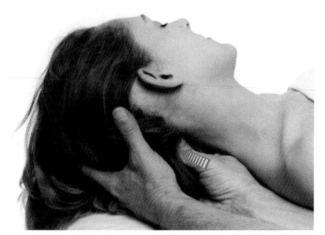

Figure 3-59 Compression of suboccipital muscles

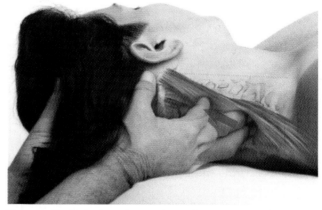

Figure 3-60 Stripping of posterior neck muscles with fingertips

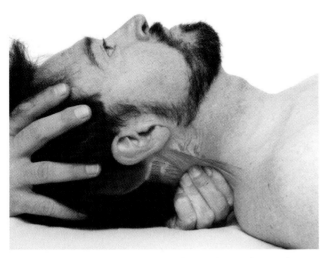

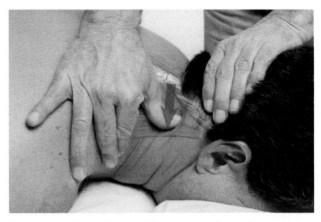

Figure 3-61 Cross-fiber stroking of posterior neck muscles with fingertips

Figure 3-62 Cross-fiber stroking on posterior neck muscles with the thumb

- Standing at the client's head and facing the neck, hold the head steady with the far hand.
- Place your fingertips on the far side of the client's neck and the tip of your thumb on the cervical spine at the base of the skull.
- Pressing firmly into the tissue, slide your thumb across the neck muscles toward your fingers (Fig. 3-62). (Note: At the base of the skull, direct your pressure partially against the occipital bone.)

- Shift your hand down the neck an inch or two and repeat the process; repeat until you reach the base of the neck.
- Move to the opposite side of the client and repeat the procedure on the other side.

REFERENCE

1. Simons DG, Travell JG, Simons LS: Travell & Simons' Myofascial Pain and Dysfunction: The Trigger Point Manual, Vol.1, Ed. 2. Baltimore: Lippincott Williams & Wilkins, 1999, pages 261-263, 354, 436, 809-812.

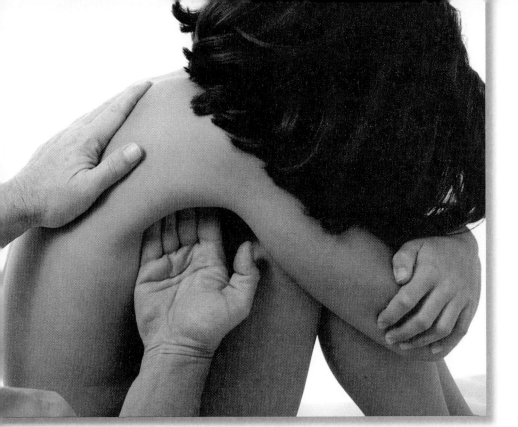

The Shoulder, Chest, and Upper Back

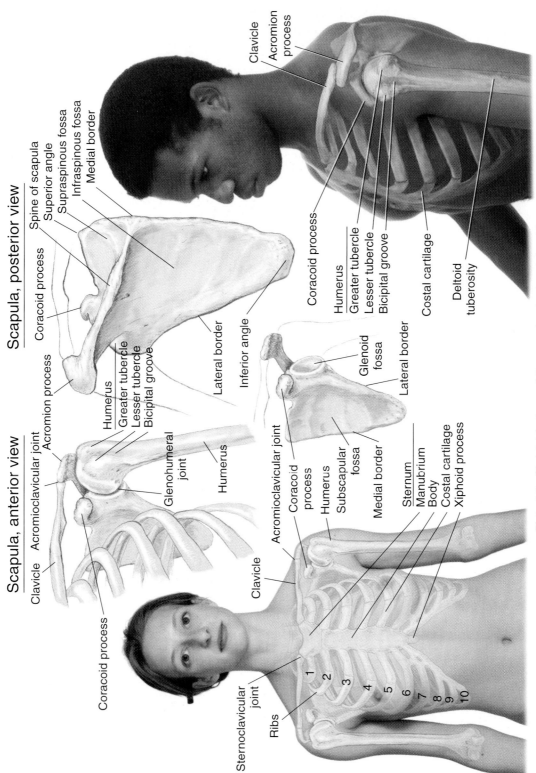

Scapula, posterior view

Spine of scapula
Superior angle
Supraspinous fossa
Infraspinous fossa
Medial border

Coracoid process

Acromion process

Humerus
Greater tubercle
Lesser tubercle
Bicipital groove

Lateral border

Inferior angle

Glenoid fossa

Lateral border

Coracoid process

Humerus
Greater tubercle
Lesser tubercle
Bicipital groove

Costal cartilage

Deltoid tuberosity

Clavicle
Acromion process

Scapula, anterior view

Clavicle   Acromioclavicular joint
Acromion

Glenohumeral joint

Humerus

Acromioclavicular joint

Coracoid process

Humerus

Subscapular fossa

Medial border

Sternum
Manubrium
Body
Costal cartilage
Xiphoid process

Clavicle

Coracoid process

Sternoclavicular joint

Ribs

1
2
3
4
5
6
7
8
9
10

Plate 4-1   Skeletal features of the scapula, chest and shoulder

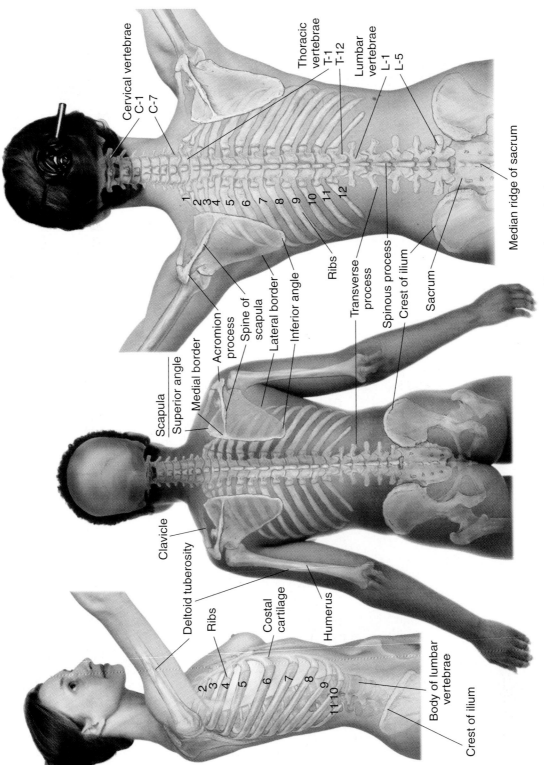

Plate 4-2 Skeletal features of the lateral chest, posterior shoulder, and upper back

Cervical vertebrae
C-1
C-7

Thoracic vertebrae
T-1
T-12

Lumbar vertebrae
L-1
L-5

Median ridge of sacrum

Scapula
Superior angle
Medial border

Acromion process
Spine of scapula
Lateral border
Inferior angle

Ribs
Transverse process
Spinous process
Crest of ilium
Sacrum

Clavicle
Deltoid tuberosity
Ribs
Costal cartilage
Humerus
Body of lumbar vertebrae
Crest of ilium

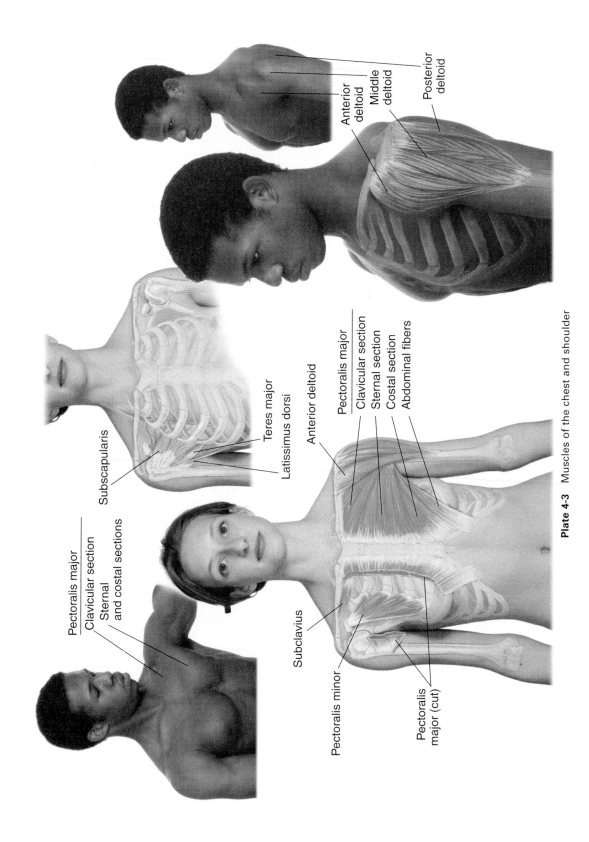

Anterior deltoid
Middle deltoid
Posterior deltoid

Subscapularis

Teres major
Latissimus dorsi

Anterior deltoid

Pectoralis major
Clavicular section
Sternal section
Costal section
Abdominal fibers

Pectoralis major
Clavicular section
Sternal
and costal sections

Subclavius

Pectoralis minor

Pectoralis
major (cut)

Plate 4-3   Muscles of the chest and shoulder

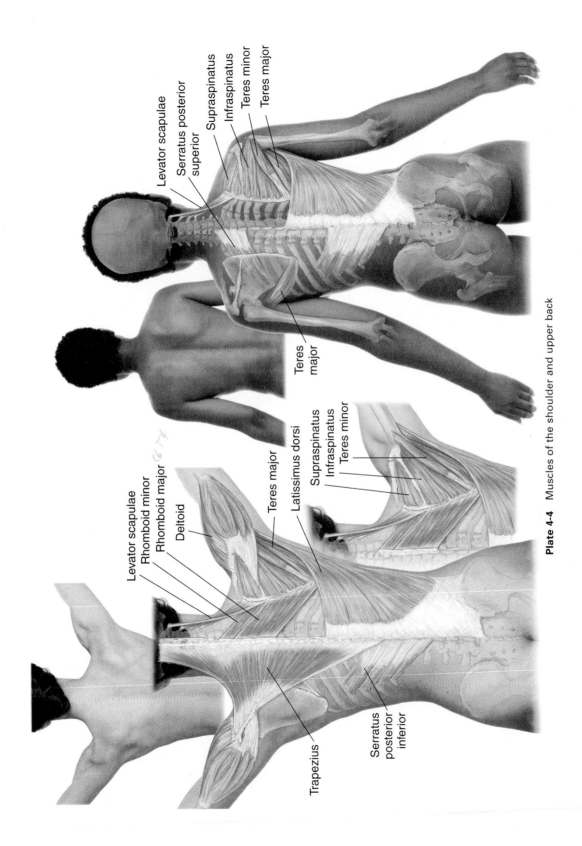

Levator scapulae
Serratus posterior superior
Supraspinatus
Infraspinatus
Teres minor
Teres major

Teres major

Levator scapulae
Rhomboid minor
Rhomboid major
Deltoid

Teres major

Latissimus dorsi
Supraspinatus
Infraspinatus
Teres minor

Trapezius

Serratus posterior inferior

Plate 4-4   Muscles of the shoulder and upper back

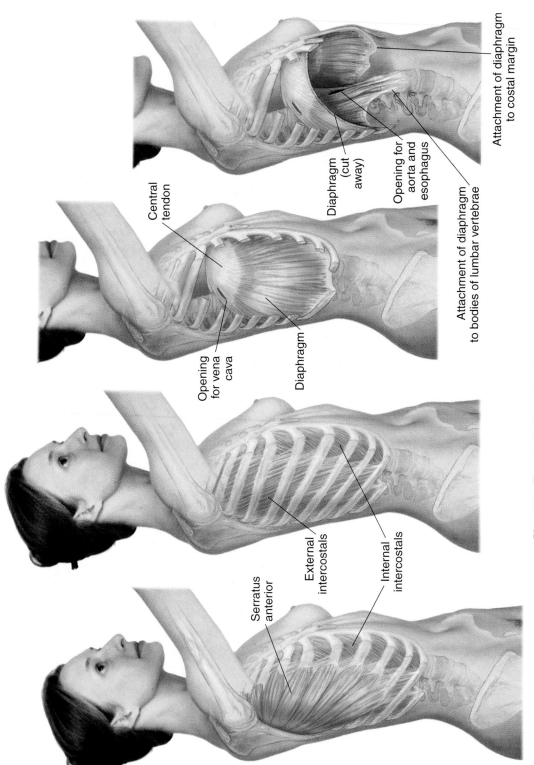

Attachment of diaphragm
to costal margin

Diaphragm
(cut
away)

Opening for
aorta and
esophagus

Attachment of diaphragm
to bodies of lumbar vertebrae

Central
tendon

Opening
for vena
cava

Diaphragm

External
intercostals

Internal
intercostals

Serratus
anterior

Plate 4-5   The principal muscles of breathing and lateral chest

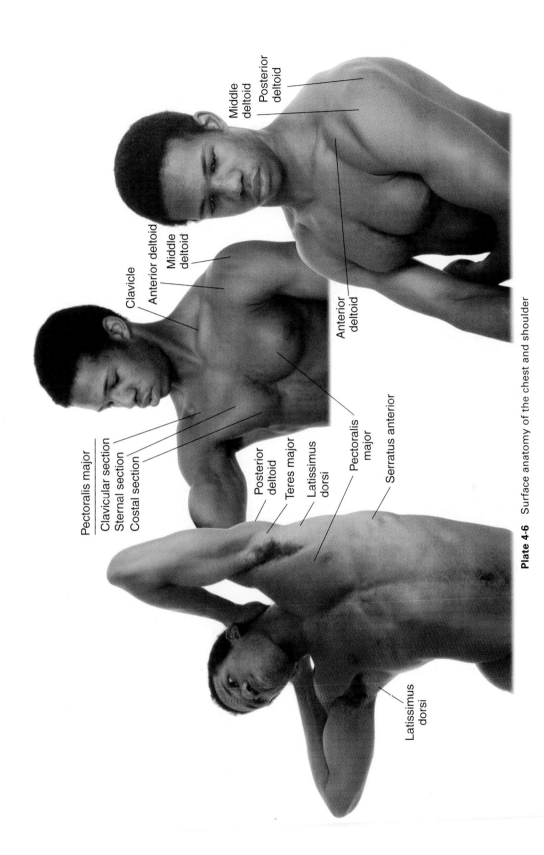

Middle
deltoid

Posterior
deltoid

Anterior
deltoid

Clavicle

Anterior deltoid

Middle
deltoid

Pectoralis major

Clavicular section

Sternal section

Costal section

Posterior
deltoid

Teres major

Latissimus
dorsi

Pectoralis
major

Serratus anterior

Latissimus
dorsi

Plate 4-6   Surface anatomy of the chest and shoulder

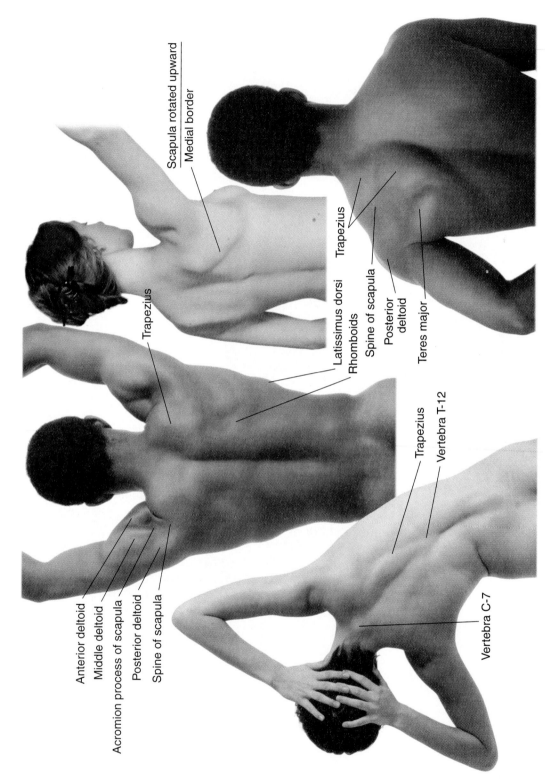

Plate 4-7   Surface anatomy of the shoulder and upper back

Scapula rotated upward
Medial border

Trapezius

Latissimus dorsi
Rhomboids
Spine of scapula
Posterior deltoid
Teres major

Trapezius

Anterior deltoid
Middle deltoid
Acromion process of scapula
Posterior deltoid
Spine of scapula

Trapezius
Vertebra T-12

Vertebra C-7

OVERVIEW OF THE REGION

The muscles of the shoulder, chest, and upper back are grouped not only because of their physical proximity but chiefly because the majority of the chest and upper back muscles are either directly involved in control of the shoulder or strongly influence it. The only muscles in this area that are not actually shoulder muscles are those of the ribs and of respiration.

Although we have already seen trapezius in Chapter 3, we need to remember that its territory is vast, covering the posterior shoulders and upper back. It plays a major role in moving and stabilizing the shoulders, and is usually involved in problems of the upper back and shoulders.

The Shoulder

Perhaps the most important thing to understand about the shoulder is that it is connected to the rest of the skeletal structure by only one joint, the **acromioclavicular joint.** Aside from this one rather tenuous connection, the entire shoulder structure, including the arm, is supported by soft tissues. While this arrangement allows considerable freedom of movement for the arm, it also renders the shoulder highly vulnerable to soft-tissue injury.

The shoulder girdle is a bony ring comprised of the *manubrium* of the sternum, the *clavicles,* and the two *scapulae.* It is an incomplete ring, since the scapulae are not joined in the back. Each side of the shoulder girdle might be compared to the boom on a sailboat (the clavicle) swinging freely from the mast (the sternum). Its considerable range of motion is limited only by the soft tissues.

Thus the shoulder combines great flexibility with great vulnerability:

■ Great flexibility, because the soft tissues (muscles, tendons, and fascia) which connect the arm and shoulder to the back, chest and neck are soft and stretchable, allowing for movement in many directions.

■ Great vulnerability, because movement too far in any direction can result in dislocation or separation of shoulder joints or injury to the soft tissues.

Shoulder Components

Two bones make up the shoulder [not counting the arm] (See Plate 4-1):

■ Anteriorly, the *clavicle,* or collarbone, which joins the arm and shoulder to the rest of the skeleton at the *manubrium* of the sternum, by means of the **sternoclavicular joints.** Posteriorly, the *scapula* or shoulderblade.

■ The clavicle has its own muscle, **subclavius,** which attaches it inferiorly to the top rib. It is a fairly simple bone, but the scapula is intricate and complex. It is rather like the famous Swiss Army knife, in that it includes several extensions that serve a variety of purposes.

The Scapula

Most of the bones in the body serve as rigid spacers, like tent poles. A few, however, instead act as anchors for soft tissues and other bones. The scapula, or shoulderblade, is one of the most important of these "anchors."

We usually think of the shoulder blade as the essentially flat, triangular bone that we can see on the surface at the back of each shoulder. This part of the scapula serves mainly as an anchor for several muscles, four of which make up the **rotator cuff** of sports injury notoriety—four muscles that help rotate the arm (**supraspinatus, infraspinatus, teres minor,** and **subscapularis**). This large section of the scapula is divided into two areas by a bony ridge running across it at a slight upward angle from the horizontal. This ridge is called the **spine of the scapula.** A muscle superior and inferior to the spine of the scapula attaches to the surface of the scapula, and muscles also attach to the spine itself.

The spine of the scapula extends beyond the flat, triangular portion to form the **acromion process.** (A **process** is an extension of a bone.) The function of the acromion process is to join with the clavicle at the **acromioclavicular joint.** It also forms a hood or roof over the joint inferior to it, the head of the **humerus,** and the tendons that pass just under it, giving them some protection.

Just inferior to the acromion process and the acromioclavicular joint, the upper outer corner of the triangular bone forms a socket for the arm. The socket is called the **glenoid fossa** (a **fossa** is a cavity or hollow), and the ball-and-socket joint where the arm bone, or humerus, fits into the glenoid fossa is called the **glenohumeral joint.** Compared to the hip joint, the glenohumeral joint is a very shallow and open ball-and-socket joint. It functions well only because of the additional protection of the acromion process and attached tendons and ligaments. Even so, dislocations of the shoulder are much more common than those of the hip—another way in which flexibility is gained at the price of vulnerability.

Finally, another process extends from the front of the superolateral corner of the scapula. This process, the **coracoid process,** serves as an anchor for muscles, such as **pectoralis minor, coracobrachialis,** and the short head of the **biceps** (these last two muscles will be presented in Chapter 5).

Since the scapula provides the socket for the arm, it must be able to move freely in all directions. It can move up or down, it can move somewhat forward and closer to the ribs, and, most importantly, it can rotate both clockwise and counterclockwise.

Six muscles hold the scapula in position and move it in these various directions:

1. Pectoralis minor
2. Rhomboid major
3. Rhomboid minor
4. Levator scapulae
5. Trapezius
6. Serratus anterior

Three other powerful muscles move the humerus:

- The **deltoid** muscle, or deltoideus, which covers the superior, anterior, posterior, and lateral aspects of the shoulder joint structure, with attachments to the spine of the scapula, the acromion process, the clavicle, and the humerus. It is often referred to as three muscles: anterior deltoid, lateral deltoid, and posterior deltoid.
- **Pectoralis major** covers the anterior chest and attaches to the humerus.
- **Latissimus dorsi** is a shoulder muscle extending from the *iliac crest* over much of the back and attaching to the humerus.

Muscles of the Ribs and Respiration

The muscles of the ribs are the *internal* and *external intercostals, serratus anterior,* and *serratus posterior superior* and *inferior.*

The mechanical and physiological aspects of the breathing process are key factors in neuromuscular integrity. Therefore, the muscles of breathing are an essential consideration in bodywork. Although other muscles assist, the primary muscle of respiration is the **diaphragm.**

ANTERIOR SHOULDER

Subclavius

sub-CLAY-vee-us

Etymology   Latin *sub*, under + *clavis*, key *(claviculus*, little key)

Overview

For such a small muscle, *subclavius* (Fig. 4-1) can refer pain over a broad expanse. It should always be treated along with the other anterior chest muscles.

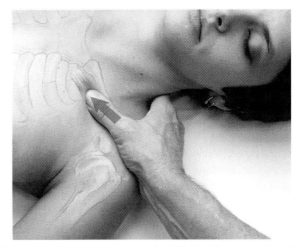

Figure 4-2   Stripping massage of subclavius (Draping option #2)

 Attachments

- Medially, to the first costal cartilage
- Laterally, to the inferior surface of the acromial end of the clavicle

 Other Muscles to Examine

- Pectoralis major and minor
- Scalenes

 Actions

- Fixes the clavicle or elevates the first rib
- Helps protract the scapula, drawing the shoulder down and forward

 Manual Therapy

STRIPPING

- The client lies supine.
- Place the thumb or fingertips on the subclavius just medial to the head of the humerus and just inferior to the clavicle.
- Pressing firmly, glide your thumb or fingertips along the muscle as far as the medial end of the clavicle (Fig. 4-2).
- This technique may also be performed with the client seated (Fig. 4-3).

 Referral Area

Laterally along the clavicle, over the front of the shoulder and upper arm, along the radial side of the forearm and into the thumb and first two fingers

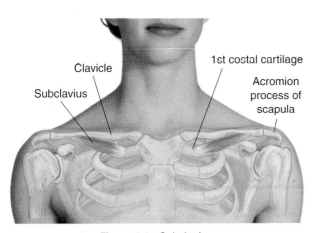

Figure 4-1   Subclavius

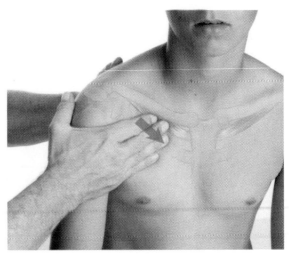

Figure 4-3   Stripping of subclavius in sitting position (Draping option #16)

Pectoralis Major

PECK-tor-AL-is MAY-jer

Etymology Latin *pectus, pectoris,* breast (chest) + *major,* larger; "the larger muscle of the breast"

Overview

Pectoralis major (Fig. 4-4) has three sections named for their attachments: *clavicular, sternal,* and *costal,* with additional fibers to the abdominal aponeurosis. The fibers of each of these sections run in different directions. The muscle crosses three joints: sternoclavicular, acromioclavicular, and glenohumeral.

Pectoralis major plays an important role in postural alignment, particularly with regard to the "head-forward" posture discussed in Chapter 3 (see pages 64-65). David G. Simons, MD, says that "the [head-forward] posture is often caused by pectoralis major MTrPs [myofascial trigger points] that pull the shoulder blades forward creating a round-shouldered posture that includes a forward positioning of the head. Correction of that posture is rarely successful for any length of time unless you correct the pec[toralis] major problem" (Simons, David G., MD, private communication, September 23, 2001).

Attachments

■ Inferiorly and medially, clavicular part, to the medial half of the clavicle; sternal and costal parts, to the anterior surface of the manubrium and the

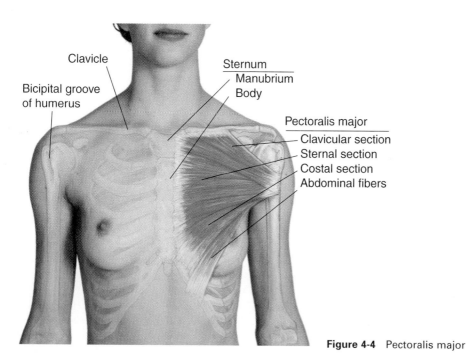

Clavicle

Bicipital groove of humerus

Sternum
Manubrium
Body

Pectoralis major
Clavicular section
Sternal section
Costal section
Abdominal fibers

Figure 4-4 Pectoralis major

body of the sternum and cartilages of the first to the sixth ribs; abdominal part, to the aponeurosis of the external oblique

- Superiorly and laterally, to the lateral lip of the bicipital groove.

Actions

Adducts, flexes, and medially rotates arm

Referral Area

In the ipsilateral (on the same side) breast and anterior chest, over the anterior shoulder, down the volar palm surface of the upper arm, over the volar surface of the forearm just below the elbow, and into the middle and ring fingers

Other Muscles to Examine

- Pectoralis minor
- Scalenes
- Sternocleidomastoid (SCM)
- Sternalis
- Subclavius
- Deltoid
- Biceps brachii
- Coracobrachialis

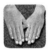

Manual Therapy

PINCER COMPRESSION
- The client lies supine.
- The therapist stands at the client's shoulder beside the head.
- Grasp the pectoralis major just medial to the humerus between the thumb and first three fingers. Squeeze the muscle firmly and wait for release (Fig. 4-5).

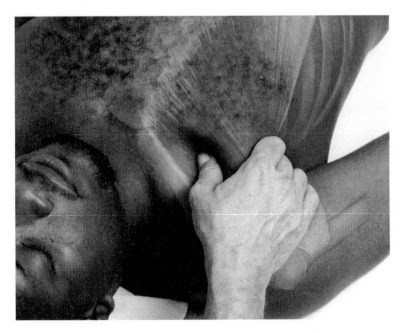

Figure 4-5 Pincer compression of pectoralis major (Draping option #2)

- Move the thumb and fingers to a position farther away from the shoulder as the muscle widens; squeeze and wait for release.
- Continue this process, moving farther along the muscle as it widens, until you have worked as much of the muscle as you can reasonably grasp.

STRIPPING
- The client lies supine.
- The therapist stands beside the client's shoulder, facing the client.
- Place the fingertips on the muscle just medial to the humerus.
- Pressing firmly into the tissue, glide the fingertips medially across the muscle to its attachments on the sternum.
- Beginning at the same spot, repeat this procedure, sliding diagonally along the muscle just inferior to the path you traced in the last movement.
- Repeat the same procedure, beginning each time at the same point, with the paths of your movement forming a fan

shape, ending with a path along the lateral edge of the muscle (Fig. 4-6).
- With a female client with developed breasts, each path should end when you reach the bulk of the breast tissue ahead of your fingers (Fig. 4-7).

COMPRESSION
- The client lies supine.
- The therapist stands beside the client facing the client's head.
- Place the hand nearest the client flat on the client's ribcage with the fingertips resting on the inferior aspect of pectoralis major.
- Press firmly into the tissue, searching for tender spots. Hold for release.
- Move the hand upward so that the fingertips are just superior to the previous spot.
- Repeat this procedure until you reach the upper aspect of the muscle.
- Start again at the lower ribcage, with your hand just medial to the original starting point. Keep moving superiorly

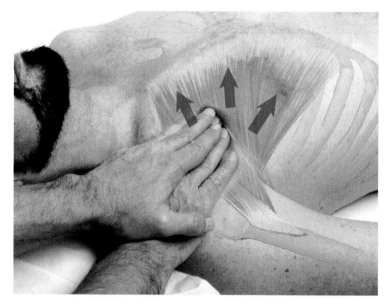

Figure 4-6 Stripping massage of pectoralis major (Draping option #2)

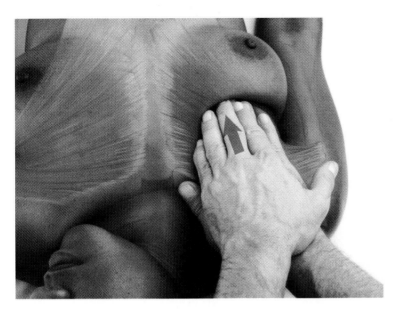

Figure 4-7 Treatment of pectoralis major in a female client (Draping option #2)

to new positions on the muscle on a slight diagonal till you reach the superior aspect.

- Continue this procedure, moving up the medial aspect of the muscle along the sternum, until you have covered the entire muscle in a fan-shaped pattern.
- With a female client with developed breasts, continue each path as far as the breast tissue allows you to remain in contact with the muscle (Fig. 4-8A). When you have worked as much of the muscle as you can from this position, move to the client's shoulder and repeat the process working inferiorly (Fig. 4-8B). You should be able to cover all the muscle tissue underlying the breast in this way.

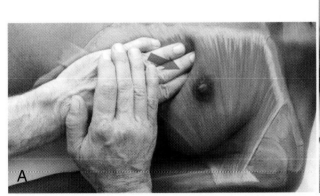
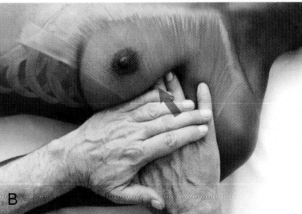

Figure 4-8 Compression of pectoralis major in a female client: medial inferior portion (A), lateral portion (B) (Draping option #3)

Pectoralis Minor

PECK-ter-AL-is MY-ner

Etymology Latin *pectus, pectoris,* breast (chest) + *minor,* smaller; "the smaller muscle of the breast."

Overview

Pectoralis minor (Fig. 4-9) anchors the scapula to the chest. It is therefore susceptible to injury from inferior motions of the arm and commonly refers pain to the arm as far as the fingertips. Pain in pectoralis minor is often accompanied by pain in the upper back muscles such as the rhomboids. Because the brachial plexus (the bundle of nerves leading to the arm) passes directly underneath the attachment to the coracoid process, tightness in pectoralis minor can entrap the nerve, causing numbness in the arm (Fig. 4-10), especially when the arm is raised.

Caution

The <u>axilla,</u> or armpit, is the area directly inferior to the *glenohumeral joint,* and lies within a cavity formed posteriorly by a bundle of muscles made up of *teres major* and *minor* and *latissimus dorsi,* and anteriorly by *pectoralis major.* Caution must be taken when working in the axilla, on account of the major brachial nerves and blood vessels that pass through the area. To avoid them, move into the axilla slowly, while maintaining constant contact with the muscle itself.

Attachments

- Inferiorly, to the third, and often the second, rib to the fifth rib at the costochondral articulations
- Superiorly, to the tip of the coracoid process of the scapula.

Actions

Rotates scapula or draws it inferiorly, or raises ribs

Referral Area

Over the anterior shoulder, into the anterior chest and along the volar surface of the arm into the last three fingers.

Other Muscles to Examine

- Pectoralis major
- Scalenes
- Sternocleidomastoid
- Rotator cuff

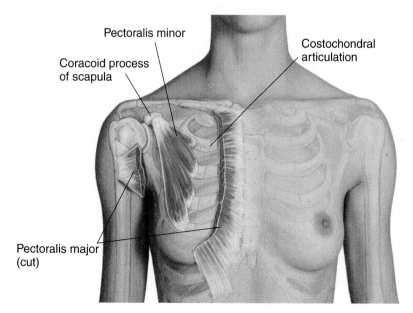

Pectoralis minor

Coracoid process of scapula

Costochondral articulation

Pectoralis major (cut)

Figure 4-9 Pectoralis minor

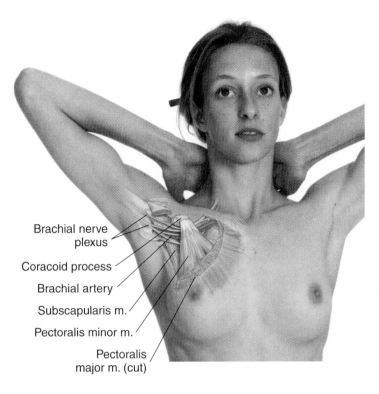

Brachial nerve plexus

Coracoid process

Brachial artery

Subscapularis m.

Pectoralis minor m.

Pectoralis major m. (cut)

Figure 4-10 Position of brachial nerves and vessels relative to pectoralis minor

Manual Therapy

STRIPPING

- The client lies supine, with the arm nearest the therapist slightly abducted and bent at the elbow.
- The therapist stands beside the client's shoulder.
- Place the fingertips on the ribcage just lateral to the pectoralis major slightly superior to the nipple, with your fingers pointing diagonally across the chest below the nipple.
- Push the fingers under the pectoralis major along the ribcage until they encounter the attachment of pectoralis minor to the fifth rib.
- Pressing your fingertips against the muscle, turn your arm and hand so that the fingertips glide along the muscle from an inferior to superior position (Fig. 4-11).
- Move your hand up to a point just below the axilla and repeat the procedure, with the fingertips finally pressing deeply into the axilla under the pectoralis major, contacting the attachment of pectoralis minor to the coracoid process (Fig. 4-12).

COMPRESSION (1)

- The client lies on the side opposite to that to be treated, with the arms raised diagonally upward. The therapist stands in front of the client at the chest.
- Place the treating hand on the ribcage with the thumb on the most inferior attachment of the muscle, in line with the nipple. The treating hand and thumb may be supported with the other hand and thumb.
- Compress the muscle with the thumb until it releases.

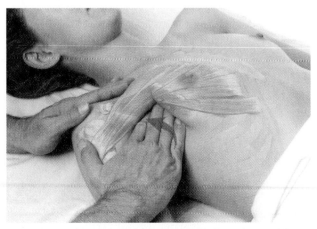

Figure 4-11 Treatment of pectoralis minor in supine position (Draping option #3)

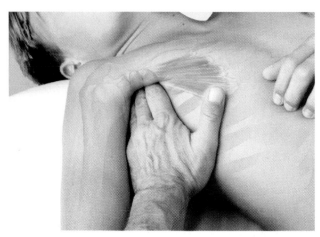

Figure 4-12 Compression of pectoralis minor attachment to coracoid process (Draping option #3)

- Shift the hand cephalad an inch or two to a new position and repeat the process.
- As you move superiorly, begin to glide the thumb laterally at each level to find tender or trigger points in all the branches of the muscle (Fig. 4-13).
- Continue this process so that the thumb gradually moves diagonally toward the coracoid process of the scapula. This movement will eventually take the thumb deep into the axilla, where you should carefully seek out the attachment to the coracoid process deep in the axilla (see Caution on page 124).

COMPRESSION (2)

- The client lies on the side opposite to that to be treated, with the arms raised diagonally upward. The therapist stands behind the client at the chest.
- Place the treating hand on the ribcage.
- Pressing pectoralis major medially with the fingertips, contact the inferior attachments of pectoralis minor at the level of the nipple and compress the muscle until it releases (Fig. 4-14A).
- Shift the hand cephalad an inch or two to a new position and repeat the process.
- As you move superiorly, begin to glide the fingertips laterally at each level to find tender or trigger points in all the branches of the muscle.
- Continue this process so that the fingertips gradually move diagonally toward the coracoid process of the scapula. This movement will eventually take the fingertips deep into the axilla (Fig. 4-14B), where you should carefully seek out the attachment to the coracoid process deep in the axilla (see Caution on page 124).
- Compression may also be performed with the thumb on a client in supine position (Fig. 4-15).

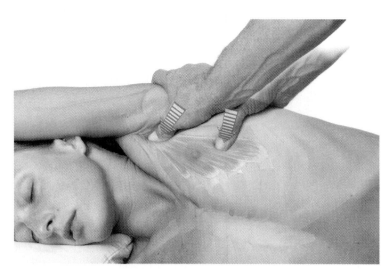

Figure 4-13 Treating pectoralis minor in sidelying position (Draping option #15)

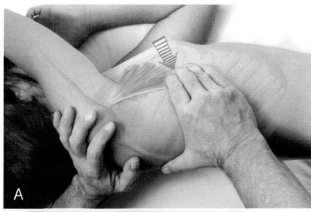

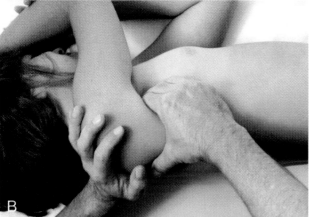

Figure 4-14 Sidelying treatment of pectoralis minor from behind client from starting position (A) to final position (B) (Draping option #15)

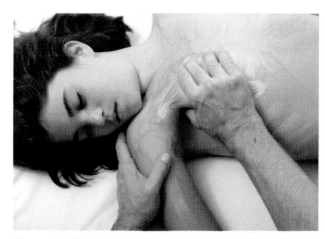

Figure 4-15 Compression of pectoralis minor with thumb (Draping option #3)

■ As the fingertips move into the axilla, turn the hand gradually so that the fingertips are pointing superiorly into the axilla, finally encountering the attachment of the muscle to the coracoid process of the scapula.

FINGERTIP COMPRESSION, CLIENT SEATED

■ The client sits upright and the therapist stands behind the client. The client's forearm on the side to be treated rests at the side, with the arm slightly abducted and rotated medially to slacken pectoralis major.

■ Place the non-treating hand on the client's shoulder contralateral (on the opposite side) to the side to be treated.

■ Place the treating hand on the client's ribcage, sliding the fingertips under pectoralis major at the level of the nipple.

■ Compress the muscle at that level, holding until release (Fig. 4-16).

■ Move the treating hand to a position just superior to the last, repeating the above procedure.

■ At each level, glide the fingertips outward to contact all the branches of the muscle.

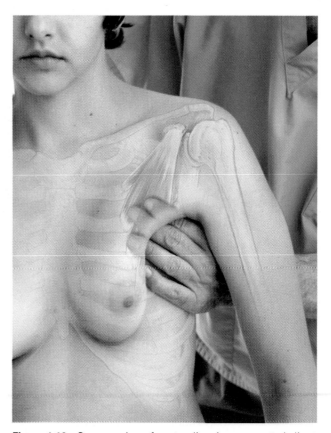

Figure 4-16 Compression of pectoralis minor on seated client (Draping option #16)

Levator Scapulae

le-VAY-ter SKAP-you-lay

Etymology Latin *levator*, raiser + *scapulae*, of the shoulderblade

Overview

After trapezius, **levator scapulae** (Fig. 4-17) is probably the most common site of pain and tightness in the neck and shoulders. It is one of the muscles most abused by the carrying of heavy backpacks and shoulder bags. It assists trapezius in raising the scapula and the rhomboids in rotating the glenoid fossa downward.

 Attachments

- Superiorly, to posterior tubercles of transverse processes of four upper cervical vertebrae
- Inferiorly, to superior angle of scapula

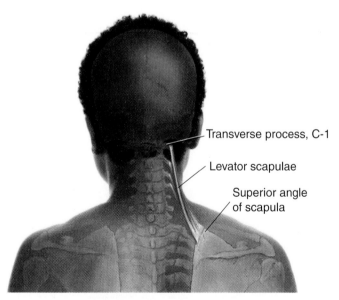

Transverse process, C-1

Levator scapulae

Superior angle of scapula

Figure 4-17 Levator scapulae

 Actions

Raises the scapula

 Referral Area

Locally over the muscle, along the medial border of the scapula, across the upper scapula to the back of the upper arm

 Other Muscles to Examine

- Rhomboids
- Trapezius
- Supraspinatus
- Posterior neck muscles

 Manual Therapy

STRIPPING (1)
- The client lies prone.
- The therapist stands at the side of the client's head to be treated, facing the shoulder.
- Place the thumb of the treating hand on the neck over the transverse processes of the cervical vertebrae.
- Pressing firmly medially and deeply, glide the thumb inferiorly along the muscle all the way to its attachment on the superior angle of the scapula (Fig. 4-18).

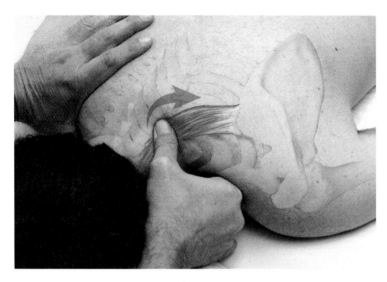

Figure 4-18 Stripping massage of levator scapulae (1) (Draping option #7)

STRIPPING (2)
- The client lies prone.
- The therapist stands at the client's side, facing diagonally toward the client's opposite shoulder.
- Place the treating hand on the near shoulder of the client with the thumb resting on the attachment of levator scapulae at the superior angle of the scapula.
- Pressing firmly medially and deeply, glide the thumb superiorly toward the neck, following the muscle all the way to its attachment to the transverse processes of the cervical vertebrae (Fig. 4-19).

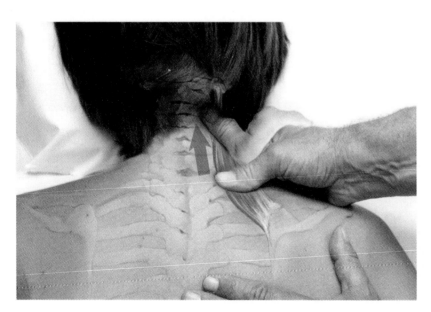

Figure 4-19 Stripping massage of levator scapulae (2) (Draping option #7)

Rhomboids Major and Minor

ROM-boydz

Etymology   Greek *rhombo,* an oblique parallelogram, but having unequal sides + *eidos,* resembling

Overview

The **rhomboids** (Fig. 4-20) are a major source of upper back pain. They rotate the scapula to lower the glenohumeral joint, and they retract the scapula. Keep in mind that they are in constant tension with the forces of the chest muscles, which pull the shoulder forward. Therefore, rhomboid tightness is almost always associated with tightness in the pectoral muscles.

Attachments

RHOMBOID MAJOR
- Above, to the spinous processes and corresponding supraspinous ligaments of the first four thoracic vertebrae
- Below, to the medial border of scapula below spine.

RHOMBOID MINOR
- Superiorly, to the spinous processes of the sixth and seventh cervical vertebrae

- Inferiorly, to the medial margin of the scapula above the spine

Actions

Draws scapula toward vertebral column; minor also draws slightly upward.

Referral Area

Along the medial border of the scapula and over the superior angle of the scapula

Other Muscles to Examine

- Serratus posterior superior
- Levator scapulae
- Thoracic paraspinal muscles

Manual Therapy

STRIPPING
- The client lies prone. The therapist stands beside the client's head, facing the client's back.
- Place the supported fingertips (or the supported thumb) just lateral to the

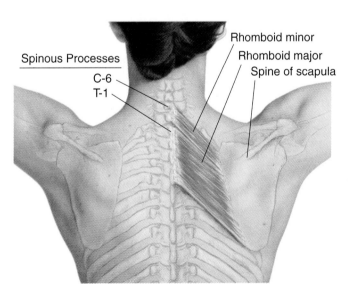

Figure 4-20   Rhomboids major and minor

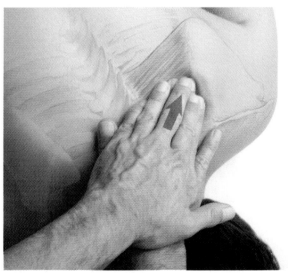

Figure 4-21   Stripping massage of the rhomboids (Draping option #7)

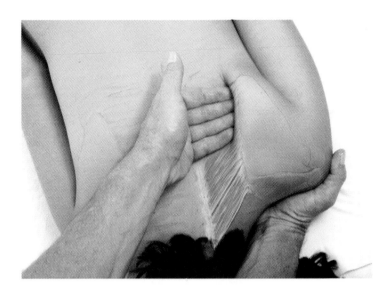

Figure 4-22 Rhomboid stretch, prone (Draping option #7)

spinous process of the sixth cervical vertebra.

- Pressing deeply, glide the fingertips (or thumb) slowly diagonally until you encounter the medial border of the scapula (Fig. 4-21).
- Place the fingertips (or thumb) at a point just below the previous starting point and repeat the above process.
- Repeat the process until you have reached the inferior angle of the scapula.

COMPRESSION/STRETCH

- The client lies prone. The therapist stands beside the client's head, facing the client's back.
- Place the fingertips at the medial border of the scapula, pointing laterally.
- With the other hand, lift the client's shoulder at the glenohumeral joint while inserting the fingertips under the scapula (Fig. 4-22).

COMPRESSION/STRETCH

- The client is seated, and the therapist sits next to the client.
- Place the hand flat on the back, the index finger aligned with the medial border of the scapula.
- With the other hand, press back on the client's shoulder at the glenohumeral joint while pressing the index finger under the medial border of the scapula (Fig. 4-23).

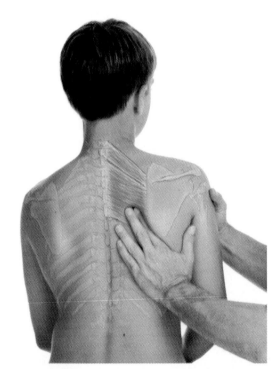

Figure 4-23 Stretch of rhomboids, client seated (Draping option #16)

Latissimus Dorsi
La-TISS-imus DOR-see

Etymology Latin *latissimus,* widest (from *latus,* wide) + *dorsi,* of the back (from *dorsum,* back)

Overview

A large and powerful muscle, **latissimus dorsi** (Fig. 4-24) allows us to pull ourselves up by the arms (or pull things down and back with the arms, e.g., paddling a canoe). It covers the lower posterior torso as trapezius covers the upper posterior torso: it extends up the back and side, and attaches to the anterior aspect of the upper arm, thus anchoring the arm to the low back and pelvis. With teres major, it forms the muscle bundle that defines the posterior border of the axilla.

Attachments

- Inferiorly, to the spinous processes of the lower five or six thoracic and the lumbar vertebrae, to the median ridge of sacrum, and to the outer lip of the iliac crest

- Superiorly, with teres major into the medial lip of the bicipital groove of the humerus.

Actions

Adducts arm, rotates it medially, and extends it

Referral Areas

- Around the inferior angle of the scapula, across the scapula to the axilla, and down the back of the arm to the last two fingers
- Over the anterior deltoid
- On the side at the waist

Other Muscles to Examine

- Serratus posterior inferior
- Teres major
- Teres minor
- Pectoralis minor
- Serratus anterior
- Interior and exterior obliques

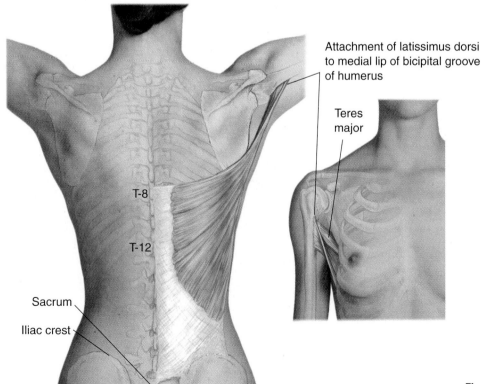

Attachment of latissimus dorsi to medial lip of bicipital groove of humerus

Teres major

T-8

T-12

Sacrum

Iliac crest

Figure 4-24 Latissimus dorsi

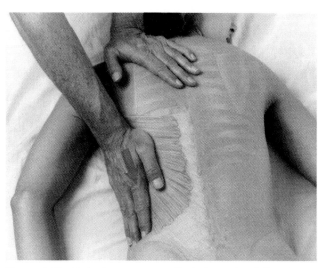

Figure 4-25 Stripping massage of latissimus dorsi (Draping option #7)

Manual Therapy

STRIPPING
- The client lies prone.
- The therapist stands at the client's head on the side to be treated.
- Place the heel of the hand (or the knuckles or supported fingertips) lateral to the lateral border of the scapula just below the axilla.

- Pressing deeply, glide the hand inferiorly all the way to the iliac crest (Fig. 4-25).
- Repeat the above process, gliding your hand to a more medial position on the iliac crest each time, then diagonally across to the spine, ending about a third of the way up the spine.

PINCER COMPRESSION
- The client may be prone or seated. The therapist stands beside the client if prone, or behind the client if seated, facing the axilla on the side to be treated.
- Grasp the bundle of muscles that form the rear border of the axilla (latissimus dorsi and teres major).
- Squeeze firmly. Explore the posterior aspect of the bundle with your thumb, compressing as needed and holding for release (Fig. 4-26). Explore the anterior aspect of the bundle with your fingertips, compressing and holding for release as needed.
- Note that there is a trigger point frequently found in the muscle near the bottom of the bundle; examine in particular for this trigger point and compress as needed. (Fig. 4-27)

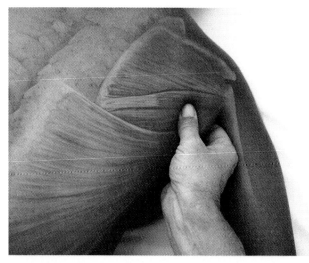

Figure 4-26 Pincer compression of latissimus dorsi (Draping option #7)

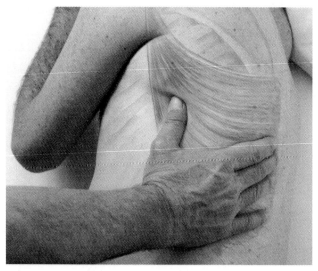

Figure 4-27 Trigger point compression in latissimus dorsi (Draping option #7)

Teres Major

TERR-ease

Etymology   Latin *teres,* round and long + *major,* greater

Overview

Teres major (Fig. 4-28) works with latissimus dorsi, exerting its force from the scapula. These two muscles form the bundle of muscle tissue that passes into the axilla from the scapula and attaches to the front of the upper humerus. This bundle forms the rear border of the armpit.

Attachments

- Medially, to the inferior angle and lower third of the lateral border of the scapula
- Laterally, to the medial border of the bicipital groove of the humerus.

Actions

Adducts and extends arm and rotates it medially.

Referral Area

Over the middle deltoid area and the dorsal forearm

Other Muscles to Examine

- Teres minor
- Middle deltoid
- Infraspinatus
- Latissimus dorsi

Manual Therapy

PINCER COMPRESSION
- The client may be prone or seated. The therapist stands beside the client if

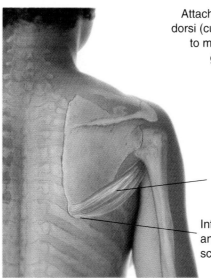

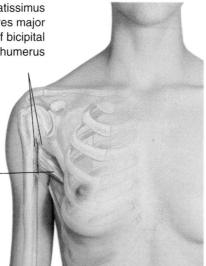

Attachment of latissimus dorsi (cut) and teres major to medial lip of bicipital groove of humerus

Teres major

Inferior angle of scapula

Figure 4-28   Teres major

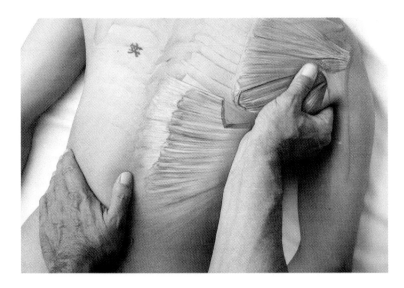

Figure 4-29 Pincer compression of teres major (Draping option #7)

prone, or behind the client if seated, facing the axilla on the side to be treated.

- Grasp the bundle of muscles that form the rear border of the axilla (latissimus dorsi and teres major).
- Find teres major just superior and medial to latissimus dorsi.
- Squeeze firmly. Explore the posterior aspect of the bundle with your thumb, compressing as needed and holding for release (Fig. 4-29). Explore the anterior aspect of the bundle with your fingertips, compressing and holding for release as needed.
- Work the bundle with a kneading motion between your thumb and fingertips.

STRIPPING
- The client lies prone. The therapist stands beside the client, facing the shoulder to be treated.
- Place the thumb of the treating hand against the lateral border of the scapula near the inferior angle (Fig. 4-30).
- Pressing deeply and medially, glide the thumb superiorly toward the axilla. Continue until your thumb reaches the humerus.

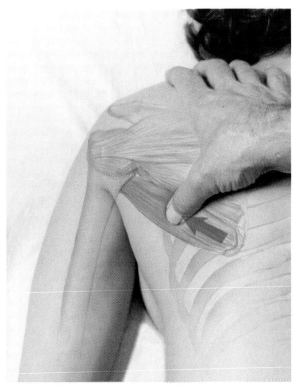

Figure 4-30 Stripping massage in teres major (Draping option #7)

Deltoid

DEL-toyd

Etymology Resembling the Greek letter *delta* (i.e., triangular)

Overview

The three aspects of the deltoid (Fig. 4-31) cap the shoulder over the head of the humerus and provide much of the force that initiates movement of the arm forward, backward, and away from the body. This three-sided arrangement makes the anterior and posterior aspects of the deltoid antagonists to each other. The middle deltoid works closely with supraspinatus in abduction. The deltoids are common problem spots, but they are easy to treat with stripping massage. Deltoid trigger points are often interpreted as bursitis (an inflammation of the bursa, the fluid filled sac that serves as a cushion underneath the muscle).

Note: the three aspects of the deltoid are often referred to as if they were three distinct muscles.

Attachments

■ Medially, to the lateral third of the clavicle, the lateral border of the acromion process, the lower border of the spine of the scapula
■ Laterally, to the lateral side of the shaft of the humerus a little above its middle (deltoid tuberosity).

Actions

Abduction, flexion, extension, and rotation of arm.

Referral Area

Radiating locally over the area of the muscle

Other Muscles to Examine

■ Rotator cuff muscles, especially infraspinatus
■ Teres major
■ Pectoralis major

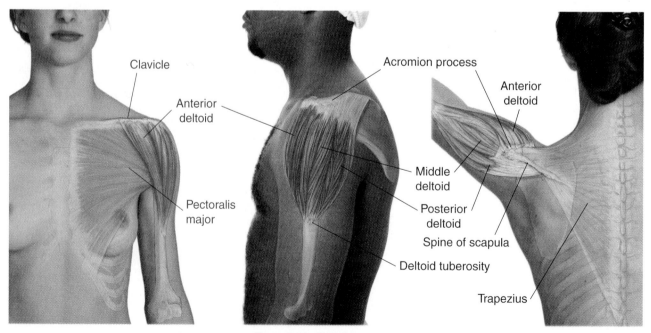

Figure 4-31 Deltoid anatomy

Manual Therapy

STRIPPING (FIG. 4-32)
- The client lies supine. The therapist stands beside the client's head, facing the shoulder to be treated.
- Place the knuckles, fingertips or thumb on the most superior aspect of the anterior deltoid at its medial border.
- Pressing deeply, glide inferiorly over the muscle to its attachment on the humerus.

- Reposition the hand laterally and repeat this procedure, moving onto the lateral deltoid and turning the hand as necessary.
- Continue repeating this procedure with the hand moving underneath the shoulder onto the posterior deltoid and pressing upward, until the entire deltoid has been treated.
- You may treat the posterior deltoid when the client is lying prone.

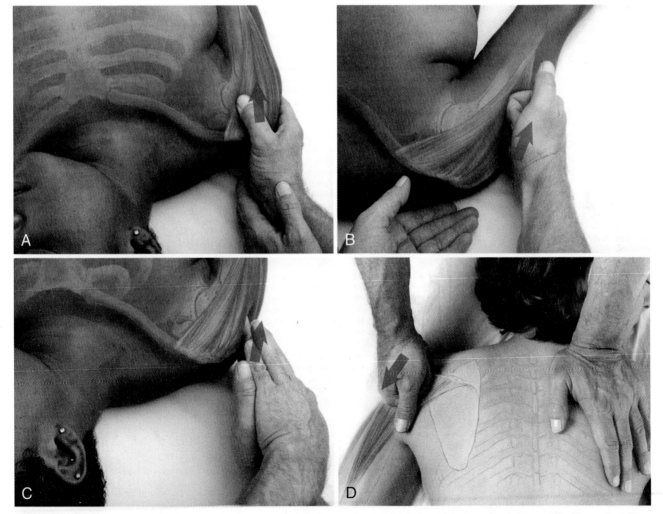

Figure 4-32 Stripping massage of all aspects of the deltoid: (from left) anterior (A), middle (knuckles) (B), middle (fingertips) (C), and posterior (D) (Draping options #2, #7)

THE ROTATOR CUFF

The *rotator cuff* is probably best known for its frequent injury in athletes, particularly baseball pitchers and football quarterbacks, because of the demands made on it by forceful throwing. The rotator cuff takes its name from the "cuff" of tendons of these four muscles that attach side by side at the head of the humerus. The traditional acronym for remembering the rotator cuff muscle is **SITS: supraspinatus, infraspinatus, teres minor,** and **subscapularis.**

Supraspinatus

SOUP-ra-spin-ATE-us

Etymology Latin *supra*, above + *spina*, spine; "above the spine (of the scapula)"

Overview

Supraspinatus (Fig. 4-33) is a surprisingly small muscle given the demands that are made on it. It functions with the middle deltoid in abduction of the arm, but most of its problems arise from its job as stabilizer of the glenohumeral joint. It is active in this capacity during all rotator cuff activities, such as holding a heavy weight in the hand, or working with the arms raised. People who carry heavy objects such as suitcases or even heavy briefcases are likely to have problems with supraspinatus. Repetitive motions also cause rotator cuff problems, such as using a computer mouse for long periods of time.

 Attachments

■ Medially, to the supraspinous fossa of scapula
■ Laterally, to the greater tubercle of the humerus.

 Actions

Initiates abduction of arm

 Referral Area

Over the shoulder, over the middle deltoid area, and down the radial aspect of the arm

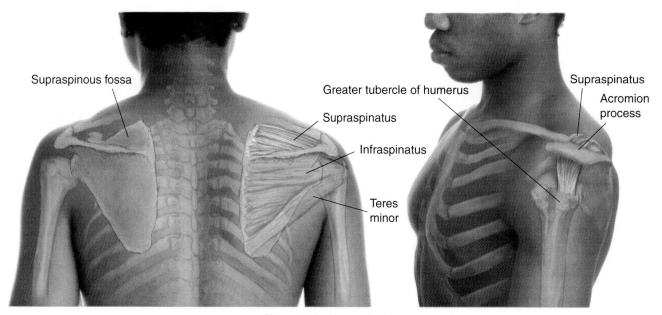

Supraspinous fossa

Greater tubercle of humerus

Supraspinatus

Infraspinatus

Teres minor

Supraspinatus

Acromion process

Figure 4-33 Supraspinatus

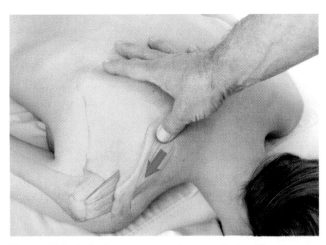

Figure 4-34   Stripping massage of supraspinatus (Draping option #7)

Other Muscles to Examine

- Middle deltoid
- Other rotator cuff muscles, especially infraspinatus

Manual Therapy

STRIPPING

- The client lies prone. The therapist stands beside the client's head on the side to be treated.
- Place the thumb of the treating hand on the medial end of the muscle at the superior angle of the scapula (Fig. 4-34).

- Pressing deeply and inferiorly, move the thumb laterally along the muscle, pressing it into the trough formed by the spine of the scapula, until your thumb is stopped by the acromion process.
- This procedure may also be done with the fingertips or elbow (Fig. 4-35).

COMPRESSION

- The client may be prone or seated. The therapist stands beside the client.
- The client's hand on the side to be treated is placed behind the client's back at the waist to internally rotate the shoulder (Fig. 4-36A).
- Press the thumb deeply through the middle deltoid just under the acromion process until you encounter the attachment of the supraspinatus tendon to the head of the humerus. Hold for release (Fig. 4-36B).

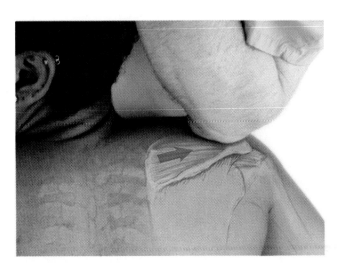

Figure 4-35   Stripping of supraspinatus with elbow (Draping option #7)

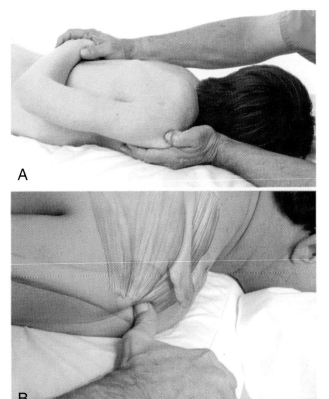

A

B

Figure 4-36   Compression of supraspinatus attachment (Draping option #7)

Infraspinatus

IN-fra-spin-ATE-us

Etymology Latin *infra*, below + *spina*, spine, hence "below the spine (of the scapula)"

Overview

Infraspinatus (Fig. 4-37) is a lateral rotator and a stabilizer of the glenohumeral joint during arm movements. It is a common trouble spot, most often referring pain to the outer aspect of the upper arm from trigger points along the scapular spine and the medial border of the scapula.

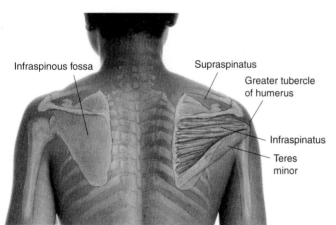

Infraspinous fossa

Supr-aspinatus

Greater tubercle of humerus

Infraspinatus

Teres minor

Figure 4-37 Infraspinatus

Attachments

- Medially, to the infraspinous fossa of the scapula
- Laterally, to the greater tubercle of humerus

Actions

Extends the arm and rotates it laterally

Referral Area

Along the medial border of the scapula, over the middle and/or anterior deltoid area, and down the radial aspect of the arm into the first two or three fingers

Other Muscles to Examine

- Deltoids
- Other rotator cuff muscles
- Biceps brachii
- Coracobrachialis

Manual Therapy

STRIPPING (1)

- The client lies prone. The therapist stands at the client's shoulder opposite

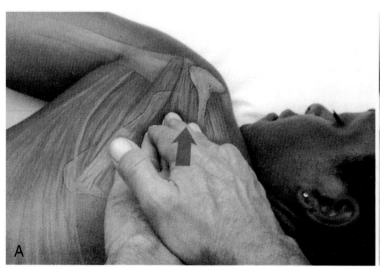

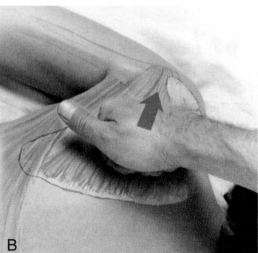

Figure 4-38 Stripping massage of infraspinatus with fingertips (A) and knuckles (B) (Draping option #7)

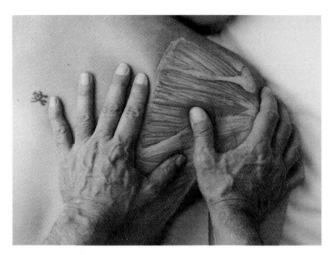

Figure 4-39 Stripping massage of infraspinatus from inferior angle (Draping option #7)

the side to be treated, facing the shoulder to be treated.

- Place the fingertips (Fig. 4-38A), knuckles (Fig. 4-38B), or supported thumb on the muscle at the medial border of the scapula just below the root of the scapular spine.
- Pressing deeply, glide laterally along the muscle just inferior to the spine of the scapula all the way to the attachment on the posterior aspect of the head of the humerus.
- Place the hand just inferior to the prior starting point and repeat the above procedure. Continue along the scapula inferiorly, shifting the angle as neces-

sary, until the entire muscle has been treated.

STRIPPING (2)
- The client lies prone. The therapist stands at the client's side, facing the scapula.
- Place the thumb on the scapula at the inferior angle.
- Pressing firmly into the muscle, glide the thumb up the lateral border of the scapula (Fig. 4-39) to the spine, then follow the muscle to the humerus.
- Either of the two procedures above may also be performed with the elbow (Fig. 4-40).

COMPRESSION
- The client lies prone. The therapist stands by the client's shoulder to be treated, facing the shoulder.
- Place the thumb on the muscle at its medial edge just inferior to the root of the spine of the scapula and press deeply.
- Repeat the procedure shifting the position of your thumb laterally, holding for release as necessary.
- When you have reached the lateral edge of the scapula, begin shifting the position of your thumb inferiorly along the lateral border of the scapula in the same way until you reach the inferior angle of the scapula (Fig. 4-41).

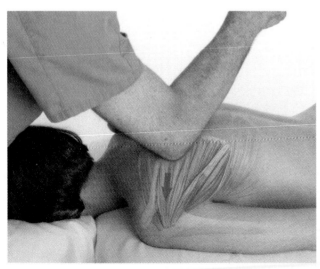

Figure 4-40 Stripping of infraspinatus with the elbow (Draping option #7)

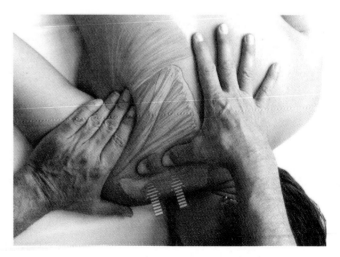

Figure 4-41 Compression of infraspinatus (Draping option #7)

Teres Minor

TERR-ease

Etymology Latin *teres,* round and smooth

Overview

Teres minor (Fig. 4-42) is essentially an adjunct muscle to infraspinatus. It has the same function and, when it has trigger points, refers to the same area (outer aspect of the upper arm).

Attachments

- Medially, to the upper two-thirds of the lateral border of scapula
- Laterally, to the greater tubercle of the humerus just below the infraspinatus

Actions

Adducts arm and rotates it laterally

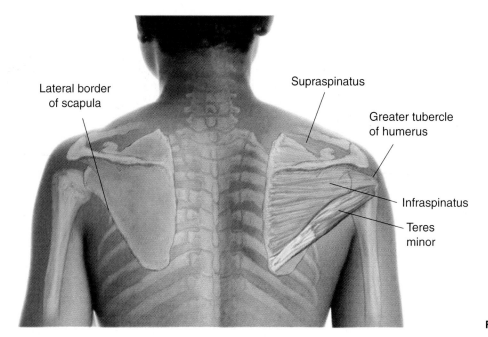

Lateral border of scapula

Supraspinatus

Greater tubercle of humerus

Infraspinatus

Teres minor

Figure 4-42 Teres minor

Referral Area

Over the outer, upper arm

Other Muscles to Examine

- Other rotator cuff muscles, especially infraspinatus
- Teres major
- Middle deltoid

Manual Therapy

STRIPPING
- The client lies prone. The therapist stands at the client's side to be treated, facing the client's shoulder.
- Use the thumb to find the muscle around the midpoint of the lateral edge of the scapula, between teres major and infraspinatus (Fig. 4-43).
- Pressing deeply with the supported thumb, glide along the muscle all the way to its attachment on the posterior aspect of the humerus.

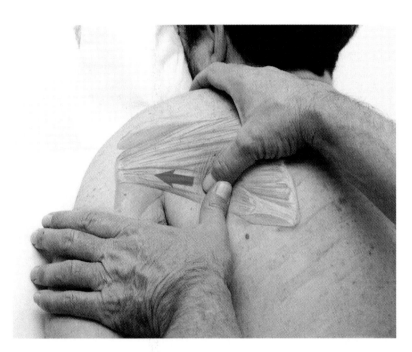

Figure 4-43   Stripping massage of teres minor (Draping option #7)

Subscapularis

SUB-SCAP-you-LAIR-iss

Etymology   Latin *sub,* under + *scapula,* shoulderblade

Overview

Subscapularis (Fig. 4-44) is a medial rotator of the shoulder and a stabilizer of the glenohumeral joint. It is stressed in heavy or repetitive lifting. An inability to raise the arm fully overhead can be a sign of a tight subscapularis.

Attachments

■ Medially, to the subscapular fossa
■ Laterally, to the lesser tubercle of humerus.

Actions

Rotates arm medially

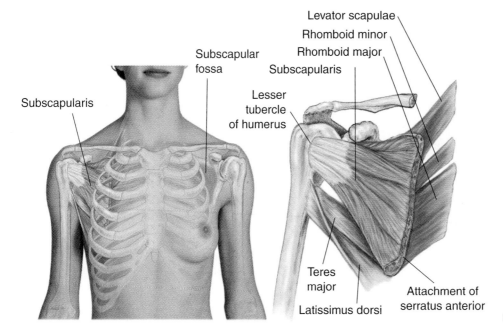

Figure 4-44   Subscapularis

Referral Area

Over the scapula, behind the axilla, along the posterior arm, and into the wrist

Other Muscles to Examine

- Other rotator cuff muscles
- Teres major

Manual Therapy

STRIPPING (1)

- The client lies prone. The therapist stands at the client's side, facing the shoulder to be treated.

- Abduct the client's arm, bending it at the elbow, and internally rotating it (palm up), to about 45°.
- Place the non-treating hand on the medial border of the scapula, pressing the scapula laterally and superiorly.
- Place the fingertips of the treating hand under the muscle bundle forming the rear boundary of the axilla, pressing medial to the bundle into subscapularis. (Fig. 4-45)
- Pressing firmly into the muscle, glide the fingertips from the superior to the inferior aspect of the muscle (or vice versa, according to what works best for you), covering as much of the muscle as possible.

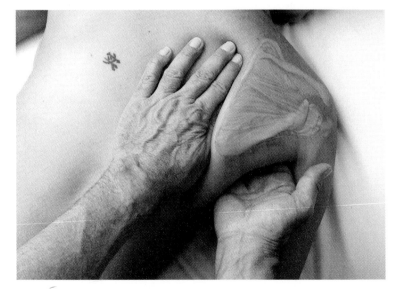

Figure 4-45 Stripping massage of subscapularis (1) (Draping option #7)

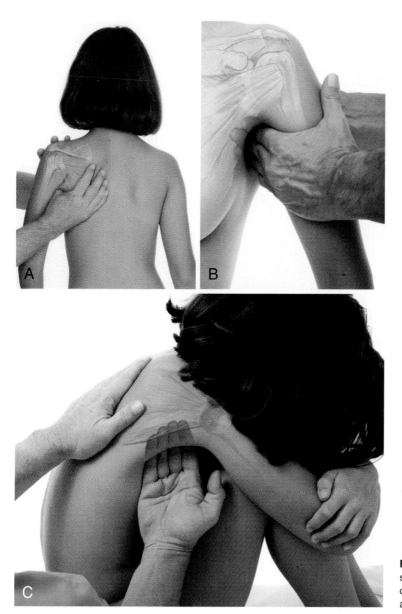

Figure 4-46 Accessing subscapularis with client seated: with thumb (A), with fingertips (B), with client's hips and knees flexed and arms wrapped around knees (C) (Draping option #16)

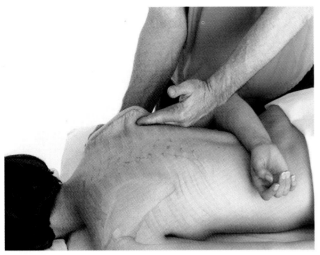

Figure 4-47 Compression of inferior aspect of subscapularis (Draping option #7)

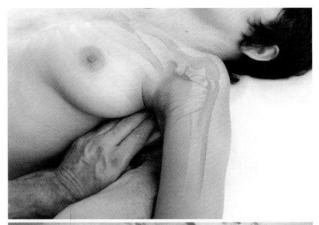

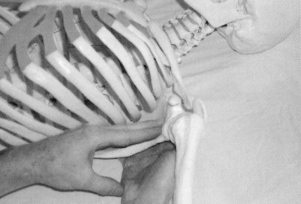

Figure 4-48 Stripping massage of subscapularis (2) (Draping option #3)

- This technique may also be performed with the client sitting on the side of the table, using the thumb (Fig. 4-46A) or the fingertips (Fig. 4-46B), or with legs drawn up and arms wrapped around legs(Fig. 4-46C).

COMPRESSION
- To reach the inferior portion of the muscle, bend the client's arm at the elbow 45° behind the back.
- Lift the shoulder with your far hand.
- Insert the fingertips of your near hand underneath the inferior angle of the scapula and press upward. (Fig. 4-47)

STRIPPING (2)
- The client lies supine with the arm abducted. The therapist stands at the client's side, facing the shoulder.

- Place the far hand under the client's scapula with the fingertips hooked over the medial border, pulling the scapula laterally.
- With the fingertips of the near hand, press firmly just under the axilla into the underside of the scapula. (Fig. 4-48)
- Glide the fingertips slowly inferiorly or superiorly along the muscle.

MUSCLES OF THE RIBS

Serratus Anterior

serr-RATE-us an-TIER-ee-yore

Etymology   Latin *serra,* saw + *anterior,* more toward the front

Overview

Serratus anterior (Fig. 4-49) works with the pectoral muscles and opposes the rhomboids. It can produce pain in the side of the chest and down the arm in a pattern similar to that of pectoralis minor, and it is most easily treated along with that muscle.

 Attachments

- Inferiorly, to the center of the lateral aspect of the first eight to nine ribs
- Superiorly, to the superior and inferior angles and intervening medial margin of scapula

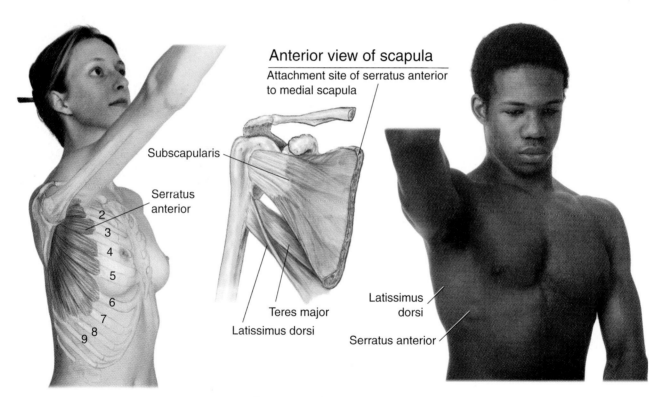

Anterior view of scapula
Attachment site of serratus anterior to medial scapula

Subscapularis

Serratus anterior

2
3
4
5
6
7
8
9

Teres major
Latissimus dorsi

Latissimus dorsi
Serratus anterior

Figure 4-49   Serratus anterior

Actions

Rotates the scapula and pulls it forward; elevates the ribs

Referral Area

To the side of the chest at the middle of the rib cage, down the ulnar aspect of the arm to the last two fingers, and just medial to the inferior angle of the scapula

Other Muscles to Examine

- Latissimus dorsi
- Teres major
- Pectoralis minor
- Rhomboids

Manual Therapy

STRIPPING

- The client lies on the side contralateral to that to be treated. The therapist stands in front of the client's chest.
- Place one hand on the side of the client's ribcage, with the fingers lying over the scapula and the thumb resting on the ninth rib.
- Pressing deeply, glide the thumb in an arc toward the scapula until it reaches the inferior angle.
- Shift the thumb one rib superiorly and repeat the process (Fig. 4-50), each time ending slightly more superiorly on the lateral border of the scapula. As you encounter the bundle of muscles that forms the posterior boundary of the axilla, let your thumbs slip under the bundle to the scapula.

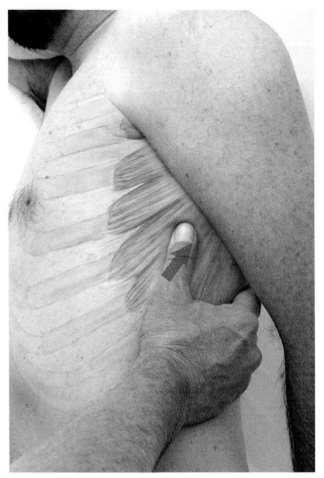

Figure 4-50 Stripping massage of serratus anterior in sidelying position (Draping option #15)

Serratus Posterior Inferior

serr-RATE-us poss-TIER-ee-yore
in-FEAR-ee-yore

Etymology Latin *serra*, saw + *posterior*, toward the back + *inferior*, lower

Overview

Serratus posterior inferior (Fig. 4-51) assists in rotation and extension of the trunk, and assists in respiration. Its most common trigger point radiates locally.

Attachments

- Medially and inferiorly, with latissimus dorsi, from the spinous processes of the two lower thoracic and two or three upper lumbar vertebrae

- Laterally and superiorly, to the lower borders of the last four ribs

Actions

Draws lower ribs backward and downward

Referral Area

Radiating locally over the muscle

Other Muscles to Examine

- Quadratus lumborum
- Iliocostalis thoracis
- Psoas major
- Rectus abdominis
- Pyramidalis
- Diaphragm

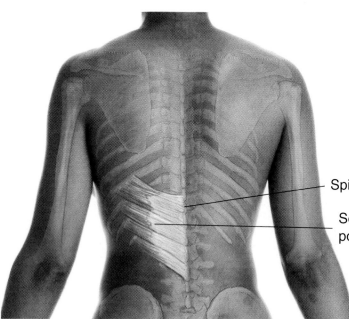

Spinous process, T-11

Serratus posterior inferior

Figure 4-51 Serratus posterior inferior

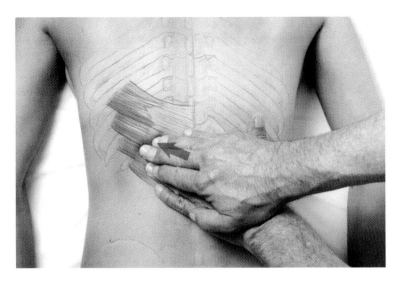

Figure 4-52   Stripping massage of serratus posterior inferior (Draping option #7)

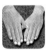 **Manual Therapy**

STRIPPING

- Client lies supine; therapist stands at client's hips on side contralateral to that to be treated.
- Place your supported fingertips at the upper lumbar vertebrae.
- Press deeply into muscle, moving the fingertips diagonally (inferiorly and laterally) over the lower two ribs.

- Move the fingertips up to the lowest two thoracic vertebrae and repeat (Fig. 4-52).
- In place of the fingertips, the thumb, elbow, or knuckles may be used.

COMPRESSION

- Palpate the area over the muscle with thumb or supported fingertip until the client reports a sharp, radiating pain.
- Compress that point with the thumb or elbow until the pain eases (Fig. 4-53).

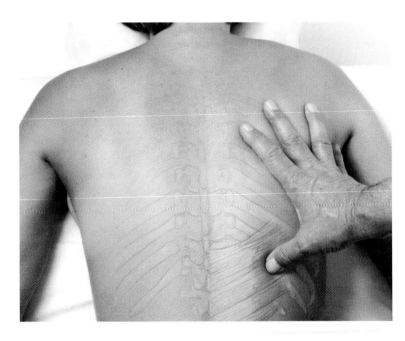

Figure 4-53   Compression of trigger point in serratus posterior inferior with thumb (Draping option #7)

Muscles of Breathing

Many, if not most, people do not breathe properly. There are many theories about why people learn improper breathing skills, but they are beyond the scope of this book. Nevertheless, the clinical massage therapist is in an excellent position to enable clients to relearn breathing skills.

Two things are necessary: first, the therapist should work on the muscles of respiration so that they are free of constrictions and trigger points, have good muscle tone, and can move freely. Second, the therapist should teach the client good breathing skills and urge the client to practice them outside of therapy.

Most people tend to breathe from the neck, shoulders, and upper chest, allowing the upper rib cage to expand while tightening the abdominal muscles. This habit is called "paradoxical breathing," because the abdomen is contracted rather than expanded. In proper breathing, the sternum, lower rib cage, and abdomen expand. This skill is called "diaphragmatic breathing."

Diaphragmatic breathing draws air more deeply into the lungs and increases breathing efficiency. It requires less effort and is far more efficient than "upper chest" breathing, is more relaxing, and increases respiratory endurance. Professional singers and musicians learn diaphragmatic breathing, and it will improve the quality of the voice. The latter advantage can be observed not only in opera singers, but in the lusty cry of a baby!

Begin by evaluating the client's breathing practices. Although the shoulders rise slightly and the upper chest expands somewhat, the ex-pansion should take place from the bottom up, rather than from the top down. The upper chest and shoulders should be pushed slightly upward by the expansion of the inferior rib cage, rather than pulled upward by the scalenes. If the breathing motion expands the abdomen and lower rib cage, followed by a moderate expansion of the upper chest and a slight rise in the shoulders, the client is breathing properly, and you need only work the respiratory muscles to loosen and relax them. However, if the abdomen contracts, the shoulders rise significantly, and the upper chest expands pronouncedly, you'll need to teach proper breathing mechanics to the client.

Manual Therapy

INITIAL ASSESSMENT
- The client may stand (Fig. 4-54), sit, or lie supine (Fig. 4-55).
- Ask the client to take a deep breath while you observe the shoulders, chest, and abdomen.
- If the client is breathing paradoxically, you will see the shoulders rise pronouncedly, the upper chest expand markedly, and the abdomen contract (Fig. 4-54A) (Fig. 4-55A).
- If the client is breathing diaphragmatically, you will see the abdomen and lower rib cage expand, the shoulders rise slightly, and the upper chest expand moderately (Fig. 4-54B) (Fig. 4-55B).

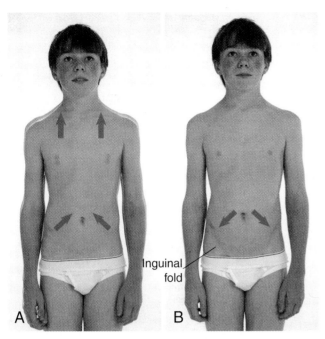

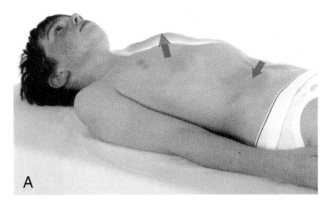

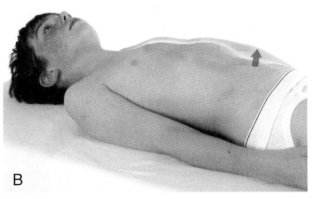

Figure 4-54   Client standing for breathing assessment: (A) paradoxical, and (B) diaphragmatic inhalation

Figure 4-55   Client supine for breathing assessment: (A) paradoxical inhalation, (B) diaphragmatic inhalation (Draping option #2)

- Note the clearer delineation of the inguinal folds (Fig. 4-54B) when the abdomen expands, and the flattening of the inguinal folds on contraction.
- Before proceeding to teach breathing, release the entire breathing apparatus with myofascial work on the chest and manual therapy of the muscles of breathing. First, examine the diaphragm. Place your hand on the abdomen with the fingers pointing superiorly just at the edge of the first rib. As the client exhales, press your fingers under the costal arch in a superior direction (Fig. 4-56). Repeat on the opposite side. Tightness or pain indicates constriction and probable trigger point activity in the breathing mechanism that can cause pain and prevent comfortable respiration.

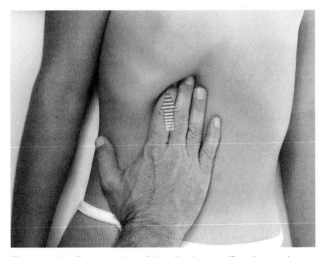

Figure 4-56   Examination of the diaphragm (Draping option #2)

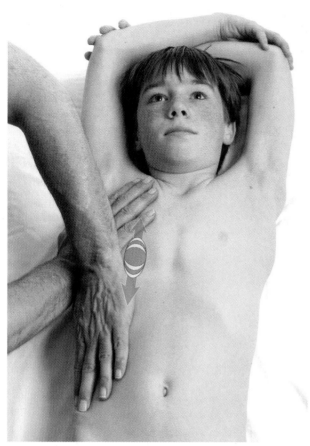

Figure 4-57   Myofascial release of the chest (1) (Draping option #2)

MYOFASCIAL RELEASE OF THE CHEST (1)

- Have the supine client raise her or his arms overhead.
- Place one hand flat on the client's chest just medial to the axilla, with your fingers pointing superiorly. Cross the other hand over the first hand and place it flat on the chest just inferior to the first hand, the fingers pointing inferiorly (Fig. 4-57).
- Let your hands sink gently into the tissue until you feel the underlying superficial fascia. Press the two hands gently away from each other, stretching the fascia. Hold until you feel that the fascia has released.
- Shift your hands medially by a hand's width and repeat the process.
- Repeat the procedure as far as the sternum, then move to the other side of the client and repeat.
- On female clients with developed breasts, discontinue this procedure at the breasts and continue on the medial side.

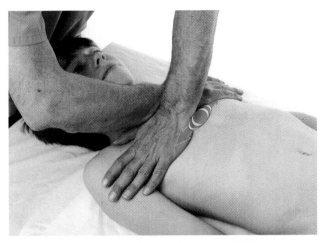

Figure 4-58 Myofascial release of the chest (2) (Draping option #2)

MYOFASCIAL RELEASE OF THE CHEST (2)

■ Stand at the client's head.
■ Place one hand flat on the client's chest with the heel of the hand resting on the sternum just below the manubrium, the fingers pointing laterally.
■ Cross the other hand over and place it next to the first, the fingers pointing laterally in the other direction (Fig. 4-58).
■ Let your hands sink gently into the tissue until you feel the underlying superficial fascia. Press the two hands gently away from each other, stretching the fascia. Hold until you feel that the fascia has released.
■ Shift your hands inferiorly by a hand's width and repeat the process.
■ Continue this procedure as far as the inferior end of the sternum.

FASCIAL WORK ON THE CHEST (3)

■ Place one hand flat on the client's sternum just inferior to the manubrium, with your fingers pointing inferiorly (Fig. 4-59).

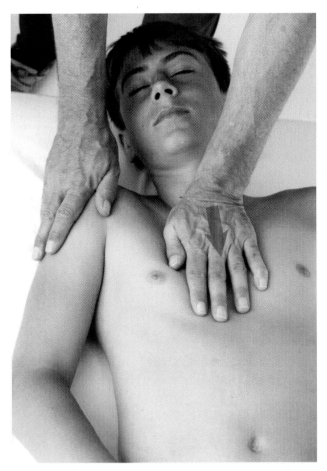

Figure 4-59 Fascial work on the chest (3) with the hand (Draping option #2)

■ Pressing firmly into the tissue, glide your hand slowly down the sternum until the heel of your hand reaches the inferior end of the sternum.

 Note: do not press on the xiphoid process. It can be broken with pressure.

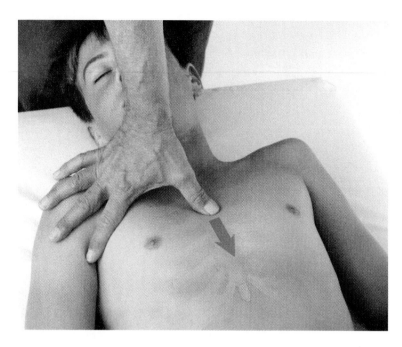

Figure 4-60   Fascial work on the chest (4) with the thumb (Draping option #2)

FASCIAL WORK ON THE CHEST (4)
- Place your thumb on the client's sternum just inferior to the manubrium.
- Pressing firmly into the tissue, glide your thumb slowly down the sternum (Fig. 4-60) until it reaches the inferior end of the sternum.

 Note: do not press on the xiphoid process. It can be broken with pressure.

FASCIAL WORK ON THE CHEST (5)
- Standing beside the supine client at chest level, place your whole hand flat on the upper chest on the contralateral side of the client's body, the heel of your hand resting on the sternum just below the manubrium.
- Pressing into the tissue primarily with the heel of your hand, glide your hand away from yourself (Fig. 4-61), following the curve of the body as far as you can reach comfortably.

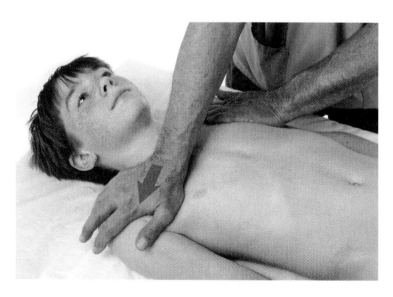

Figure 4-61   Fascial work on the chest (5) with the hand (Draping option #2)

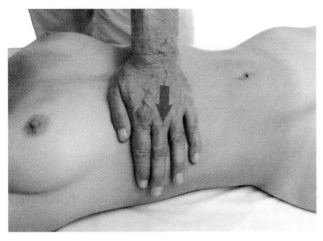

Figure 4-62 Fascial work on the chest (5) with a female client with developed breasts (Draping option #2)

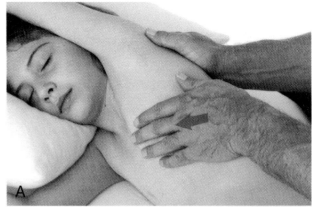

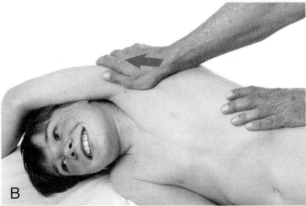

Figure 4-63 Fascial work on the chest (6) with client in sidely-ing position: (A) starting position, (B) over shoulder (Draping option #15)

- Shift your hand by a hand's width inferiorly on the chest and repeat the process, continuing to the inferior rib cage.
- In the case of female clients with developed breasts, perform this procedure as far as the breast area, then continue on the chest below the breast (Fig. 4-62).

FASCIAL WORK ON THE CHEST (6)
- The client is in sidelying position.
- The therapist stands behind the client at waist level.
- Place one hand on the inferior rib cage, iliac crest, or back, to stabilize the client. Place the other hand on the lateral rib cage, the fingers pointing diagonally toward the client's contralateral shoulder (Fig. 4-63A).
- Pressing deeply into the tissue with the whole palm of the hand, glide the hand diagonally over the rib cage as far as the sternum (or until breast tissue is encountered in a female client with developed breasts).

- From the same starting point, repeat the procedure to the axilla.
- From the same starting point, change hands as necessary, and repeat the procedure directly up the client's side and over the posterior border of the axilla to the deltoid area (Fig. 4-63B).
- From the same starting point, repeat the procedure over the posterior chest to the scapula.

The Diaphragm

DIE-a-fram

Greek *dia*, through + *phragma*, enclosure

Overview

The *diaphragm* (Fig. 4-64) is a dome of muscle and connective tissue separating the thoracic from the abdominal cavity. It is the primary muscle of inspiration.

 Attachments

- Anteriorly, to the sternum
- Posteriorly, to the bodies of the upper lumbar vertebrae
- Peripherally, to the costal margin
- In the center, the central tendon is penetrated by the aorta, vena cava, and esophagus
- Posteriorly the arcuate ligaments allow passage of psoas major and quadratus lumborum.

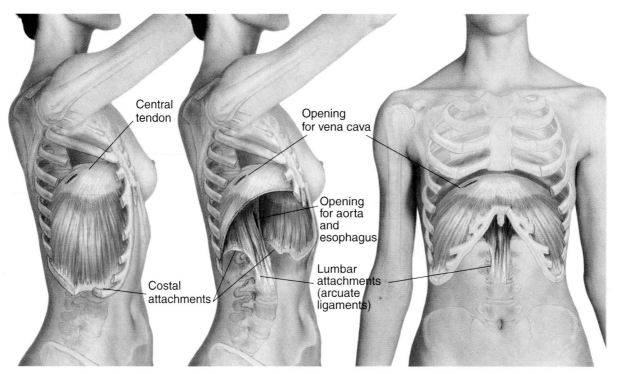

Figure 4-64   Anatomy of the diaphragm

Actions

Elevates and expands the lower costal margin and lower ribs, expanding the abdomen and lower ribcage in inspiration

 Referral Area

"Stitch in the side", chest pain, substernal pain, or pain along the lower border of the ribs

 Other Muscles to Examine

- Intercostals
- Scalenes
- Pectoralis major
- Pectoralis minor
- Rectus abdominis

 Manual Therapy

RELEASE

- Standing at the client's side at waist level, place one or both hands at the base of the opposite rib cage, with the thumb, supported thumb, or fingertips against the lowest rib.
- Ask the client to inhale deeply, then slowly exhale.
- As the client exhales, press the thumb (Fig. 4-65A), supported thumb (Fig. 4-65B), or fingertips deeply under the lower rib cage, lifting it upward and away from yourself.
- Move to the other side of the client and repeat the procedure.

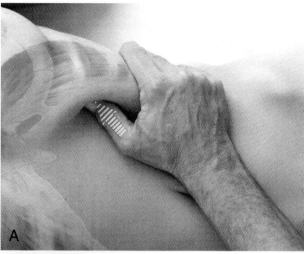

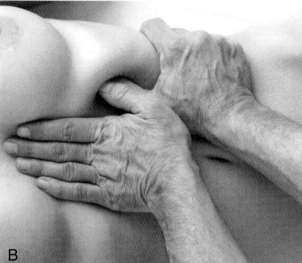

Figure 4-65 Release of diaphragm with thumb (A) or supported thumb (B) (Draping option #2)

Serratus Posterior Superior

serr-RATE-us poss-TIER-ee-yore
sue-PEER-ee-yore

Etymology   Latin *serra,* saw + *posterior,* toward the back + *superior,* higher

Overview

Serratus posterior superior (Fig. 4-66) assists in breathing by raising the ribs to which it attaches. Note that the client's arm must be raised to access its most common trigger point.

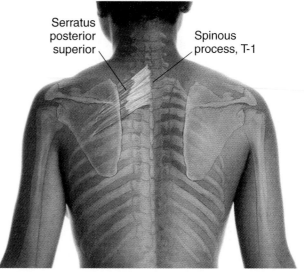

Figure 4-66   Anatomy of serratus posterior superior

Attachments

- Medially, to the spinous processes of the two lower cervical and two upper thoracic vertebrae
- Laterally, to lateral side of angles of second to fifth ribs.

Actions

Raises the second through fifth ribs to assist inhalation

Referral Area

Over the upper half of the scapula, into the anterior chest, along the dorsal and ulnar aspects of the arm to the little finger

Other Muscles to Examine

- Rhomboids
- Rotator cuff muscles
- Teres major
- Pectoralis minor
- Posterior and middle deltoids

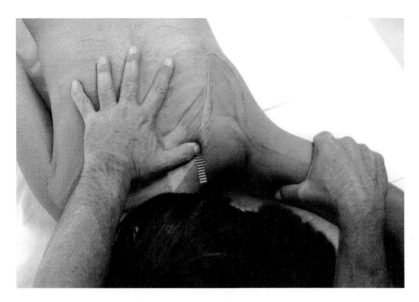

Figure 4-67 Compression of trigger point in serratus posterior superior (Draping option #7)

Manual Therapy

STRIPPING/COMPRESSION

- The client lies supine, with the arm on the side to be treated abducted and extended to rotate the superior angle of the scapula downward to expose more of the muscle. The therapist stands beside the client's head contralateral to the side to be treated.
- Place the fingertips or supported thumb just next to the spinous process of the sixth cervical vertebra. Pressing deeply, glide the hand diagonally downward as far as the scapula will permit.
- Repeat the process at the seventh cervical and first two thoracic vertebrae.
- The most common trigger point in this muscle lies in the area nearest the ribs that is uncovered by rotating the scapula. If this trigger point is present, compress and hold until it releases (Fig. 4-67).

Intercostals

In-ter-COST-als

Latin *inter*, between + *costa*, rib

Overview

The intercostals (Fig. 4-68) have both respiratory and postural functions, and their precise functions are quite complex. Essentially, they control the activity of the ribs, and thus both inspiration and thoracic rotation. Release of shortened intercostals is, therefore, an important part of work on the thorax.

Attachments

- External: Each attaches to the inferior border of one rib and passes obliquely in an inferior and anterior direction to the superior border of the rib below.
- Internal: Each attaches to the inferior border of one rib and passes obliquely in an inferior and posterior direction to the upper border of the rib below.
- Note: The external intercostals do not extend all the way to the costal cartilages except between the lowest ribs. In their place is fascia.
- External intercostals contract during inspiration; internal intercostals contract during expiration. Both also maintain tension to resist mediolateral

movement, and are active in rotation of the thoracic spine.

Referral Area

Locally, tending to extend anteriorly

Other Muscles to Examine

- Diaphragm
- Serratus posterior inferior
- Serratus anterior
- Pectoralis major
- Pectoralis minor
- Rectus abdominis
- Transversus abdominis
- External and internal obliques

Manual Therapy

Anterior Treatment

Lower Intercostals
STRIPPING
- The client lies supine.
- Standing beside the client at chest level, place your thumb at the juncture of the eighth and ninth ribs at the costal cartilage on the opposite side of the body.
- Pressing between the ribs and following the curve of the ribs, glide your

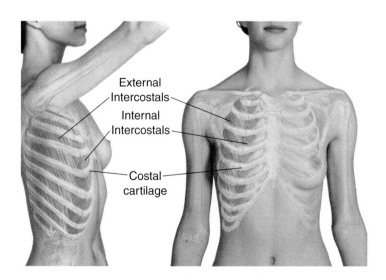

External Intercostals

Internal Intercostals

Costal cartilage

Figure 4-68 Anatomy of the intercostals

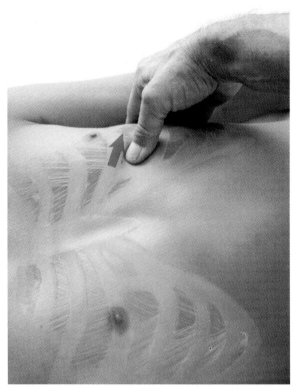

Figure 4-69 Stripping massage of intercostals (Draping option #2)

thumb slowly as far as you can comfortably reach.

- Shift your thumb superiorly to the next intercostal space and repeat the process (Fig. 4-69).
- As you move into the area occupied by the pectoralis major, and the breasts in women, continue your motion only as

far as you are able to feel the intercostal space (Fig. 4-70).

- Move to the other side of the client and repeat the process.

STRETCH

- The client lies supine.
- Stand next the client at chest level. Have the client raise the near arm overhead, reaching toward the opposite shoulder.
- Place your hand nearest the client's head on the client's axillary region, maintaining an upward pressure.
- Place your other hand over the client's lower rib cage on the side, maintaining a downward pressure.
- Ask the client to breathe deeply. As the client inhales, use the rib cage hand to resist the elevation of the ribs.
- As the client exhales, press downward on the ribs, and have the client reach toward the opposite shoulder (Fig. 4-71).
- Repeat for two or three cycles, then move to the other side of the client and repeat the entire process.

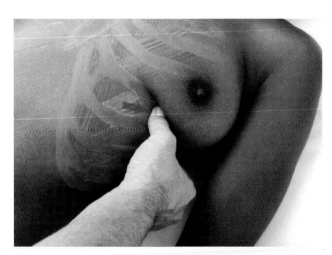

Figure 4-70 Stripping massage of intercostals in a female client (Draping option #2)

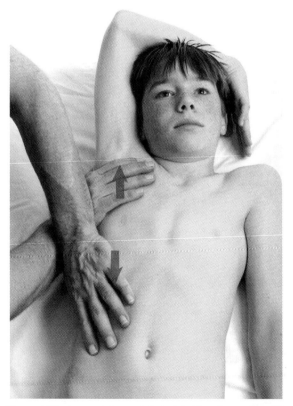

Figure 4-71 Lower intercostal stretch (Draping option #2)

Upper Intercostals
STRETCH

- Stand at the head of the client, who is supine with the hand on the side to be treated raised overhead.
- Place one hand under the client's back on the posterior superior ribs.
- Place the other hand on the client's upper rib cage.
- Ask the client to take slow, deep breaths. Pull the posterior ribs superiorly (toward you) with hand underneath the client; push the anterior ribs inferiorly (away from you) with the hand on the client's chest (Fig. 4-72).
- Maintain this pressure through five or six breathing cycles, or until you feel release in the rib cage.
- Repeat on the other side.

Posterior Treatment

Posterior trigger points in the intercostals tend to refer anteriorly, and should be located and treated individually with compression.

TEACHING DIAPHRAGMATIC BREATHING

Once all the muscles of the breathing apparatus have been released, the client is ready to learn diaphragmatic breathing skills without muscular re-

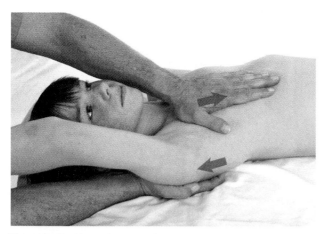

Figure 4-72 Upper intercostal stretch (Draping option #2)

strictions. Proceed slowly and patiently; a good rapport with the client is essential. The process will seem awkward and ungainly at first, like any new activity.

The client should experience expansion of the lower rib cage and the abdomen, then be encouraged to let the expansion move deeply into the pelvic basin. The learning process is kinesthetic, of course, and you can best teach it by placing your hand successively on the lower rib cage, the middle abdomen, and the lower abdomen, and asking the client to direct the breathing expansion into your hand as it lies on each of these areas. Remember that these sensations are new to the client. Be encouraging, patient, and supportive, reinforcing every step in the desired direction.

 Manual Therapy

- The client may stand, sit, or lie supine.
- Ask the client to place her or his hands behind the head to neutralize involvement of the shoulders.
- Standing beside the supine client, place one hand (Fig. 4-73A) on the lower anterior rib cage. Alternatively, standing or sitting beside the standing or seated client, place one hand on the lower anterior and the other on the lower posterior rib cage (Fig. 4-74).
- Ask the client to inhale slowly and deeply through the nose, concentrating on breathing into your anterior hand. Continue this until you feel movement in the rib cage (Fig. 4-73B). Verbally reinforce any movement you feel.
- Place one hand on the client's upper abdomen covering the umbilicus (Fig. 4-73C). If the client is standing or seated, place the other hand on the same area of the client's back. Ask the client to inhale slowly and deeply through the nose, concentrating on breathing into your hands. Continue this until you feel the abdomen expand (Fig. 4-73D). Verbally reinforce any movement you feel.

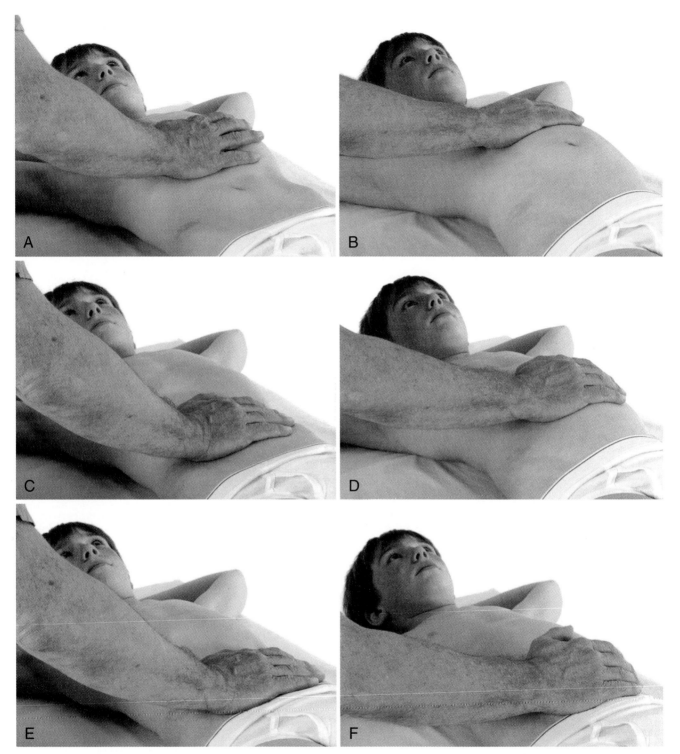

Figure 4-73 Teaching diaphragmatic breathing with client supine: (A) rib cage neutral, (B) rib cage expanded, (C) middle abdomen neutral, (D) middle abdomen expanded, (E) lower abdomen neutral, (F) lower abdomen expanded (Draping option #2)

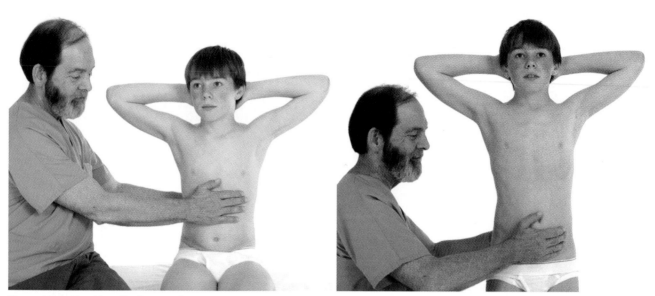

Figure 4-74 Teaching diaphragmatic breathing with client standing or seated, with the therapist's hands placed on anterior and posterior rib cage or abdomen

■ Place your hand on the lower abdomen just above the pubis (Fig. 4-73E). If the client is standing or seated (Fig. 4-74), place the other hand at the top of the client's sacrum. Ask the client to inhale slowly and deeply through the nose, concentrating on breathing into your hands. Continue this until you feel the abdomen expand (Fig. 4-73F). Verbally reinforce any movement you feel.

Some people catch on very quickly, while others find it more challenging, so work patiently. Urge the client to practice these skills at home. Assure the client that this style of breathing, once mastered, will be far more comfortable and relaxing than his or her previous style.

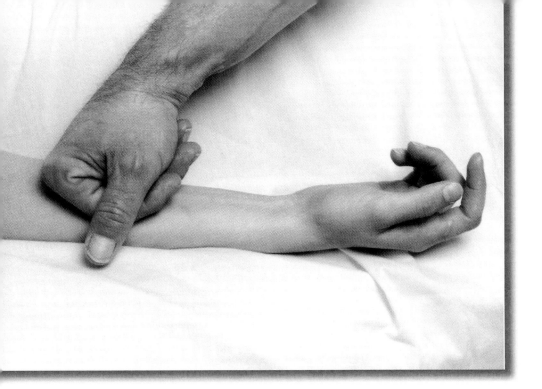

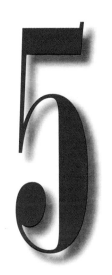

The Arm and Hand

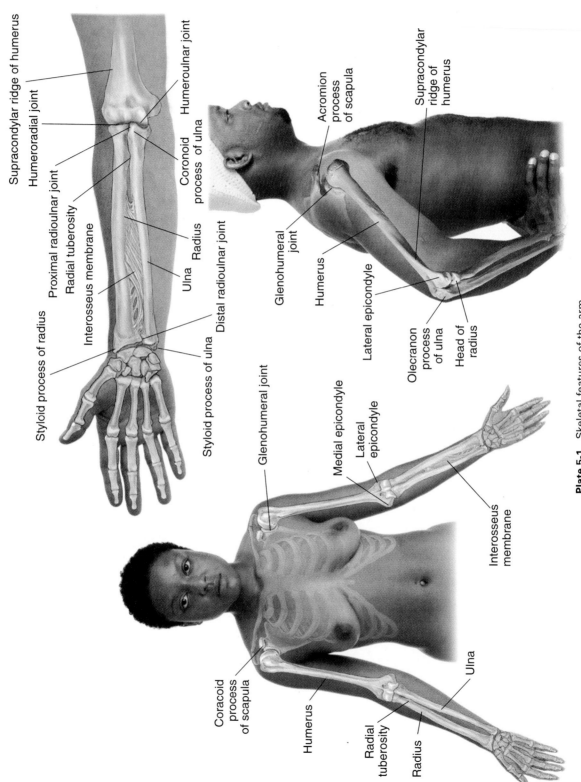

Plate 5-1 Skeletal features of the arm

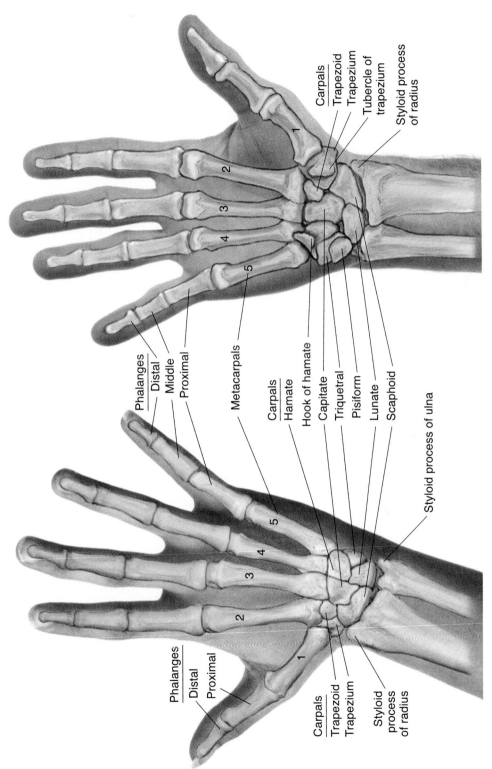

Plate 5-2 Skeletal features of the hand and wrist

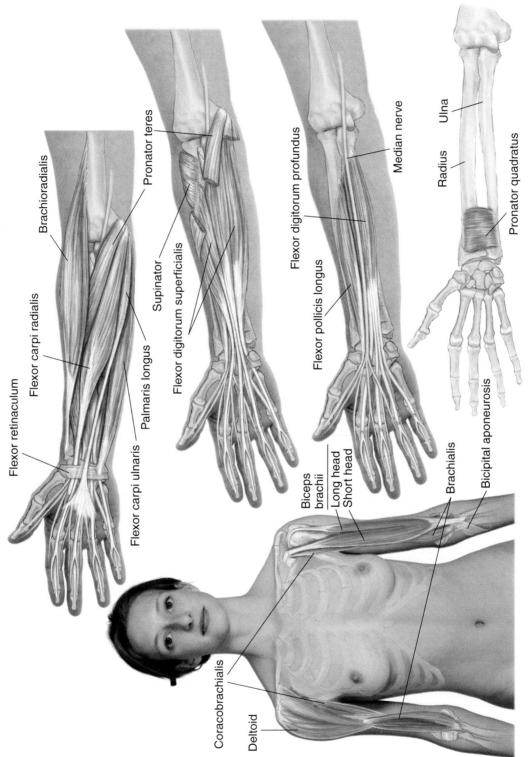

Plate 5-3 Muscles of the anterior arm and forearm

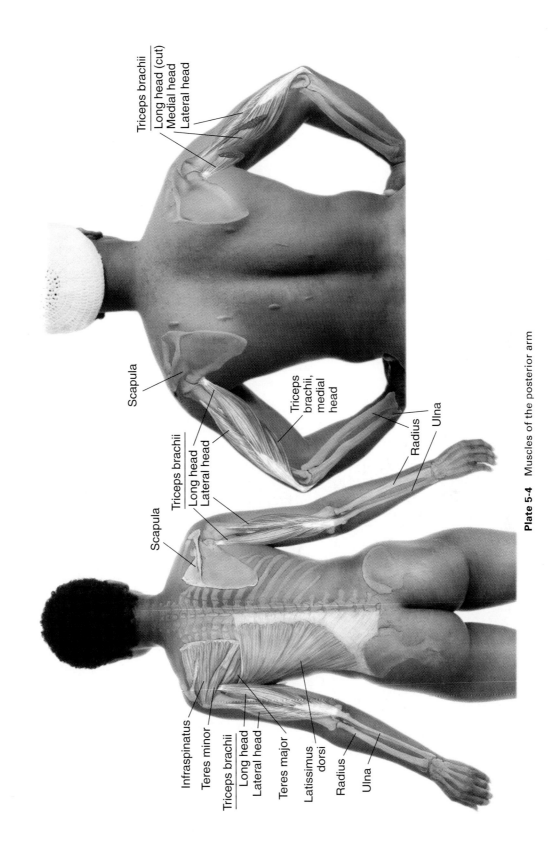

Triceps brachii
Long head (cut)
Medial head
Lateral head

Scapula

Triceps brachii, medial head

Radius

Ulna

Scapula

Triceps brachii
Long head
Lateral head

Infraspinatus

Teres minor

Triceps brachii
Long head
Lateral head

Teres major

Latissimus dorsi

Radius

Ulna

Plate 5-4 Muscles of the posterior arm

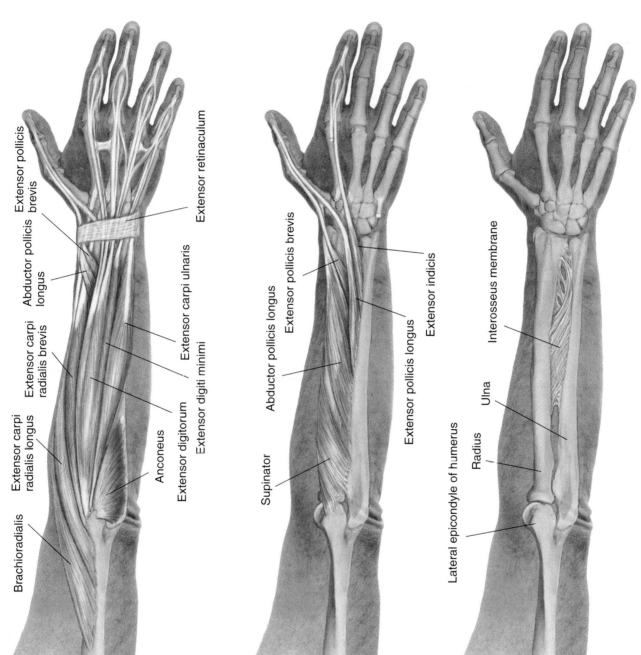

Extensor pollicis brevis

Abductor pollicis longus

Extensor retinaculum

Extensor carpi radialis brevis

Extensor carpi ulnaris

Extensor digiti minimi

Extensor carpi radialis longus

Anconeus

Extensor digitorum

Brachioradialis

Supinator

Abductor pollicis longus

Extensor pollicis brevis

Extensor indicis

Extensor pollicis longus

Lateral epicondyle of humerus

Radius

Ulna

Interosseus membrane

Plate 5-5   Muscles of the posterior forearm

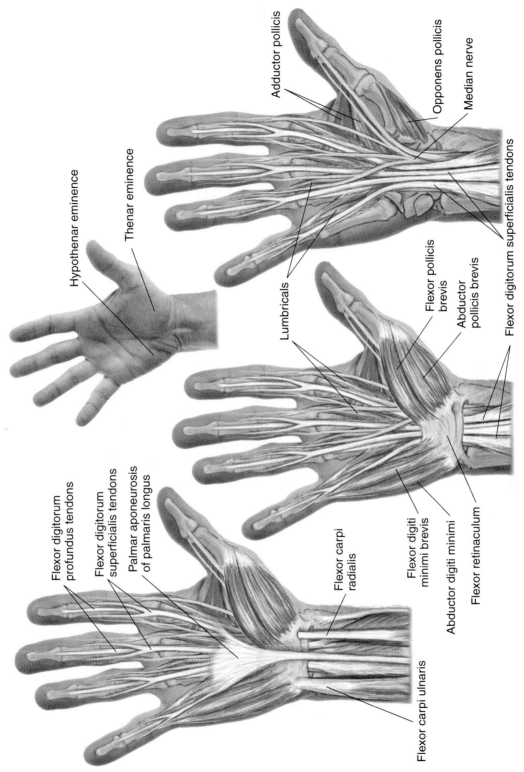

Adductor pollicis

Opponens pollicis

Median nerve

Flexor digitorum superficialis tendons

Hypothenar eminence

Thenar eminence

Lumbricals

Flexor pollicis brevis

Abductor pollicis brevis

Flexor digitorum profundus tendons

Flexor digitorum superficialis tendons

Palmar aponeurosis of palmaris longus

Flexor carpi radialis

Flexor digiti minimi brevis

Abductor digiti minimi

Flexor retinaculum

Flexor carpi ulnaris

Plate 5-6 Superficial muscles of the palmar (anterior) hand

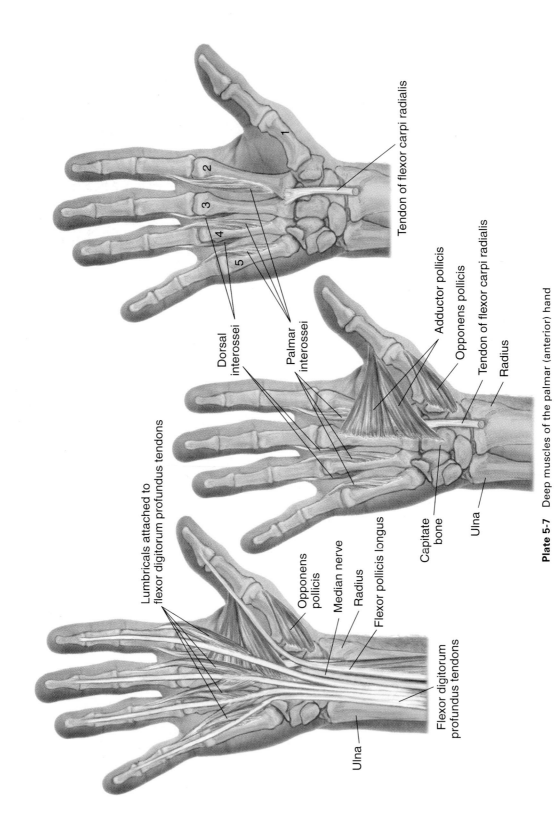

1
2
3
4
5

Tendon of flexor carpi radialis

Dorsal interossei

Palmar interossei

Adductor pollicis
Opponens pollicis
Tendon of flexor carpi radialis
Radius

Lumbricals attached to flexor digitorum profundus tendons

Opponens pollicis
Median nerve
Radius
Flexor pollicis longus

Capitate bone
Ulna

Flexor digitorum profundus tendons

Ulna

Plate 5-7 Deep muscles of the palmar (anterior) hand

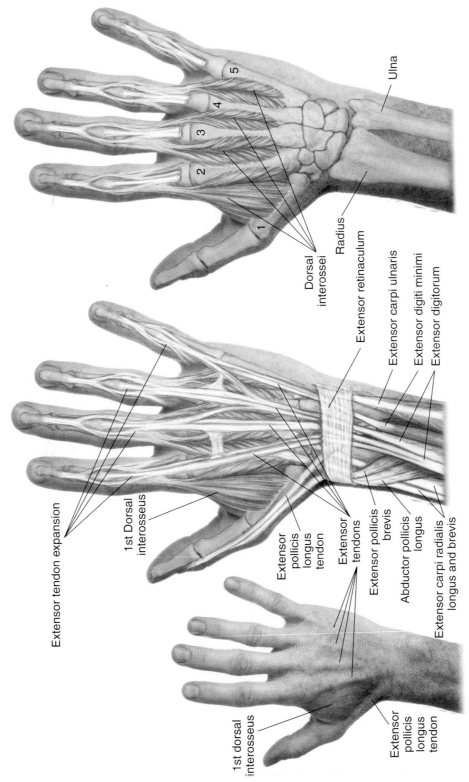

Ulna

Radius

Dorsal
interossei

Extensor retinaculum

Extensor carpi ulnaris

Extensor digiti minimi

Extensor digitorum

Extensor tendon expansion

1st Dorsal
interosseus

Extensor
pollicis
longus
tendon

Extensor
tendons

Extensor pollicis
brevis

Abductor pollicis
longus

Extensor carpi radialis
longus and brevis

1st dorsal
interosseus

Extensor
pollicis
longus
tendon

Plate 5-8   Muscles of the dorsal (posterior) hand

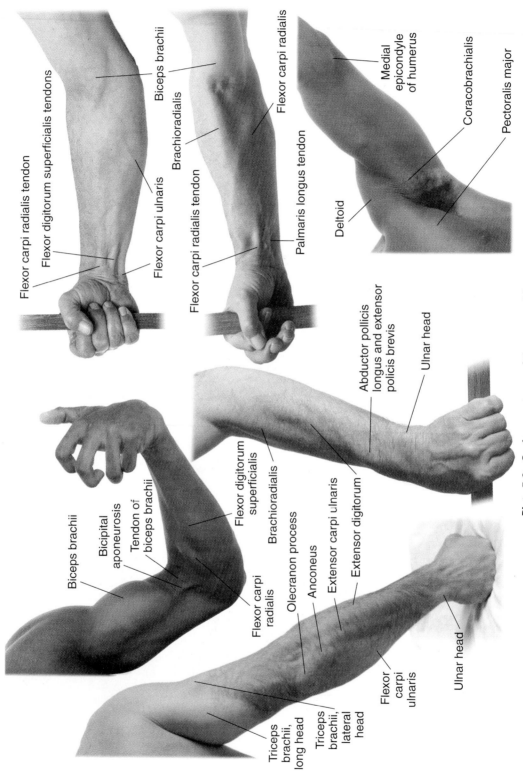

Plate 5-9 Surface anatomy of the arm and forearm

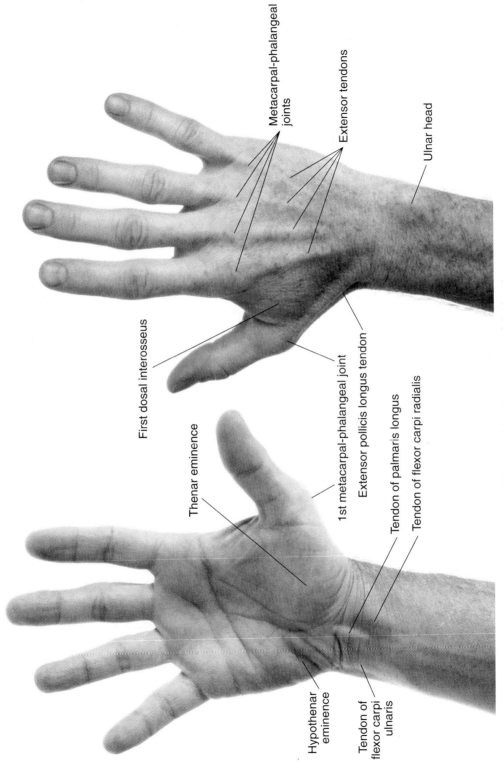

Metacarpal-phalangeal joints

Extensor tendons

Ulnar head

First dosal interosseus

Thenar eminence

1st metacarpal-phalangeal joint

Extensor pollicis longus tendon

Tendon of palmaris longus

Tendon of flexor carpi radialis

Hypothenar eminence

Tendon of flexor carpi ulnaris

Plate 5-10 Surface anatomy of the hand

OVERVIEW OF THE REGION

Pain in the arm and hand presents a clinical challenge, because it can originate in so many different places. Nerve entrapments at the cervical roots, thoracic outlet, pectoralis minor attachment to the coracoid process, or in the arm itself, including the wrist, may be responsible for arm or hand pain. Arm or hand pain may also be referred from trigger points in the muscles of the neck, shoulder, upper arm, or forearm. An assessment of arm or hand pain must include these possibilities.

In anatomy, the word "arm" (Latin *brachium*) is reserved for what we normally call the upper arm. The term "forearm" is used to denote the lower arm. The arm consists of a single bone, the **humerus**, which articulates with the scapula via the **glenohumeral joint**. We have already seen the muscles that cross the glenohumeral joint from the scapula in Chapter 4. The muscles that reside on the humerus and cross the glenohumeral joint are:

- biceps brachii
- triceps brachii
- coracobrachialis

The elbow consists of two joints: the **humeroradial** and **humeroulnar** joints. The muscles crossing this pair of joints are:

- biceps brachii
- triceps brachii
- brachialis
- anconeus
- brachioradialis

The forearm allows not only flexion and extension in relation to the humerus, but also rotation of the radius around the ulna, called **supination** (lateral or upward rotation) and **pronation** (medial or downward rotation). These movements take place through motion at the humeroradial joint and the **proximal** and **distal radioulnar joints**. Rotation is accomplished primarily by **biceps brachii, supinator, pronator quadratus,** and **pronator teres**.

Distally, the radius and ulna articulate with the carpal bones of the wrist and with each other at the **distal radioulnar joint**.

One wrist structure that deserves special clinical attention is the **carpal tunnel**, formed by the carpal bones deep and on either side, and the **flexor retinaculum** superficially. This tunnel permits passage of the flexor tendons and the median nerve to the hand (see Fig. 5-32, p. 204). When these tendons become inflamed and swollen, they compress the median nerve, producing pain and numbness in the radial aspect of the hand, known as **carpal tunnel syndrome**.

The muscles that cross the wrist are the flexors and extensors of the hand and fingers, which will be addressed in some detail in this chapter.

NOTE: Directional terms used in this chapter include **"volar"** to indicate the anterior aspect of the forearm, and **"palmar"** to indicate the anterior aspect of the hand in anatomical position. The opposite of both these terms is **"dorsal"** or posterior.

Etymology

- Latin *vola,* palm of the hand or sole of the foot
- Latin *palma,* palm of the hand
- Latin *dorsum,* back

MUSCLES OF THE UPPER ARM

Biceps Brachii

BI-seps BRAY-kee-eye

Etymology   Latin *biceps,* two-headed + *brachii,* of the arm
Note: in anatomical terminology, the Latin word *brachium* and the English word *arm* refer technically to the upper arm and do not include the forearm.

Overview

Biceps brachii (Fig. 5-1) crosses two joints: the glenohumeral and the elbow. It resides on the humerus but has no attachments to it. Although we think of it as the flexor of the elbow, biceps brachii is also the most powerful supinator of the forearm.

Attachments

- Proximally, the long head from supraglenoid tuberosity of scapula, the short head from coracoid process
- Distally, to the tuberosity of radius and antebrachial fascia by the bicipital aponeurosis

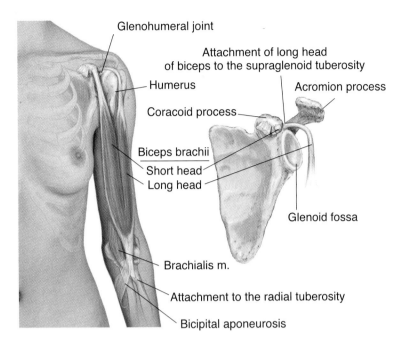

Figure 5-1 Anatomy of biceps brachii

Glenohumeral joint

Attachment of long head of biceps to the supraglenoid tuberosity

Humerus

Acromion process

Coracoid process

Biceps brachii
Short head
Long head

Glenoid fossa

Brachialis m.

Attachment to the radial tuberosity

Bicipital aponeurosis

Action

Flexes the elbow and supinates the forearm

Referral Area

Over the area of the muscle itself, to the inner aspect of the elbow, to the area of the middle deltoid, and to the area just proximal to supraspinatus

Other Muscles to Examine

- Brachialis
- Supinator
- Brachioradialis
- Middle deltoid
- Rotator cuff muscles

Manual Therapy

STRIPPING
- The client lies supine.
- The therapist stands beside the client at the hip.
- Place the knuckles on the muscle at the elbow.
- Pressing firmly into the tissue, slide the knuckles proximally along the muscle (Fig. 5-2) to the head of the humerus.

- Beginning at the same spot, repeat this procedure, following the short head medially to the axilla.

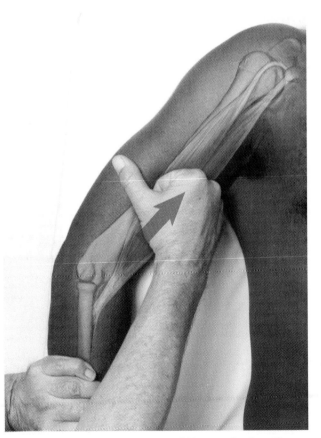

Figure 5-2 Stripping massage of biceps using knuckles

Brachialis

BRAY-kee-AL-is

Etymology Latin *brachium,* arm

Overview

Brachialis (Fig. 5-3) is a prime flexor of the elbow. Biceps brachii must be displaced to work on this muscle.

Attachments

- Proximally, to the lower two-thirds of anterior surface of humerus
- Distally, to the coronoid process of the ulna

Action

Flexes the elbow

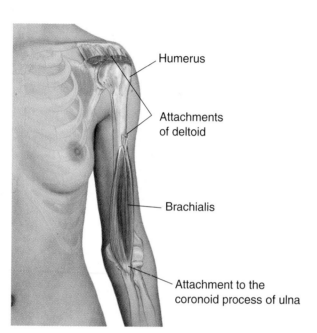

Humerus

Attachments of deltoid

Brachialis

Attachment to the coronoid process of ulna

Figure 5-3 Anatomy of brachialis

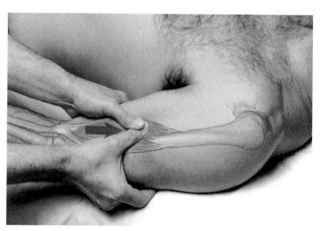

Figure 5-4 Stripping massage of brachialis using supported thumb (from lateral side)

Referral Area

To the anterior surface of the arm up to the acromion, to the anterior aspect of the elbow, and to the lateral and posterior aspect of the base of the thumb.

Other Muscles to Examine

- Biceps brachii
- Supinator
- Brachioradialis
- Opponens pollicis
- Adductor pollicis

Manual Therapy

STRIPPING
- The client lies supine.
- The therapist stands beside the client at the hip.
- Place the thumb on the lateral aspect of the distal extent of brachialis just proximal to the elbow, pushing biceps brachii medially out of the way.
- Pressing firmly into the tissue, slide the thumb along brachialis (Fig. 5-4) to its attachment on the humerus just distal to the attachment of the middle deltoid.
- Repeat the stroke on the medial side of the muscle (Fig. 5-5), continuing about halfway up the humerus.

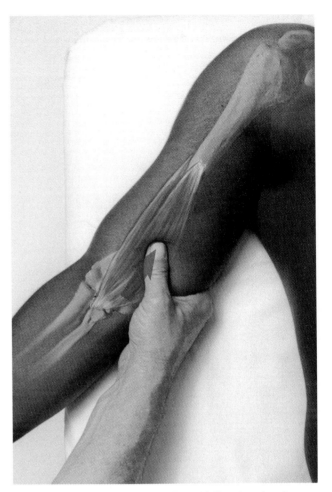

Figure 5-5 Stripping massage of brachialis using thumb (from medial side)

Triceps Brachii

TRY-seps BRAY-kee-eye

Etymology Latin *triceps,* three-headed + *brachii,* of the arm

Overview

Two of the three heads of triceps brachii (Fig. 5-6) cross only the elbow joint, while the long head crosses both the elbow and shoulder joints. This muscle opposes biceps brachii and brachialis. Its trigger points can cause pain in an area ranging from the neck to the fingers.

Attachments

Proximally:

- long or scapular head: to the infraglenoid tubercle at the lateral border of scapula inferior to the glenoid fossa
- lateral head: to the lateral and posterior surface of humerus below greater tubercle a medial head: to the distal posterior surface of humerus

Distally, to the olecranon of ulna

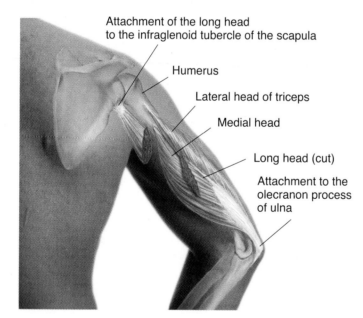

Attachment of the long head
to the infraglenoid tubercle of the scapula

Humerus

Lateral head of triceps

Medial head

Long head (cut)

Attachment to the
olecranon process
of ulna

Figure 5-6 Anatomy of triceps brachii

Action

Extends elbow

Referral Area

To the dorsal surface of the arm proximally over the back of the shoulder and distally to the back of the hand into the fourth and fifth fingers; also over the volar surface of the forearm and just proximal to the elbow.

Other Muscles to Examine

- All the muscles of the arm and forearm
- Rotator cuff muscles
- Pectoralis minor
- Pectoralis major

Manual Therapy

STRIPPING
- The client lies supine.
- The therapist stands beside the client at the waist.
- Place the thumb, knuckles, or fingertips on the muscle just proximal to the olecranon process.
- Pressing firmly into the tissue, slide the thumb, knuckles, or fingertips (Figs. 5-7 and 5-8) along the muscle to the attachment of the posterior deltoid.

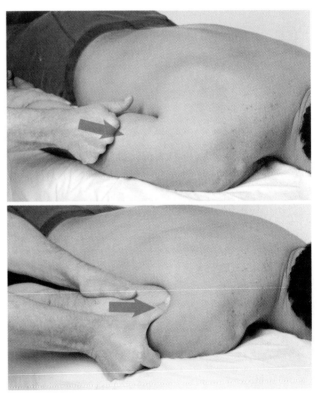

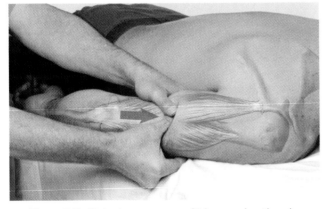

Figure 5-7   Stripping massage of triceps using thumbs

Figure 5-8   Stripping massage of triceps using knuckles and thumb

Anconeus (Fig. 5-9)

ang-KO-knee-us, an-KO-knee-us

Etymology   Latin *ancon,* from Greek *ankon,* elbow

Overview

Anconeus is a small muscle that assists triceps brachii in elbow extension. Its pain referral zone is local.

Attachments

- Proximally, to the posterior aspect of the lateral condyle of the humerus
- Distally, to the olecranon process and the posterior surface of the ulna

Action

Extends elbow

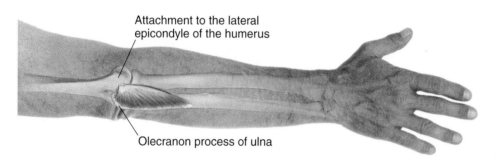

Attachment to the lateral epicondyle of the humerus

Olecranon process of ulna

Figure 5-9   Anatomy of anconeus, dorsal (posterior) view

Referral Area

Area over the lateral condyle of humerus

Other Muscles to Examine

- Triceps brachii
- Scalenes
- Supraspinatus
- Serratus posterior superior

Manual Therapy

STRIPPING

- The client may be in any position that makes the dorsal aspect of the elbow easily accessible.
- Place the thumb on the proximal posterior aspect of the ulna just distal to the olecranon.
- Pressing firmly into the tissue, slide the thumb along the muscle (Fig. 5-10) diagonally to its attachment on the lateral epicondyle of the humerus (a very short distance!).

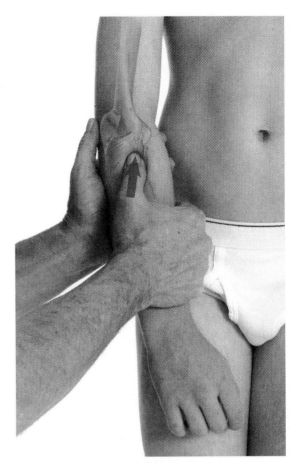

Figure 5-10 Stripping massage of anconeus

Coracobrachialis (Fig. 5-11)

KOR-a-ko-BRAKE-ee-AL-is

Etymology From *coracoid* (Greek *korakodes,* like a raven's beak, from *korax,* raven + *eidos,* resemblance) + Latin *brachialis,* relating to the arm *(brachium).*

Overview

Coracobrachialis is one of three muscles that attach to the coracoid process of the scapula, and that maintain the complex, three-way interaction of the arm, scapula, and chest (rib cage). The other two muscles are biceps brachii and pectoralis minor.

Attachments

- Proximally, to the coracoid process of the scapula
- Distally, to the middle of the medial border of the humerus

Actions

- Adducts and flexes the humerus
- Resists downward dislocation of shoulder joint.

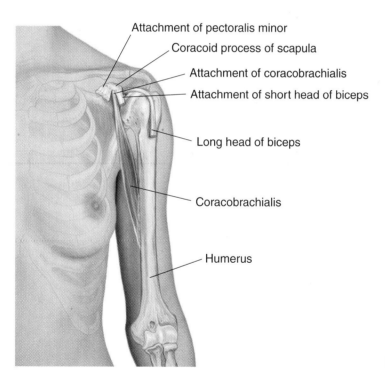

Attachment of pectoralis minor

Coracoid process of scapula

Attachment of coracobrachialis

Attachment of short head of biceps

Long head of biceps

Coracobrachialis

Humerus

Figure 5-11 Anatomy of coracobrachialis

Referral

To the posterior aspect of the upper arm, forearm, and hand, and to the area of the middle and anterior deltoid

Other Muscles to Examine

- All the muscles of the arm and forearm
- Rotator cuff muscles
- Deltoids

Manual Therapy

STRIPPING AND COMPRESSION

- The client lies supine. The therapist stands at the client's side, facing the client's head. The therapist holds the arm to be treated at the elbow with the non-treating hand.
- With the treating hand (i.e., the hand nearest the client), grasp the upper arm from the medial side in such a way that the thumb can comfortably extend along the medial side of the humerus.
- Press the thumb under biceps brachii to the medial side of the humerus about halfway up the humerus, seeking the distal attachment of coracobrachialis. Hold for release.
- Glide the thumb proximally along the muscle, holding for release where tenderness is found (Fig. 5-12).
- The thumb will finally follow the muscle deep into the axilla to the upper attachment to the coracoid process.

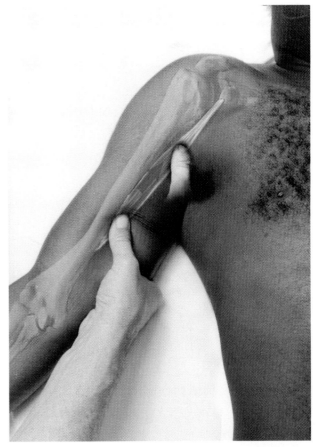

Figure 5-12   Stripping and compression of coracobrachialis using thumb

 In working in the axilla, take care to maintain contact with the muscle, and avoid the nerves and blood vessels that pass under the coracoid process into the arm.

MUSCLES OF THE FOREARM AND HAND

Supinator

SOUP-in-ay-ter

Etymology Latin *supinare,* to bend backwards or place on back (*supinus,* supine)

Overview

Supinator (Fig. 5-13) assists biceps brachii in its supinating function. Supinator is deep, but can be worked by compression through the superficial muscles.

Attachments

■ Proximally, to the lateral epicondyle of humerus radial collateral and annular ligaments, and to the supinator ridge of ulna
■ Distally, to the anterior and lateral surface of radius

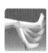

Action

Supinates the forearm

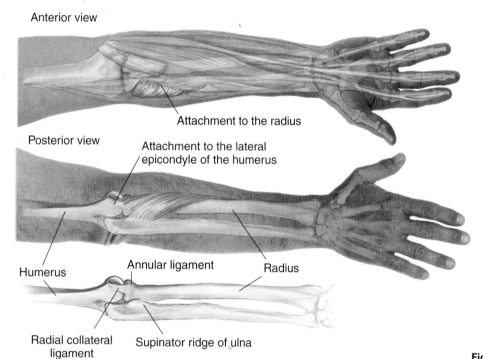

Anterior view

Attachment to the radius

Posterior view

Attachment to the lateral epicondyle of the humerus

Humerus   Annular ligament   Radius

Radial collateral ligament   Supinator ridge of ulna

Figure 5-13 Anatomy of supinator

Referral Area

To the volar elbow and over the lateral epicondyle, and to the dorsal side of the hand at the base of the thumb and index finger

Other Muscles to Examine

- Infraspinatus
- Subclavius
- Scalenes
- Brachialis
- Anconeus
- Brachioradialis
- Extensors of the hand

Manual Therapy

COMPRESSION
- The client lies supine.
- The therapist stands beside the client at the hip.
- Holding the forearm in pronation, place the thumb of the other hand on the ulnar side of the large extensor bundle just distal to the elbow.
- Displace the extensor bundle laterally to press into the interosseous space.
- Press firmly into the tissue, looking for tender spots. Hold for release (Fig. 5-14).

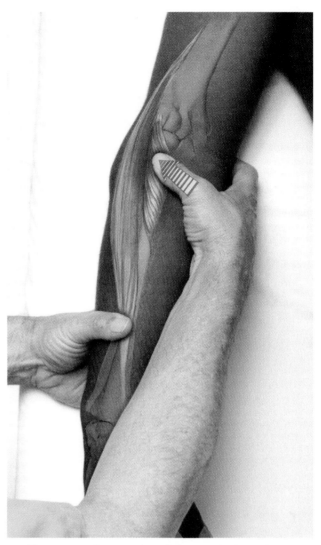

Figure 5-14 Compression of trigger point in supinator

Pronator Teres

PRO-nay-ter TER-ease

Etymology   Latin, *pronare*, to bend forward + *teres*, round, smooth, from *terere*, to rub

Overview

Pronator teres (Fig. 5-15) is matched to supinator in size and opposing action. Like supinator, it lies deep but can be compressed through the muscles superficial to it.

 Attachments

■ Proximally, the superficial (humeral) head from the common flexor origin on the medial epicondyle of the humerus, deep (ulnar) head from the medial (ulnar) side of the coronoid process of the ulna
■ Distally, to the middle of the lateral surface of the radius

 Action

■ Pronates forearm
■ Assists elbow flexion

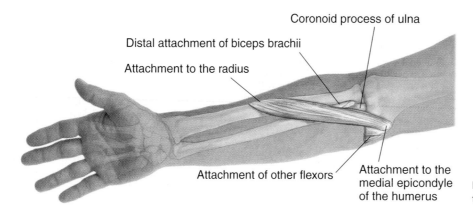

Coronoid process of ulna

Distal attachment of biceps brachii

Attachment to the radius

Attachment of other flexors

Attachment to the medial epicondyle of the humerus

Figure 5-15 Anatomy of pronator teres, volar (anterior) view

Referral Area

Over the radial edge of the volar forearm, especially to the wrist, and into the base of the thumb

Other Muscles to Examine

- Scalenes
- Infraspinatus
- Subclavius

Manual Therapy

STRIPPING
- The client lies supine.
- The therapist stands beside the client at the hip.
- Holding the arm with the volar side up, place the thumb on the center of the forearm just distal to the crease of the elbow (Fig. 5-16).
- Pressing firmly into the tissue, glide the thumb in a proximal and ulnar direction across the crease of the elbow to the attachment on the medial epicondyle of the humerus.

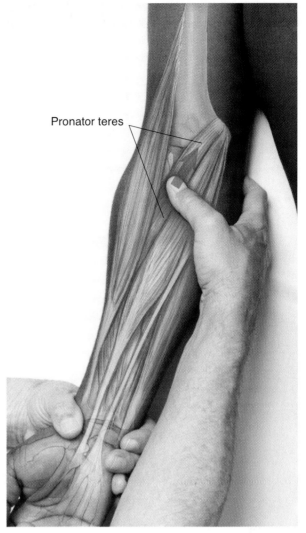

Pronator teres

Figure 5-16   Stripping of pronator teres

Pronator Quadratus

PRO-nay-ter qua-DRAY-tus

Etymology Latin, *pronare,* to bend forward + *quadratus,* four-sided

Overview
No trigger points have been documented for pronator quadratus (Fig. 5-17), but it is included here for completeness.

Attachments

- Medially, to the distal fourth of anterior surface of ulna
- Laterally, to the distal fourth of anterior surface of radius

Action

Pronates forearm

Referral Area

Not applicable

Other Muscles to Examine

Not applicable

Manual Therapy

Not applicable

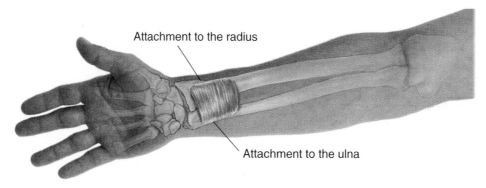

Attachment to the radius

Attachment to the ulna

Figure 5-17 Anatomy of pronator quadratus, volar (anterior) view

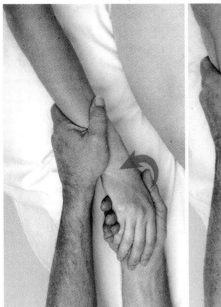
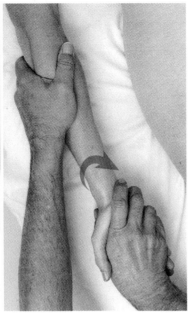

Figure 5-18 Stretching the pronator and supinator muscles

Manual Therapy for the Pronator and Supinator Muscles

STRETCH AND MOBILIZATION

- The client lies supine.
- The therapist stands beside the client at the hip.
- With the hand that is further from the client, grasp the client's forearm just proximal to the wrist.

- With the hand that is nearer the client, grasp the client's hand as if shaking hands.
- Turn the hand firmly into supination, then into pronation.
- Shift the other hand to the middle of the forearm and repeat the stretch.
- Shift the other hand to just distal to the elbow and repeat the stretch (Fig. 5-18).

Brachioradialis

BRAY-key-oh-ray-dee-AL-is

Etymology Latin *brachium,* arm + *radialis,* adjective from *radius,* spoke of a wheel

Overview

Because the distance of both its attachments from the elbow give it considerable leverage compared to most muscles, brachioradialis (Fig. 5-19) is a very powerful and efficient flexor of the elbow.

Attachments

- Proximally, to the lateral supracondylar ridge of humerus

- Distally, to the front of the base of the styloid process of the radius

Action

Flexes elbow and returns forearm to a neutral position from supination or pronation

Referral Area

Radial surface of elbow, dorsal surface of hand between thumb and index finger, radial surface of forearm

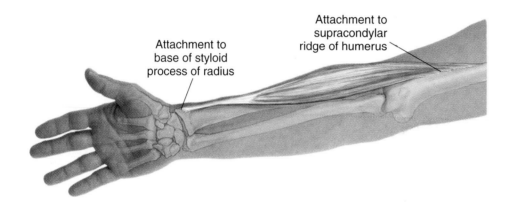

Attachment to base of styloid process of radius

Attachment to supracondylar ridge of humerus

Figure 5-19 Anatomy of brachioradialis

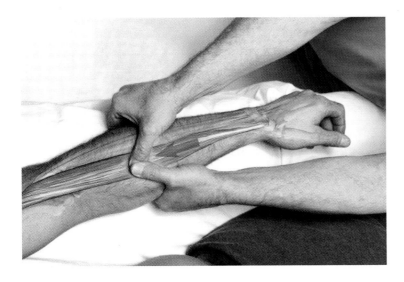

Figure 5-20 Stripping of brachioradialis with supported thumb

 Other Muscles to Examine

- Infraspinatus
- Supraspinatus
- Scalenes
- Subclavius

 Manual Therapy

STRIPPING
- The client lies supine.
- The therapist stands beside the client at the hip.
- Using the supported thumb, find the brachioradialis at its attachment near the distal end of the radius.
- Pressing firmly into the tissue, glide the thumb (Fig. 5-20) proximally along the muscle across the elbow to its attachment on the humerus.

EXTENSORS OF THE HAND, WRIST, AND FINGERS

Overview

The muscles that extend the hand and fingers cover the dorsal aspect of the forearm. Along with the flexors on the volar forearm, they stabilize the wrist during hand movements. They can be treated effectively as a group with deep massage. For this reason, manual therapy for them will be covered at the end of the descriptions of all the individual extensors.

 Referral Area

Dorsal surface of hand

 Other Muscles to Examine

- Subscapularis
- Infraspinatus
- Coracobrachialis
- Brachialis

 Manual Therapy

See Manual Therapy for the Extensors, below.

Extensor Carpi Radialis Brevis (Fig. 5-21)

ex-TEN-ser CAR-pie ray-dee-AL-is BREV-is

Etymology Latin *extensor*, extender + *carpi*, of the wrist + *radialis*, adjective from *radius*, spoke of a wheel + *brevis*, short

 Attachments

- Proximally, to the lateral epicondyle of humerus
- Distally, to the base of the third metacarpal bone

 Action

Extends and abducts wrist radially

Extensor Carpi Radialis Longus (Fig. 5-22)

ex-TEN-ser CAR-pie ray-dee-AL-is LONG-gus

Etymology Latin *extensor*, extender + *carpi*, of the wrist + *radialis*, adjective from *radius*, spoke of a wheel + *longus*, long

 Attachments

- Proximally, to the lateral supracondylar ridge of humerus
- Distally, to the back of base of second metacarpal bone

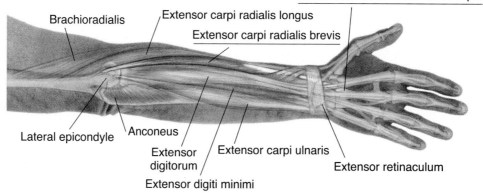

Figure 5-21 Anatomy of extensor carpi radialis brevis, dorsal (posterior) view

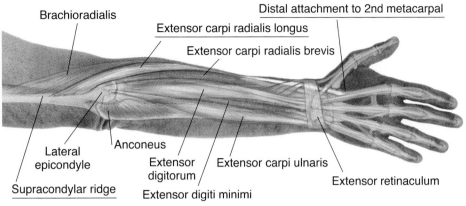

Brachioradialis

Extensor carpi radialis longus

Distal attachment to 2nd metacarpal

Extensor carpi radialis brevis

Lateral epicondyle

Anconeus

Extensor digitorum

Extensor carpi ulnaris

Extensor retinaculum

Supracondylar ridge

Extensor digiti minimi

Figure 5-22 Anatomy of extensor carpi radialis longus, dorsal (posterior) view

Action

Extends and deviates wrist radially

Referral Area

Surface of elbow, radial aspect of dorsal hand, dorsal forearm

Other Muscles to Examine

- Extensor carpi radialis brevis
- Supinator
- Extensor indicis
- Brachialis
- Infraspinatus
- Serratus posterior superior
- Scalenes

Manual Therapy

See Manual Therapy for the Extensors, below.

Extensor Carpi Ulnaris (Fig. 5-23)

ex-TEN-ser CAR-pie ul-NAR-is

Etymology Latin *extensor,* extender + *carpi,* of the wrist + *ulnaris,* adjective from *ulna,* elbow or arm

Attachments

- Proximally, to the lateral epicondyle of humerus (humeral head) and posterior border of proximal ulna (ulnar head)
- Distally, to the base of the fifth metacarpal bone

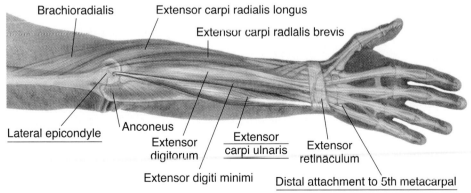

Brachioradialis

Extensor carpi radialis longus

Extensor carpi radialis brevis

Lateral epicondyle

Anconeus

Extensor digitorum

Extensor carpi ulnaris

Extensor retinaculum

Extensor digiti minimi

Distal attachment to 5th metacarpal

Figure 5-23 Anatomy of extensor carpi ulnaris, dorsal (posterior) view

Action

Extends and deviates wrist ulnarly

Referral Area

Ulnar surface of wrist

Other Muscles to Examine

- Subscapularis
- Serratus posterior superior

Manual Therapy

See Manual Therapy for the Extensors, below.

Extensor Digiti Minimi (Fig. 5-24)

ex-TEN-ser DIH-jih-tea MIH-nih-mee

Etymology   Latin *extensor*, extender + *digiti*, of the finger + *minimi*, smallest

Attachments

- Proximally, to the lateral epicondyle of the humerus
- Distally, to the dorsum of the proximal, middle, and distal phalanges of little finger

Action

Extends the fifth finger at the metacarpophalangeal joint and interphalangeal (IP) joints

Manual Therapy

See Manual Therapy for the Extensors, below.

Extensor Digitorum (Fig. 5-25)

ex-TEN-ser dih-jih-TOR-um

Etymology   Latin *extensor*, extender + *digitorum*, of the fingers

Attachments

- Proximally, to the lateral epicondyle of humerus
- Distally, by four tendons into the base of the proximal and middle and base of the distal phalanges or four fingers

Action

Extends four fingers at the metacarpophalangeal joints and interphalgeal (IP) joints

Manual Therapy

See Manual Therapy for the Extensors, below.

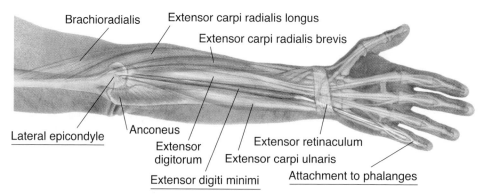

Figure 5-24   Anatomy of extensor digiti minimi, dorsal (posterior) view

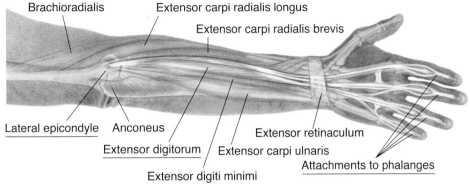

Brachioradialis
Extensor carpi radialis longus
Extensor carpi radialis brevis
Lateral epicondyle
Anconeus
Extensor digitorum
Extensor digiti minimi
Extensor carpi ulnaris
Extensor retinaculum
Attachments to phalanges

Figure 5-25 Anatomy of extensor digitorum, dorsal (posterior) view

Extensor Indicis (Fig. 5-26)

ex-TEN-ser IN-dis-sis

Etymology Latin *extensor,* extender + *indicis,* of the forefinger

Attachments

- Proximally, to the dorsal surface of the ulna and interosseous membrane
- Distally, to the dorsal extensor aponeurosis of index finger

Action

Extends the forefinger at the metacarpophalangeal joint

Referral Area

Dorsal surface of the hand to the dorsal forefinger

Other Muscles to Examine

- Coracobrachialis
- Subclavius

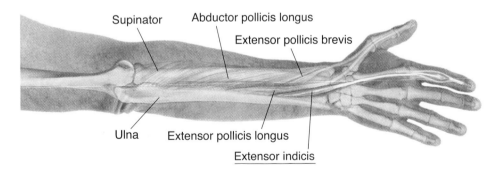

Supinator
Abductor pollicis longus
Extensor pollicis brevis
Ulna
Extensor pollicis longus
Extensor indicis

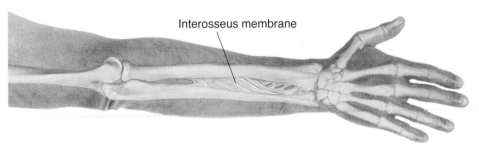

Interosseus membrane

Figure 5-26 Anatomy of extensor indicis, dorsal (posterior) view

Manual Therapy

See Manual Therapy for the Extensors, below.

Extensor Pollicis Brevis (Fig. 5-27)

ex-TEN-ser PAHL-iss-iss BREV-iss

Etymology Latin *extensor,* extender + *pollicis,* of the thumb + *brevis,* short

Attachments

- Proximally, to the dorsal surface of radius and interosseous membrane
- Distally, to the base of proximal phalanx of thumb

Action

Extends and abducts the thumb

Referral Area

Not applicable

Other Muscles to Examine

Not applicable

Manual Therapy

See Manual Therapy for the Extensors, below.

Extensor Pollicis Longus (Fig. 5-28)

ex-TEN-ser PAHL-iss-iss LONG-gus

Etymology Latin *extensor,* extender + *pollicis,* of the thumb + *longus,* long

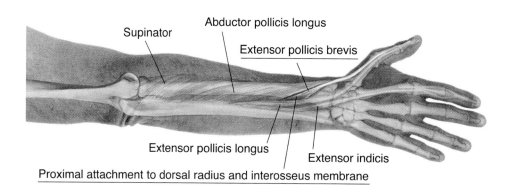

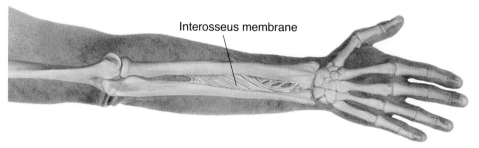

Figure 5-27 Anatomy of extensor pollicis brevis, dorsal (posterior) view

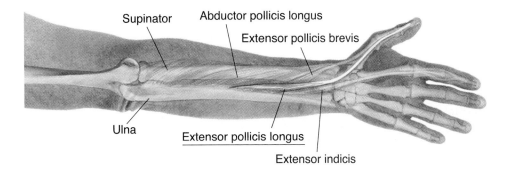

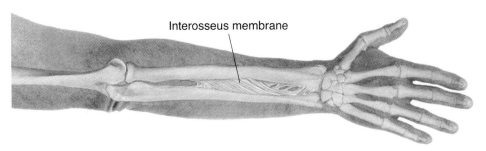

Figure 5-28 Anatomy of extensor pollicis longus, dorsal (posterior) view

 Attachments

- Proximally, to the posterior surface of the ulna and middle third of the interosseous membrane
- Distally, to the base of distal phalanx of thumb at the interphalangeal joint

 Action

Extends distal phalanx of thumb

 Referral Area

Not applicable

 Other Muscles to Examine

Not applicable

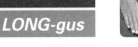

Abductor Pollicis Longus (Fig. 5-29)

ab-DUCK-ter PAHL-iss-iss LONG-gus

Etymology Latin *abductor,* that which draws away from + *pollicis,* of the thumb + *lungus,* long

 Attachments

- Proximally, to posterior surfaces of radius and ulna and the interosseous membrane
- Distally, to the lateral side of the base of the first metacarpal bone

 Action

Abducts and assists in extending thumb

 Referral Area

Not applicable

 Other Muscles to Examine

Not applicable

 Manual Therapy

See Manual Therapy for the Extensors, below.

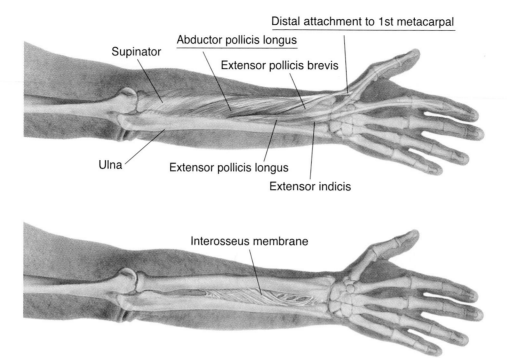

Distal attachment to 1st metacarpal

Abductor pollicis longus

Supinator

Extensor pollicis brevis

Ulna

Extensor pollicis longus

Extensor indicis

Interosseus membrane

Figure 5-29 Anatomy of abductor pollicis longus, dorsal (posterior) view

Manual Therapy for the Extensors of the Hand, Wrist, and Fingers

Stripping Massage of Individual Extensor Muscles

- The client lies supine with the forearm and hand pronated and slightly flexed at the elbow.
- The therapist stands beside the client at the hip.
- With the non-treating hand, hold the client's hand to steady the arm and wrist.

- Place the thumb on the wrist next to the head of the ulna.
- Pressing firmly into the tissue, glide the thumb proximally (Fig. 5-30) to the lateral epicondyle of the humerus.
- Shifting the thumb to a point slightly farther toward the radius, repeat this movement, sliding along a line parallel to the last motion to the distal humerus.
- Repeat the same procedure, following parallel lines, until the whole extensor (dorsal) aspect of the forearm has been covered.

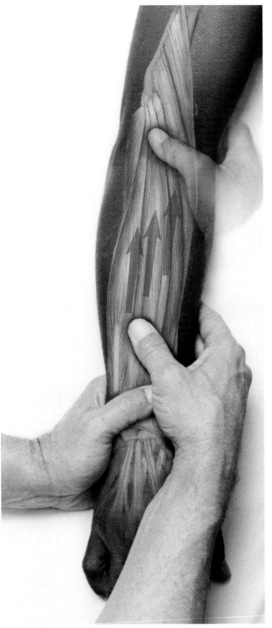

Figure 5-30 Stripping massage of the extensors using the thumb

Stripping Massage of the Extensor Group

- The client lies supine.
- The therapist stands beside the client at the hip.
- Place the knuckles or the heel of the hand on the dorsal wrist.
- Pressing firmly into the tissue, glide the knuckles (Fig. 5-31) or heel of the hand slowly along the muscle group across the elbow to the distal humerus.

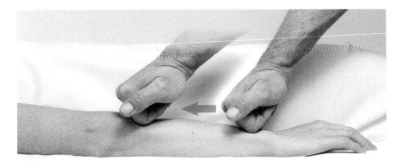

Figure 5-31 Stripping massage of the extensor muscles using the knuckles

FLEXORS OF THE HAND, WRIST, AND FINGERS

Overview

Most of the tendons of the flexors of the hand, wrist, and fingers pass through the carpal tunnel, a passage formed by the carpal bones and the flexor retinaculum. When these tendons are swollen, they can entrap and irritate the median nerve, causing carpal tunnel syndrome. Keeping the flexor muscles in the forearm relaxed can help prevent this condition. Like the extensors, the flexors can be massaged deeply as a group. Manual therapy will follow individual descriptions of all the muscles.

Flexor Retinaculum (Transverse Carpal Ligament) (Fig. 5-32)

FLEX-er ret-in-ACK-yu-lum

Etymology Latin *flexor*, bender + *retinaculum*, band or halter (from *retinere*, to hold back)

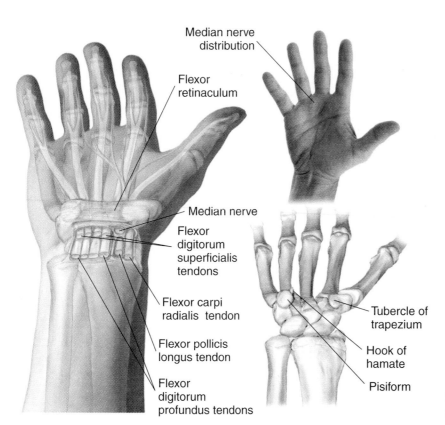

Figure 5-32 Carpal tunnel and flexor retinaculum, volar (anterior) view

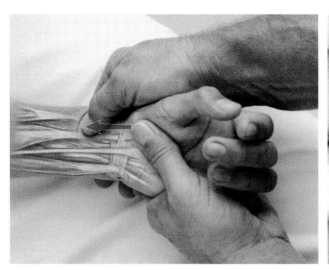
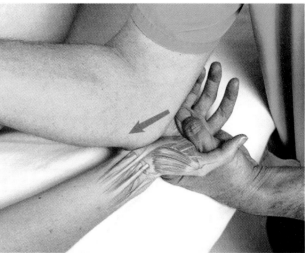

Figure 5-33 Stretching the flexor retinaculum using the thumb and elbow

Action

Binds down the flexor tendons of the digits, the flexor carpi radialis tendon, and the median nerve, creating the carpal tunnel

Manual Therapy

DEEP CROSS-FIBER STROKING
- The client lies supine with the volar aspect of the forearm facing up.
- Place the thumb or elbow on the palmar surface of the hand about an inch distal to the wrist.
- Slide proximally in a series of parallel lines (Fig. 5-33) shifting gradually from one side of the volar wrist to the other to stretch the retinaculum.

Palmaris Longus

pal-MAR-is LONG-gus

Etymology Latin *palmaris,* relating to the palm + *longus,* long

Overview

Palmaris longus (Fig. 5-34) is the only hand flexor whose tendon lies superficial to the flexor retinaculum. It stands out prominently when the hand is cupped and flexed at the wrist.

Attachments

- Proximally, to the medial epicondyle of the humerus
- Distally, to the flexor retinaculum of the wrist and palmar fascia

Action

- Tenses palmar fascia
- Flexes the hand at the wrist
- Flexes the forearm

Referral Area

Prickling pain along the volar surface of the forearm and concentrated in the palm

Other Muscles to Examine

All other flexors in the forearm
Pronator teres
Serratus anterior
Pectoralis major and minor

Manual Therapy

See Manual Therapy for the Flexors, below.

Flexor Carpi Radialis (Fig. 5-35)

FLEX-er CAR-pie ray-dee-AL-iss

Etymology Latin *flexor,* bender + *carpi,* of the wrist + *radialis,* adjective from *radius,* spoke of a wheel

Attachments

- Proximally, to the common flexor origin of the medial epicondyle of humerus
- Distally, to the anterior surface of the base of the second and third metacarpal bones

Action

Flexes wrist and abducts wrist radially

Referral Area

Middle of the volar wrist toward the radial side

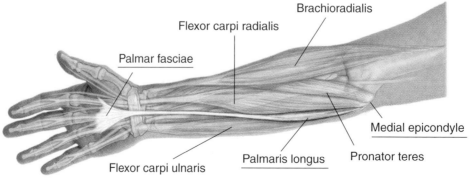

Figure 5-34 Anatomy of palmaris longus, volar (anterior) view

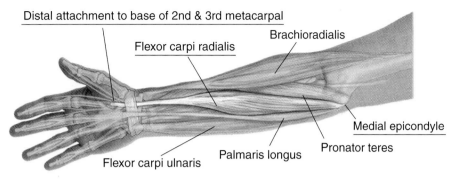

Distal attachment to base of 2nd & 3rd metacarpal

Flexor carpi radialis

Brachioradialis

Medial epicondyle

Pronator teres

Palmaris longus

Flexor carpi ulnaris

Figure 5-35 Anatomy of flexor carpi radialis, volar (anterior) view

Other Muscles to Examine

Pronator teres

Manual Therapy

See Manual Therapy for the Flexors, below.

Flexor Carpi Ulnaris (Fig. 5-36)

FLEX-er CAR-pie ul-NAR-iss

Etymology   Latin *flexor*, bender + *carpi*, of the wrist + *ulnaris*, adjective from *ulna*, elbow or arm

Attachments

- Proximally, the humeral head of the muscle to the medial epicondyle of humerus, ulnar head of the muscle to the olecranon process and upper three-fifths of posterior border of ulna
- Distally, to the pisiform bone, the pisometacarpal ligament, and base of the fifth metacarpal

Action

Flexes wrist and deviates wrist ulnarly

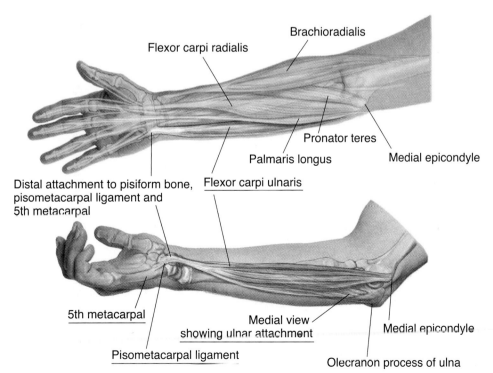

Flexor carpi radialis

Brachioradialis

Pronator teres

Palmaris longus

Medial epicondyle

Distal attachment to pisiform bone, pisometacarpal ligament and 5th metacarpal

Flexor carpi ulnaris

5th metacarpal

Medial view showing ulnar attachment

Medial epicondyle

Pisometacarpal ligament

Olecranon process of ulna

Figure 5-36 Anatomy of flexor carpi ulnaris, volar (anterior) and ulnar (medial) view

Referral Area

Ulnar and volar wrist

Other Muscles to Examine

Pectoralis minor
Serratus posterior superior

Manual Therapy

See Manual Therapy for the Flexors, below.

Flexor Digitorum Profundus (Fig. 5-37)

FLEX-er dih-jih-TOR-um pro-FUN-dus

Etymology Latin *flexor,* bender + *digitorum,* of the fingers + *profundus,* deep

Attachments

- Proximally, to the anterior surface of upper third of ulna and interosseous membrane
- Distally, by four tendons into the base of distal phalanx of each finger

Action

Flexes distal interphalangeal joint of four fingers

Referral Area

Not applicable

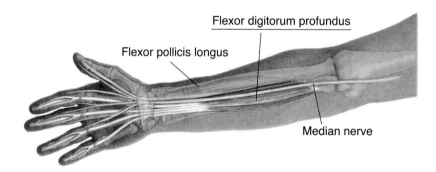

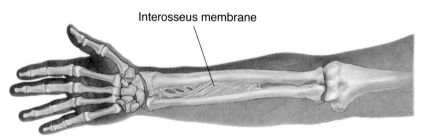

Figure 5-37 Anatomy of flexor digitorum profundus, volar (anterior) view

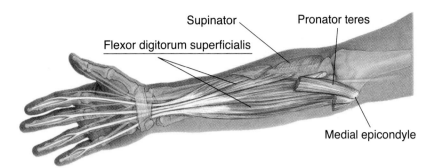

Supinator

Pronator teres

Flexor digitorum superficialis

Medial epicondyle

Figure 5-38   Anatomy of flexor digitorum superficialis, volar (anterior) view

 Other Muscles to Examine

Not applicable

 Manual Therapy

See Manual Therapy for the Flexors, below.

Flexor Digitorum Superficialis (Fig. 5-38)

FLEX-er dih-jih-TOR-um SOUP or fishy Alice

Etymology   Latin *flexor*, bender + *digitorum*, of the fingers + *superficialis*, superficial

 Attachments

■ Proximally, the humeroulnar head to the medial epicondyle of the humerus, the medial border of the coronoid process, and a tendinous arch between these points, the radial head to the anterior oblique line and middle third of the lateral border of the radius

■ Distally, by four split tendons, passing to either side of the profundus tendons, into sides of middle phalanx of each finger

 Action

Flexes proximal interphalangeal joint of the fingers

 Referral Area

Not applicable

 Other Muscles to Examine

Not applicable

 Manual Therapy

See Manual Therapy for the Flexors, below.

Flexor Pollicis Longus (Fig. 5-39)

FLEX-er PAHL-iss-iss LONG-gus

Etymology   Latin *flexor,* bender + *pollicis,* of the thumb + *longus,* long

Attachments

- Proximally, to the anterior surface of the middle third of the radius and interosseous membrane
- Distally, to the distal phalanx of the thumb

Action

Flexes distal phalanx of thumb at interphalangeal joint

Referral Area

Through the palmar aspect of the thumb to the tip

Other Muscles to Examine

- Scalenes
- Subclavius

Manual Therapy

See Manual Therapy for the Flexors, below.

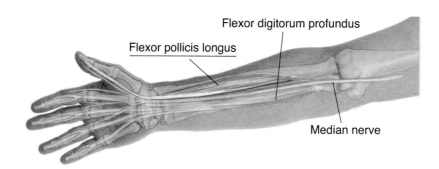

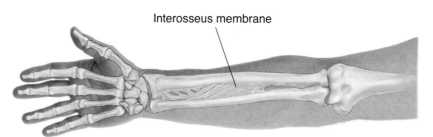

Figure 5-39   Anatomy of flexor pollicis longus, volar (anterior) view

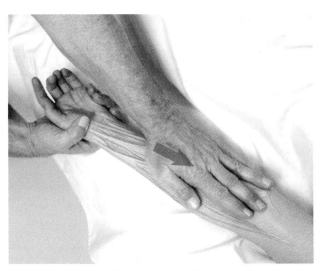

Figure 5-40 Moving compression of the flexors

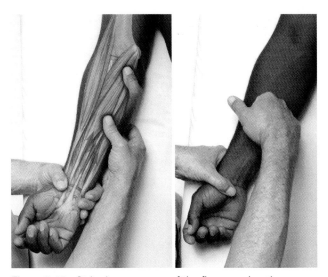

Figure 5-41 Stripping massage of the flexors using the thumb and the knuckles

 Manual Therapy for the Flexor Muscles of the Hand, Wrist, and Fingers

Stripping Massage of the Flexor Group
- The client lies supine.
- The therapist stands beside the client at the hip.
- With the non-treating hand, hold the client's hand to stabilize the arm.
- Place the knuckles or the heel of the hand on the volar wrist.
- Pressing firmly into the tissue, slide the knuckles or heel of the hand slowly along the muscle group (Fig. 5-40) across the elbow onto the distal end of biceps brachii.

Stripping Massage of Individual Extensor Muscles
- The client lies supine.
- The therapist stands beside the client at the hip.
- With the non-treating hand, hold the client's hand to stabilize the arm.
- Place the thumb, knuckles, or fingertips on the wrist just to the ulnar side of and proximal to the distal end of the radius.
- Pressing firmly into the tissue, slide the thumb, knuckles, or fingertips (Fig. 5-41) proximally along the radius to the volar aspect of the lateral epicondyle of the humerus.
- Beginning at a point slightly nearer the center of the wrist, repeat this movement, sliding along a line parallel to the last motion and ending at the base of biceps brachii.
- Repeat the same movement, following parallel lines, until the whole flexor (volar) aspect of the forearm has been covered (the last movement should be along the ulna).

MUSCLES IN THE HAND

Muscles of the Thumb

One of the distinguishing characteristics of homo sapiens is the opposable thumb, and we use it intensively, as every massage therapist certainly knows. Soreness, tender points, and trigger points in the thumb muscles due to overuse are quite common. Pain in the thumb area can also be a symptom of carpal tunnel syndrome, so careful examination and thorough treatment of both the thumb muscles and the muscles of the forearm are important.

The principal muscles of the thumb (abductor pollicis and opponens pollicis) comprise the **thenar eminence,** commonly called the ball of the thumb, the thick, muscular bundle of muscles at the base of the thumb just distal to the wrist.

Adductor Pollicis (Fig. 5-42)

ad-DUCK-ter POL-ly-sis

Etymology Latin *adductor (ad,* to or toward + *ducere,* to lead), that which draws toward + *pollex,* thumb

Attachments

By two heads:
- The transverse head from the shaft of the third metacarpal
- The oblique head from the front of the base of the second metacarpal, the trapezoid and capitate bones
- Both heads to the ulnar side of base of proximal phalanx of thumb

Action

Adducts thumb at carpometacarpal joint

Referral Area

The base of the thumb on both the palmar and dorsal sides

Other Muscles to Examine

- Opponens pollicis
- Supinator
- Brachioradialis
- Brachialis
- Infraspinatus
- Subclavius
- Scalenes

Manual Therapy

See Manual Therapy for the Palmar Thumb Muscles, below

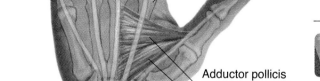

3rd metacarpal
2nd metacarpal
Adductor pollicis
Transverse head
Oblique head
Trapezoid bone
Capitate bone
Flexor pollicis longus and tendon
Tendons of flexor digitorum profundus

Figure 5-42 Anatomy of adductor pollicis

Flexor Pollicis Brevis (Fig. 5-43)

FLEX-er PAHL-iss-iss BREV-iss

Etymology   Latin *flexor,* bender + *pollicis,* of the thumb + *brevis,* short

Attachments

- Proximally, superficial portion to the trapezium and the flexor retinaculum of the wrist, deep portion from ulnar side of first metacarpal bone
- Distally, to the base of the proximal phalanx of the thumb

Action

Flexes proximal phalanx of thumb

Referral Area

Not applicable

Other Muscles to Examine

Not applicable

Manual Therapy

See Manual Therapy for the Palmar Thumb Muscles, below.

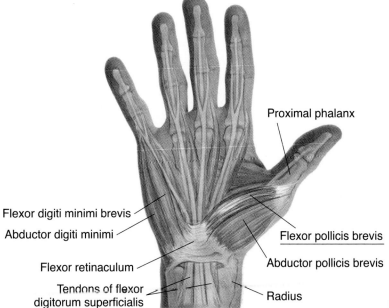

Flexor digiti minimi brevis

Abductor digiti minimi

Flexor retinaculum

Tendons of flexor digitorum superficialis

Proximal phalanx

Flexor pollicis brevis

Abductor pollicis brevis

Radius

Figure 5-43   Anatomy of flexor pollicis brevis

Abductor Pollicis Brevis (Fig. 5-44)

ab-DUCK-ter POL-ly-sis BREV-iss

Etymology Latin *abductor (ab,* from + *ducere,* to lead), that which draws away from + *pollex,* thumb

Attachments

- Proximally, to the tubercle of the trapezium and flexor retinaculum
- Distally, to the base of the radial side of the proximal phalanx of the thumb

Action

Abducts thumb at the carpometacarpal joint

Referral Area

None

Other Muscles to Examine

Not applicable

Manual Therapy

None

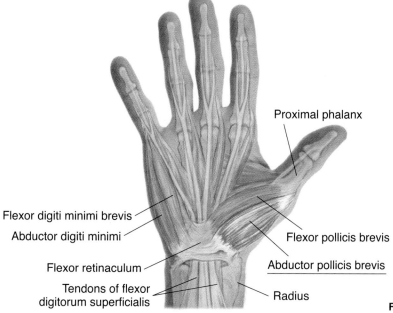

Flexor digiti minimi brevis

Abductor digiti minimi

Flexor retinaculum

Tendons of flexor digitorum superficialis

Proximal phalanx

Flexor pollicis brevis

Abductor pollicis brevis

Radius

Figure 5-44 Anatomy of abductor pollicis brevis

Opponens Pollicis (Fig. 5-45)

op-POE-nens POL-ly-sis

Etymology   Latin *opponere,* to place against, oppose

Attachments

- Proximally, to the ridge of the trapezium and flexor retinaculum
- Distally, to the radial side of the full length of the shaft of the first metacarpal bone

Action

Puts the thumb in opposition to the other fingers by drawing the base of the thumb toward the palm at the carpometacarpal joint

Referral Area

Lateral surface of thumb, wrist at the head of the radius

Other Muscles to Examine

- Adductor pollicis
- Infraspinatus
- Brachialis
- Subscapularis
- Subclavius
- Scalenes
- Serratus posterior superior

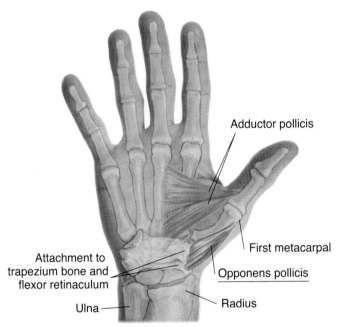

Adductor pollicis

First metacarpal

Opponens pollicis

Attachment to trapezium bone and flexor retinaculum

Ulna

Radius

Figure 5-45   Anatomy of opponens pollicis

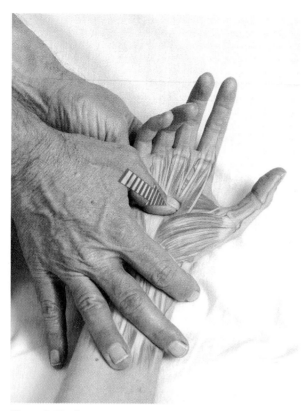

Figure 5-46 Compression of trigger point in opponens pollicis

Manual Therapy for the Palmar Thumb Muscles

TRIGGER POINT COMPRESSION
- Holding the client's hand with the palm up, use the other thumb to search for a trigger point on the thenar eminence near the base (Fig. 5-46).
- Compress with the thumb and hold for release.

STRIPPING
- The client may be in any position that gives easy access to the palm of the hand.
- Holding the hand firmly with the palm facing you, place your supported or unsupported thumb at the base of the thenar eminence (Fig. 5-47).
- Pressing firmly, slide your thumb radially to the first carpophalangeal joint.
- Repeat this procedure (Fig. 5-48) on a line just distal and parallel to the first.
- Continue until the whole thenar eminence has been treated.

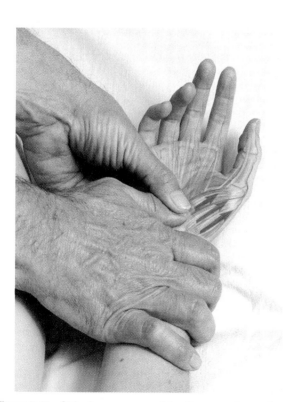

Figure 5-47 Stripping massage of the thenar eminence beginning at opponens pollicis (with supported thumb)

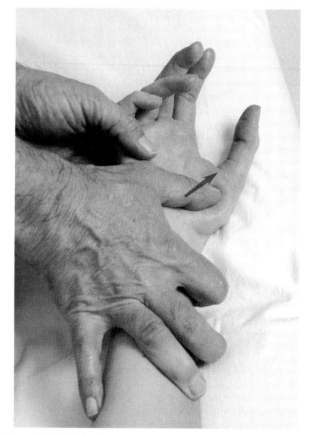

Figure 5-48 Stripping massage of the muscles of the thenar eminence (with unsupported thumb)

Interosseus Muscles of the Hand

IN-ter-OSS-see-us

Etymology   Latin *inter*, between + *os*, bone

Overview

The palmar interosseous muscles adduct the fingers toward the midline, the dorsal interosseous muscles abduct the fingers from the midline.

Attachments

Dorsal interosseous muscles (four) (Fig. 5-49):

- Proximally, to the sides of adjacent metacarpal bones
- Distally, to the base of the proximal phalanges and extensor expansion, first on radial side of second digit, sec-ond on radial side of third digit, third on ulnar side of third digit, fourth on ulnar side of fourth digit

Palmar interosseous muscles (three) (Fig. 5-50):

- Proximally, to the palmar surface of second, fourth, and fifth metacarpal bones
- Distally, the first palmar interosseous muscle into the base of the ulnar side of the second digit, the second and third palmar interosseous muscles into radial sides of fourth and fifth digits.

Action

Dorsal: abduct second and third digits from the axis of the third digit and adduct third and fourth digits

Palmar: adduct second, fourth, and fifth digits toward axis of the third digit

Referral Area

Edges of corresponding fingers

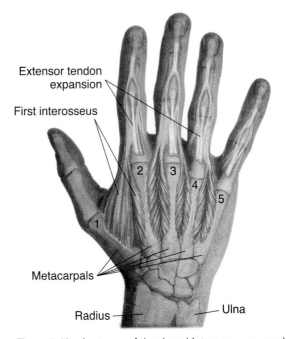

Figure 5-49   Anatomy of the dorsal interosseous muscles

Other Muscles to Examine

- Infraspinatus
- Scalenes
- Subclavius
- Pectoralis major
- Pectoralis minor
- Coracobrachialis
- Serratus anterior

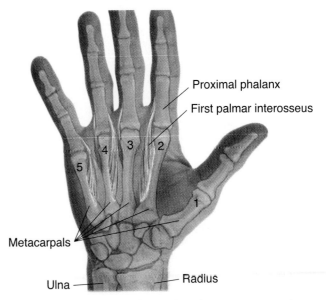

Figure 5-50   Anatomy of the palmar interosseous muscles

Manual Therapy of Palmar Interosseous Muscles of the Hand

STRIPPING

- The client lies supine. (The client may also be seated, or in any position that makes the palmar aspect of the hand accessible.)
- The therapist stands beside the client at the shoulder.
- Place the thumb on the palm of the hand between the 1st and 2nd metacarpophalangeal joints.
- Pressing firmly into the tissue, slide the thumb distally between the first and second fingers to the thenar eminence.
- Repeat this procedure between each pair of metacarpals (Fig. 5-51), shifting the thumb ulnarly, until the entire hand has been treated.

 Manual Therapy of Dorsal Interosseous Muscles of the Hand

STRIPPING

- The client lies supine. (The client may also be seated, or in any position that allows access to the dorsal aspect of the hand.)
- The therapist stands beside the client at the hips.
- Hold and stabilize the client's hand with your non-treating hand.
- Place the thumb on the dorsal aspect of the hand between the 1st and 2nd metacarpals (i.e., between the thumb and forefinger) just next to the metacarpophalangeal joint.
- Pressing firmly into the tissue, slide the thumb proximally between the thumb and forefinger (Fig. 5-52) to the end of the tissue.
- Repeat this procedure between each pair of metacarpals until the entire hand has been treated (Fig. 5-53).

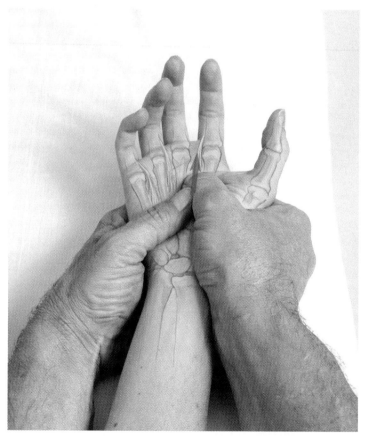

Figure 5-51 Stripping massage of palmar interosseous muscles between 2nd and 3rd metacarpals

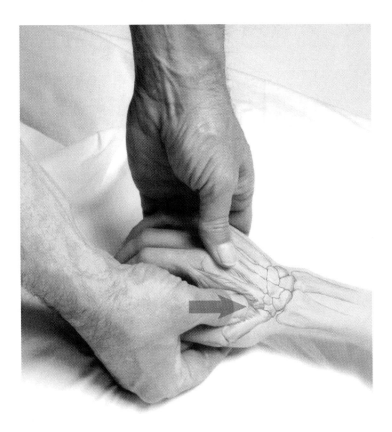

Figure 5-52 Stripping massage of first dorsal interosseous muscle

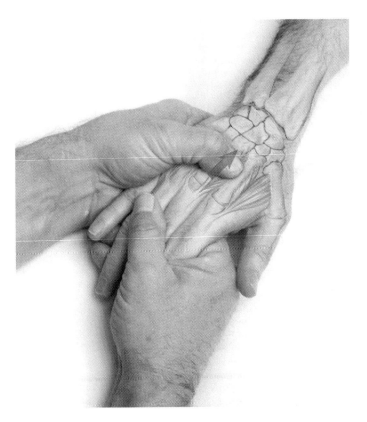

Figure 5-53 Stripping massage of dorsal interosseous muscles

Lumbrical Muscles of the Hand (Fig. 5-54)

LUM-bri-cal

Etymology Latin *lumbricus,* earthworm

The lumbricals work with the interossei in refining actions of the fingers, particularly in strong grasping. They are unusual in that they attach only to tendons, rather than bones.

Attachments

Proximally
- The two lateral (radial): from the radial side of the tendons of the flexor digitorum profundus going to the second and third digits
- The two medial (ulnar): from the adjacent sides of the second and third, and third and fourth tendons

Distally
- To the radial side of extensor tendon on dorsum of each of the four fingers at the proximal phalanges

Action

Flex metacarpophalangeal joint and extend the proximal and distal interphalangeal joint.

Referral Area

No specific trigger points have been documented in the lumbrical muscles. They are included here for completeness.

Other Muscles to Examine

None

Manual Therapy

These muscles are treated with the interossei, above.

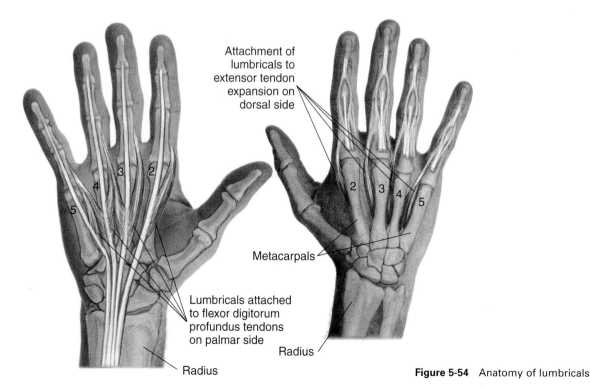

Figure 5-54 Anatomy of lumbricals

Flexor Digiti Minimi Brevis (Fig. 5-55)

FLEX-er DIJ-it-tea MIN-im-me BREV-is

Etymology   Latin *flexor,* flexor + *digiti,* of the finger + *minimi,* smallest + *brevis,* short

Attachments

- Proximally, to the hamulus of the hamate bone
- Distally, to the ulnar side of the proximal 5th phalanx

Action

Flexes the proximal phalanx of the fifth digit

Referral Area

No trigger points have been documented for this muscle.

Other Muscles to Examine

None

Manual Therapy

Not applicable

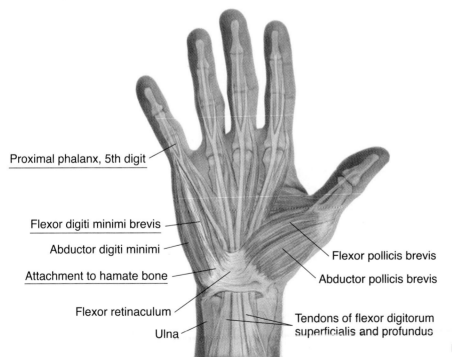

Proximal phalanx, 5th digit

Flexor digiti minimi brevis

Abductor digiti minimi

Attachment to hamate bone

Flexor retinaculum

Ulna

Flexor pollicis brevis

Abductor pollicis brevis

Tendons of flexor digitorum superficialis and profundus

Figure 5-55   Anatomy of flexor digiti minimi brevis

Abductor Digiti Minimi

ab-DUCK-ter DIJ-it-tea MIN-im-me

Etymology   Latin *abductor (ab,* away from + *ducere,* to lead), that which draws away + *digiti,* of the finger + *minimi,* smallest

Overview

If there were a sixth digit, abductor digiti minimi (Fig. 5.56) would be half of its dorsal interosseous muscle. It typically develops a trigger point at the center of the belly, palpable on the dorsal side.

Attachments

■ Proximally, to the pisiform bone and pisohamate ligament
■ Distally, to the ulnar side of the base of the proximal 5th phalanx

Action

Abducts proximal phalanx of and flexes the fifth digit

Referral Area

Lateral and dorsal aspects of the little finger

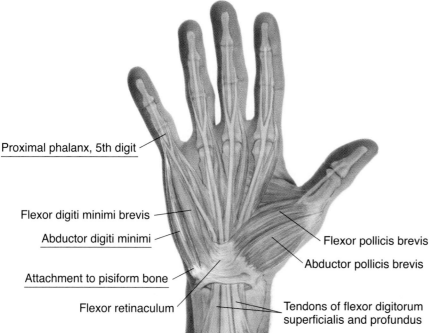

Proximal phalanx, 5th digit

Flexor digiti minimi brevis

Abductor digiti minimi

Attachment to pisiform bone

Flexor retinaculum

Flexor pollicis brevis

Abductor pollicis brevis

Tendons of flexor digitorum superficialis and profundus

Figure 5.56 Anatomy of abductor digiti minimi

Other Muscles to Examine

- Pectoralis minor
- Serratus posterior superior
- Latissimus dorsi
- Triceps brachii
- Flexor digitorum

Manual Therapy

Pincer Compression

- The client is in any position that allows access to the ulnar edge of the hand.
- With the non-treating hand, hold and stabilize the client's hand.
- Using the thumb and index finger, explore the dorsal aspect of abductor digiti minimi looking for tender spots (Fig. 5-57).
- Hold for release.

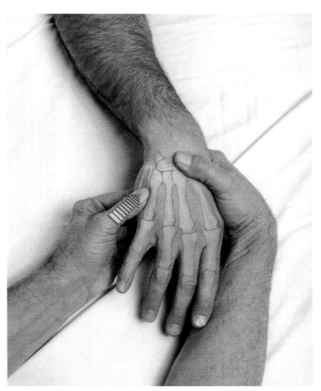

Figure 5-57 Pincer compression of trigger point in abductor digiti minimi

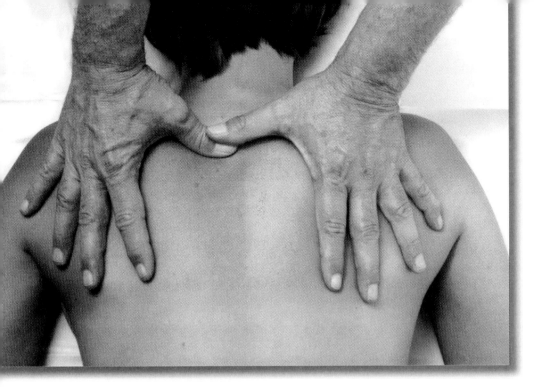

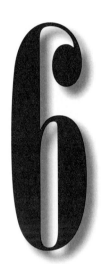

"The spinal column is a long bunch of bones. The head sits on the top, and you sit on the bottom."

—A child, on a test

The Vertebral Column

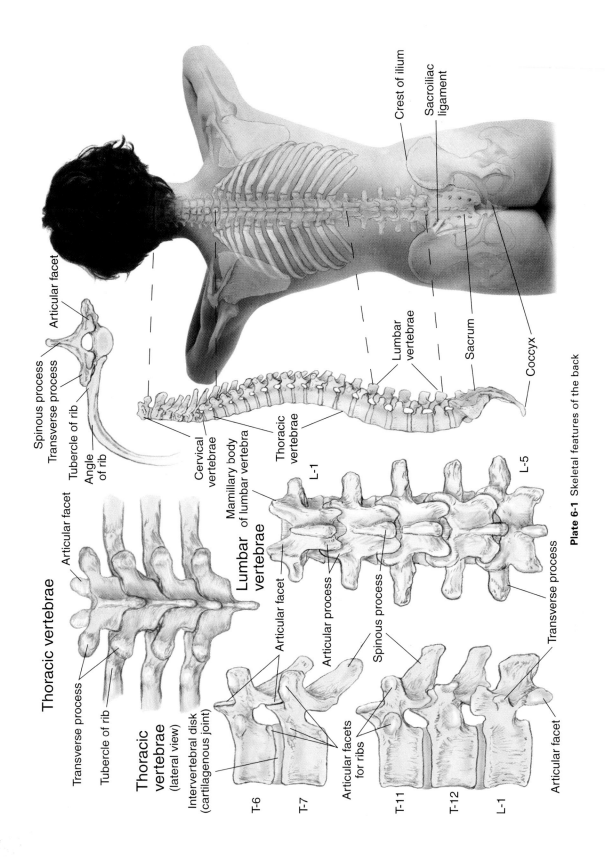

Plate 6-1 Skeletal features of the back

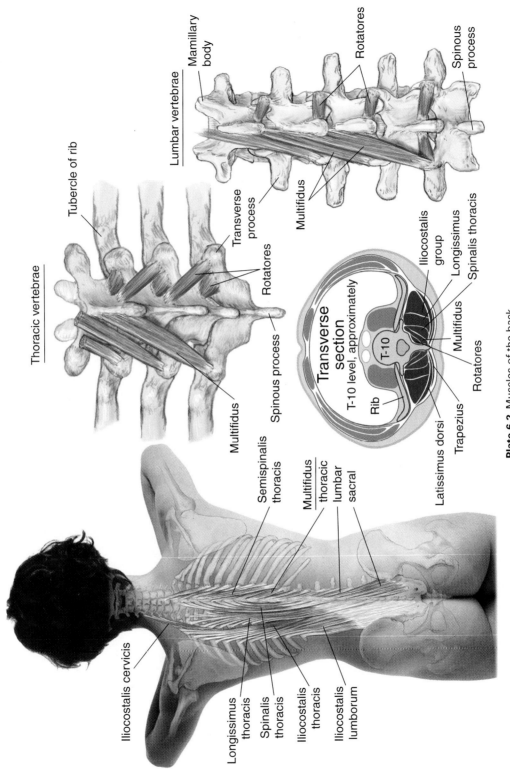

Mamillary body

Rotatores

Spinous process

Lumbar vertebrae

Transverse process

Multifidus

Tubercle of rib

Thoracic vertebrae

Transverse process

Rotatores

Iliocostalis group

Longissimus

Spinalis thoracis

Multifidus

Rotatores

Trapezius

Latissimus dorsi

Rib

T-10

Transverse section
T-10 level, approximately

Multifidus

Spinous process

Semispinalis thoracis

Multifidus
thoracic
lumbar
sacral

Iliocostalis cervicis

Longissimus thoracis

Spinalis thoracis

Iliocostalis thoracis

Iliocostalis lumborum

Plate 6-2 Muscles of the back

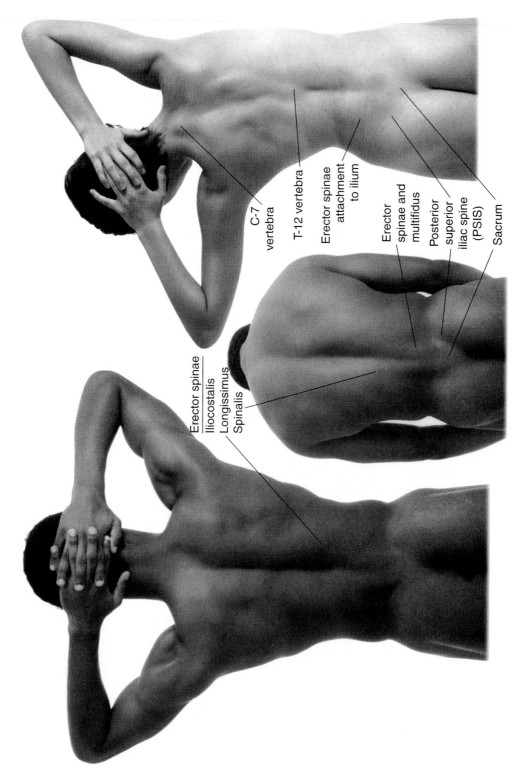

C-7 vertebra

T-12 vertebra

Erector spinae attachment to ilium

Erector spinae and multifidus

Posterior superior iliac spine (PSIS)

Sacrum

Erector spinae
Iliocostalis
Longissimus
Spinalis

Plate 6-3 Surface anatomy of the back

OVERVIEW OF THE REGION

The vertebral column, or spine, is divided into five regions:

■ The cervical spine, with seven vertebrae (C1 through C7)
■ The thoracic spine, with twelve vertebrae and attached ribs (T1 through T12)
■ The lumbar spine, with five vertebrae (L1 through L5)
■ The sacrum, with five fused vertebrae
■ The coccyx, usually consisting of four vertebrae

Though similar in basic structure and function, the vertebrae vary considerably in size and shape in the different regions, the cervical vertebrae being the smallest and the lumbar vertebrae being the largest.

At birth the spine has a single posterior curvature forming the typical "C" shape of the newborn infant. As the child begins to hold the head erect, sit up, and learn to stand, additional spinal curvatures develop. The five regions of the adult spine include four normal curvatures. The cervical and lumbar regions have an anterior curvature while the thoracic, sacral and coccygeal regions retain their original posterior curvature. Excessive increases or decreases in these curves (**kyphosis, lordosis**) threatens postural integrity, and their restoration and maintenance is one of the aims of posturally oriented bodywork.

There are two types of joints between most of the vertebrae of the spine:

■ Cartilaginous joints between the broad vertebral body of adjoining vertebrae, comprised of fibrocartilage surrounding a gel-filled disk that supports most of the weight
■ Synovial facet joints between articular processes that guide most of the movement

There are two facet joints on each side, articulating with the facets of the two adjoining vertebrae. In addition, the thoracic vertebrae also articulate with the ribs and accordingly have facets for those joints.

These joints and the variations in shape between vertebrae of different regions determine the type and range of movement of the spine. These movements are:

■ Anterior flexion
■ Lateral flexion (sometimes called lateral bending)
■ Extension (and hyperextension)
■ Rotation

The cervical region is the only one capable of the full range of spinal movement. All other regions are limited in one or more movements. The spinous processes of the thoracic vertebrae are angled sharply in an inferior direction and prevent hyperextension of this region in most individuals. The planes of the articular facets of the lumbar region are nearly vertical and thus limit rotation. Since the vertebrae are usually fused in the sacrum and coccyx by eighteen to thirty years of age (and for all practical purposes much earlier), there is no movement possible within those regions, although they do move relative to adjoining regions. Note that the coccyx is joined to the sacrum by ligaments, and can move in relation to it in response to pressure.

Comment

The directional terms **"cephalad"** (toward the head) and **"caudad"** (toward the tail, i.e., coccyx) are used in this chapter.

Etymology
■ Greek *kephal,* head
■ Latin *cauda,* tail

It is helpful to do some general work on the back before treating specific areas in order to stimulate local blood flow and relax the superficial musculature. This may include effleurage, petrissage, kneading, and percussion, but be careful not to use excessive lubrication, as it will hinder work in specific areas afterwards. One helpful technique for preparatory treatment of the back is myofascial stretching (see Chapter 1, page 12).

Manual Therapy

MYOFASCIAL STRETCHING
FOR THE BACK

- The client lies supine.
- The therapist stands beside the client at the torso.
- Place the hand nearest the client's head flat on the lumbar area lateral to the vertebrae with the fingers over the iliac crest just lateral to the sacrum.
- Crossing the other hand over or under the first, place it flat on the thoracic area over the lowest three or four ribs.
- Let your hands sink into the tissue until you feel contact with the superficial fascia.
- Press the hands in opposite directions, with enough downward pressure to engage and stretch the superficial fascia (Fig. 6-1).

- Hold until you feel significant release in the fascia.
- Shift both hands laterally (toward yourself) by one hand's width and repeat the technique.
- Shift the hands cephalad, so that the caudad hand rests on the lower three or four ribs and the cephalad hand rests on the third through the sixth ribs, both hands just lateral to the vertebrae.
- Repeat the technique.
- Repeat the technique at this level shifting the hands laterally.
- Repeat the entire procedure on the opposite side.

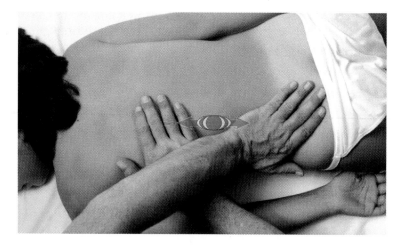

Figure 6-1 Myofascial stretch for the back (Draping option 7)

THE SUPERFICIAL PARASPINAL MUSCLES

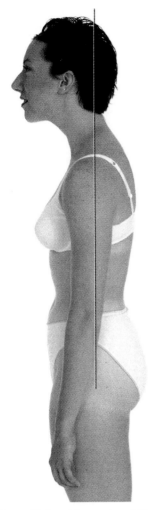

Figure 6-2   Posture with head forward and shoulders medially rotated

We need to keep two facts in mind when viewing the vertebral column in the context of the whole body:

- The center of gravity of the body is in the pelvic region, well forward of the spine.
- As we noted in Chapter 4 (page 117), the entire arm and shoulder structure is attached to the skeleton by only one joint, the sternoclavicular joint, also well forward of the spine.

The implication of these two facts is that the spine and the muscles that attach to it must maintain the integrity of the posture against a strong anterior pull. Because of the location of our eyes and the construction of our shoulders and arms, virtually everything that we human beings do requires us to move our heads, arms, and torsos forward, down, and inward. It is the task of the superficial muscles of the vertebral column (along with the muscles of the low back) to counterbalance us in such activities. Poor posture—that is, posture in which the head is carried forward of the sagittal midline, the shoulders are medially rotated, and the anterior intercostal and abdominal muscles are habitually shortened (Fig. 6.2)—places a severe strain on the superficial muscles of the spine and posterior neck, resulting in the development of active trigger points and pain. Although, according to David G. Simons, MD, "there are no hard scientific data as to when and how latent MTrPs [myofascial trigger points] start,"[1] we do know that "by correcting the postural problem the MTrP either clears up or is much more treatable."[2]

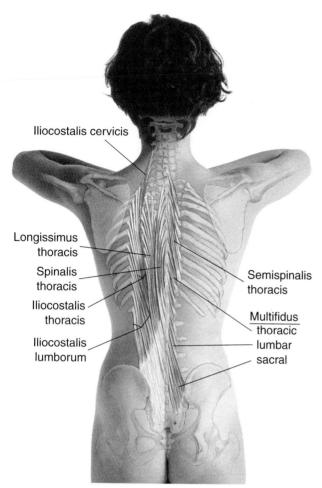

Iliocostalis cervicis

Longissimus thoracis

Spinalis thoracis

Iliocostalis thoracis

Iliocostalis lumborum

Semispinalis thoracis

Multifidus thoracic

lumbar

sacral

Figure 6-3　Anatomy of the erector spinae muscles

Erector Spinae (Fig. 6-3)
e-RECK-ter SPEE-nay

Etymology　Latin *erector,* straightener + *spinae,* of the spine

Comment

Erector spinae is a collective term for the group of muscles that extend and maintain the balance of the vertebral column and the rib cage. They also contract strongly in coughing and in straining during bowel movements.

These muscles originate from the sacrum, ilium, and the processes of the lumbar vertebrae. They are divided into three groups: **iliocostalis, longissimus,** and **spinalis.** Their branches attach to the vertebrae and ribs at ascending levels.

The Iliocostalis Group

The iliocostalis group represents the most lateral column of the erector spinae. It is comprised of three divisions: iliocostalis lumborum, iliocostalis thoracis, and iliocostalis cervicis.

Iliocostalis Lumborum (Fig. 6-4)

ILL-ee-oh-kos-TAL-is lum-BOR-um

Etymology   Latin *ilio-*, relating to the ilium + *costalis*, relating to the ribs (*costa*, rib) + *lumborum*, of the loins

Attachments

- Inferiorly, from sacrum and ilium
- Superiorly, to the inferior borders of the lower six ribs

Action

Extends, laterally flexes, and rotates lumbar vertebrae

Referral Area

Over the lumbar region into the center of the buttock

Other Muscles to Examine

Iliocostalis thoracis, longissimus, quadratus lumborum, gluteals, piriformis and other lateral hip rotators

Manual Therapy

STRIPPING
- The client lies supine.
- The therapist stands beside the client at the torso.
- Place the knuckles on the muscles at the waist of the client just lateral to the lumbar vertebrae.
- Pressing firmly into the tissue, slide the knuckles inferiorly over the sacrum to its base (Fig. 6-5).
- Repeat the procedure on the opposite side.

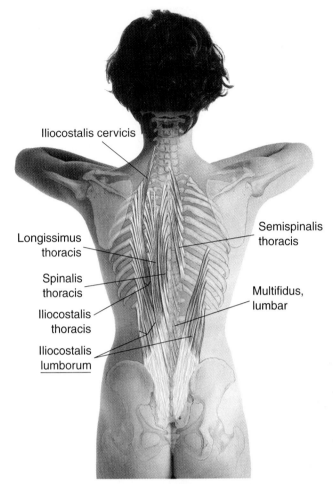

Figure 6-4   Anatomy of iliocostalis lumborum

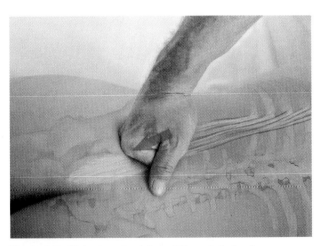

Figure 6-5   Stripping of origins of iliocostalis lumborum (Draping option 7)

Iliocostalis Thoracis (Fig. 6-6)

ILL-ee-oh-kos-TAL-is THOR-as-iss

Etymology   Latin *ilio-*, relating to the ilium + *costalis*, relating to the ribs (*costa*, rib) + *thoracis*, of the chest

Comment

Because of our extensive use of our arms and hands, our need to look down what our hands are doing, and the prevalence of poor posture, iliocostalis thoracis frequently develops painful trigger point activity in branches of the muscle that extend under the scapulae. This area just inferior and medial to the scapula is one of the most common areas in need of trigger point release. Pain here often accompanies pain in the muscles of the shoulders.

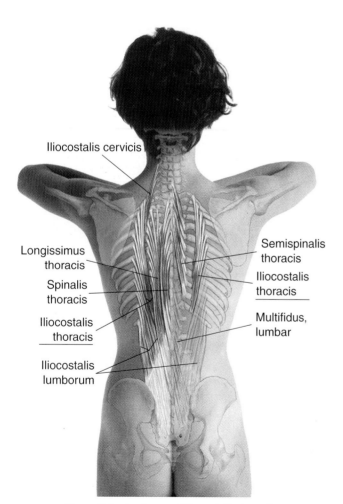

Iliocostalis cervicis

Longissimus thoracis

Spinalis thoracis

Iliocostalis thoracis

Iliocostalis lumborum

Semispinalis thoracis

Iliocostalis thoracis

Multifidus, lumbar

Figure 6-6 Anatomy of iliocostalis thoracis

Attachments

- Inferiorly, to the medial side of the inferior borders of the lower six ribs
- Superiorly, to the inferior borders of the upper six ribs

Action

Extends, laterally flexes, and rotates thoracic vertebrae

Referral Area

- Inferior angle of the scapula, inside the medial border of the scapula to the superior angle; anterior chest over the angle of the sternum and the costal arch
- Over the lumbar region, into the lateral inferior thoracic region, up across the scapula; lower ipsilateral quadrant of the abdomen

Other Muscles to Examine

- Trapezius, rotator cuff muscles, teres major, rhomboids
- Pectoralis major, intercostals
- Serratus posterior inferior, quadratus lumborum, iliocostalis lumborum
- Abdominal obliques, iliopsoas

Manual Therapy

STRIPPING
- The client lies supine.
- The therapist stands beside the client at the head.
- Palpate for a distinct muscular band running diagonally in a superolateral direction under the inferomedial border of the scapula. Explore this band just inferior to the scapula for tenderness.
- Place the supported thumb on the tender spot and press firmly into the tissue.
- Glide the thumb diagonally along the muscle to the erector bundle (Fig. 6-7).
- Beginning at the same spot, repeat this procedure two or three times.

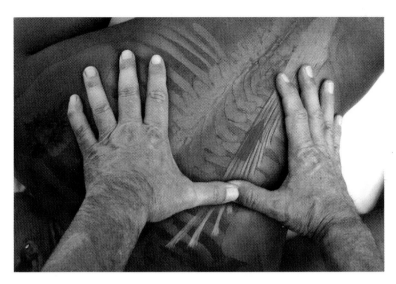

Figure 6-7 Stripping of iliocostalis thoracis with supported thumb

CROSS-FIBER STROKING
- The client lies supine.
- The therapist stands beside the client at the head.
- Place the hand (Fig. 6-8A) or the knuckles (Fig. 6-8B) on the upper back medial to the superior angle of the scapula.
- Pressing firmly into the tissue with the heel of your hand or your knuckles, slide your hand diagonally along the medial border of the scapula past the inferior angle.
- Beginning at the same spot, repeat this procedure two or three times.

CROSS-FIBER FRICTION
- The client lies supine.
- The therapist stands beside the client at the head.
- Place the fingertips or the knuckles next to the muscular band at the inferomedial border of the scapula.
- Move the fingertips or knuckles back and forth across the band at a rate of about twice per second.
- Continue until you feel release in the tissue.

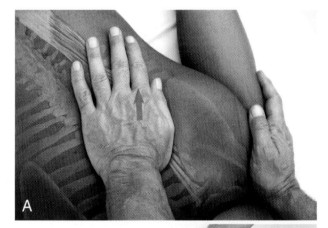

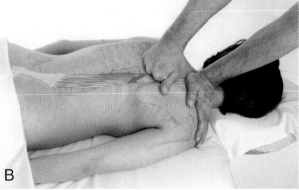

Figure 6-8 Cross-fiber stroking of iliocostalis thoracis with heel of hand (A) or knuckles (B)

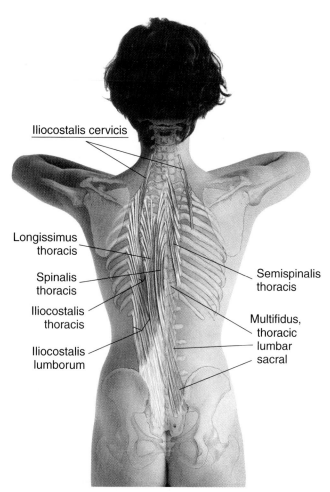

Iliocostalis cervicis

Longissimus
thoracis

Spinalis
thoracis

Iliocostalis
thoracis

Iliocostalis
lumborum

Semispinalis
thoracis

Multifidus,
thoracic
lumbar
sacral

Figure 6-9 Anatomy of iliocostalis cervicis

Iliocostalis Cervicis (Fig. 6-9)

ILL-ee-oh-kos-TAL-is SERV-iss-iss

Etymology Latin *ilio-*, relating to the ilium + *costalis*, relating to the ribs (*costa*, rib) + *cervicis*, of the neck

Attachments

- Inferiorly, to the superior borders of the upper six ribs
- Superiorly, to the transverse processes of the middle cervical vertebrae

Action

Extends, laterally flexes, and rotates cervical vertebrae

Comment

No trigger points have been recorded for this muscle; it is included here for completeness.

Longissimus Thoracis (Fig. 6.10)

long-GISS-i-mus THOR-as-iss

Etymology   Latin, *longissimus,* longest + *thoracis,* of the chest

Attachments

- Inferiorly, to the transverse processes of the lumbar vertebrae
- Superiorly, to the tips of the transverse processes of all thoracic vertebrae and the last nine or ten ribs between their tubercles and angles

Action

Extends vertebral column

Referral Area

Over the lumbar region into the superior aspect of the buttock; over the buttock to the inferior aspect

Other Muscles to Examine

- Serratus posterior inferior
- Quadratus lumborum
- Iliocostalis lumborum and thoracis
- Gluteal muscles
- Piriformis and other lateral rotators
- Hamstrings

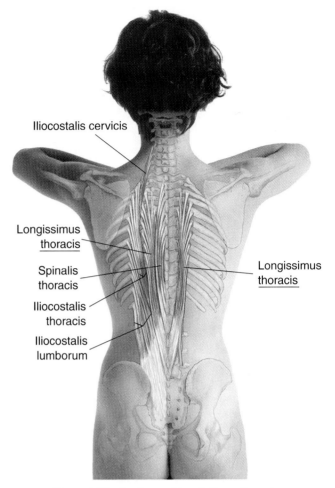

Figure 6-10   Anatomy of longissimus thoracis

Manual Therapy

See Manual Therapy for the Erector Spinae, below.

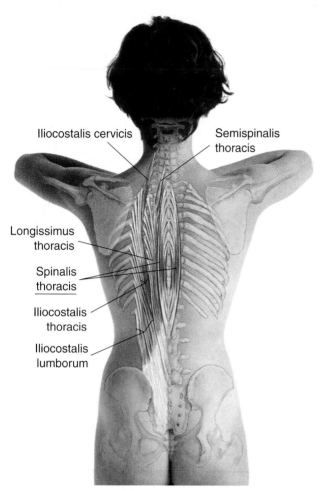

Iliocostalis cervicis

Semispinalis thoracis

Longissimus thoracis

Spinalis thoracis

Iliocostalis thoracis

Iliocostalis lumborum

Figure 6-11   Anatomy of spinalis thoracis

Spinalis Thoracis (Fig. 6-11)

spin-AL-iss THOR-as-iss

Etymology   Latin *spinalis,* relating to the spine

Attachments

■ Inferiorly, to the spinous processes of the upper lumbar and two lower thoracic vertebrae

■ Superiorly, to the spinous processes of middle and upper thoracic vertebrae

Action

Supports and extends the vertebral column

Referral Area

None recorded

Other Muscles to Examine

Not applicable

Manual Therapy

See Manual Therapy for the Erector Spinae, below.

Semispinalis Thoracis (Fig. 6-12)

SEM-i-spin-AL-iss THOR-as-iss

Etymology   Latin *semi,* half + *spinalis,* relating to the spine + *thoracis,* of the chest

Attachments

- Inferiorly, to the transverse processes of the fifth to eleventh thoracic vertebrae
- Superiorly, to the spinous processes of the first four thoracic and fifth and seventh cervical vertebrae

Action

Extends vertebral column.

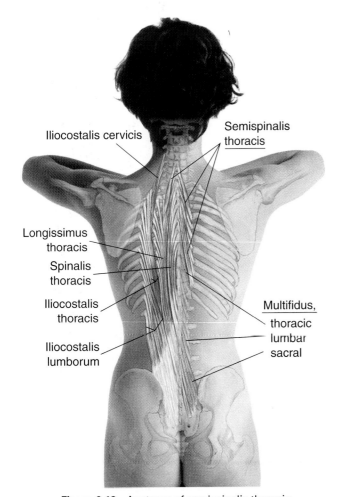

Figure 6-12   Anatomy of semispinalis thoracis

Labels: Iliocostalis cervicis; Semispinalis thoracis; Longissimus thoracis; Spinalis thoracis; Iliocostalis thoracis; Iliocostalis lumborum; Multifidus, thoracic lumbar sacral

Referral Area

None recorded

Other Muscles to Examine

Not applicable

Manual Therapy for the Erector Spinae

Because the erector spinae muscles are gathered together in a paraspinal bundle, they can most easily be treated as a group. Stripping massage may be applied in either a caudad or cephalad direction. It is helpful to do both, as different trigger points may be accessed in each direction. You may use the hand, thumb, knuckles, fingertips, or elbow.

STRIPPING
- The client lies supine.
- The therapist stands beside the client at either the head or shoulder (to work in a caudad direction) or at the hips (to work in a cephalad direction).
- Place the heel of the hand (Fig. 6-13), the supported fingertips (Fig. 6-14), the supported thumbs (Fig. 6-15), the knuckles (Fig. 6-16), or the elbow (Fig. 6-17) on the muscle bundle near C7 (to work caudad) or at the sacrum (to work cephalad).
- Pressing firmly into the tissue, slide the body part you are using along the entire length of the muscle bundle.

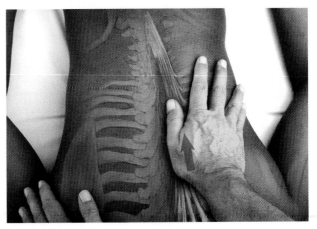

Figure 6-13   Stripping of erector spinae bundle with heel of hand (longissimus is shown)

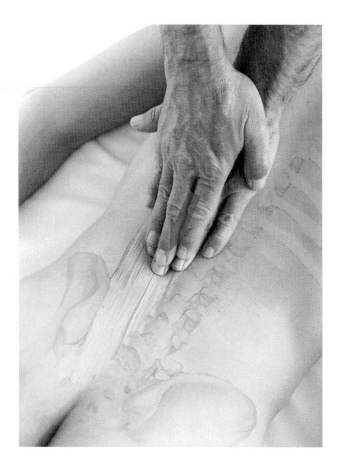

Figure 6-14 Stripping of erector spinae bundle with supported fingertips (longissimus is shown) (Draping option 7)

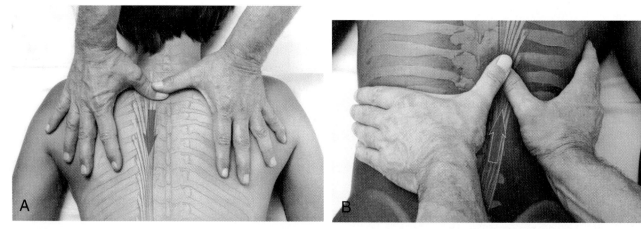

Figure 6-15 Stripping of erector spinae bundle with supported thumb both caudad and cephalad, showing longissimus. (A) starting position stripping caudad, (B) midway position stripping cephalad

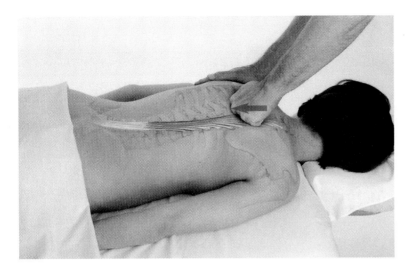

Figure 6-16 Stripping of erector spinae bundle with knuckles, showing longissimus

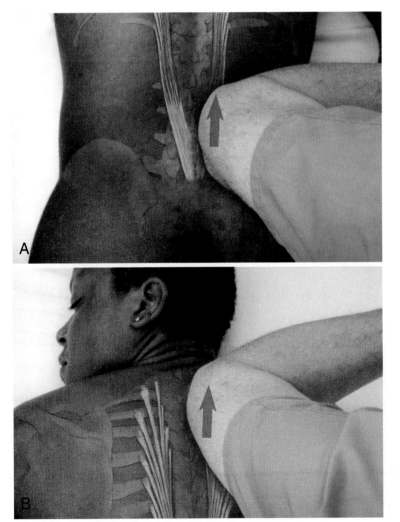

Figure 6-17 Stripping of erector spinae bundle with elbow, showing longissimus. (A) starting point, (B) ending point (Draping option 7)

THE DEEP MUSCLES OF THE VERTEBRAL COLUMN

Multifidus (Plural *Multifidi*) (Fig. 6-18)

mul-TIFF-I-duss

Etymology Latin *multi,* many + *fidus,* divided, thus "divided into many segments."

Comment

This group of muscles is located all along the vertebral column, from the cervical region to the base of the spine. The lower segments of multifidus that reach from the sacrum to the lumbar vertebrae are very strong and prominent, resembling the stays on the mast of a sailboat. In fact multifidus is one of the strongest muscles in the body. You will frequently find tenderness over the sacrum in clients with low back pain.

Attachments

- Inferiorly, from the sacrum and the sacroiliac ligament, mamillary processes of the lumbar vertebrae, transverse processes of thoracic vertebrae, and articular processes of last four cervical vertebrae
- Superiorly, into the spinous processes of all the vertebrae up to and including the axis

Action

Extends, rotates, and stabilizes the vertebral column

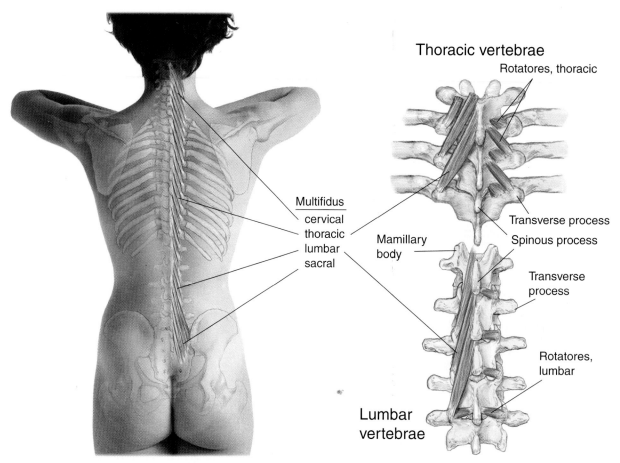

Figure 6-18 Anatomy of multifidus

Referral Area

- Between the vertebral column and the medial border of the scapula
- The region just lateral to T12 and L1, and over the lumbar region; upper lateral quadrant of the abdomen
- Over the sacrum, into the buttock along the gluteal cleft, into the posterior thigh below the buttock; lower lateral quadrant of the abdomen
- Around the coccyx

Other Muscles to Examine

- Iliocostalis thoracis, rhomboids
- Quadratus lumborum, serratus posterior inferior, iliocostalis thoracis and lumborum
- Rectus abdominis, iliopsoas

- Gluteal muscles, hamstrings
- Abdominal obliques, iliopsoas
- Levator ani

Manual Therapy

STRIPPING

- The client lies prone.
- The therapist stands at the client's side at the chest, facing caudad.
- Place the fingertips (Fig. 6-19A) or thumb (Fig. 6-19B), supported or unsupported, at the superior aspect of the sacrum just lateral to the spinal column, pointing caudad (inferiorly).
- Pressing firmly into the tissue, glide the thumb or fingertips caudad as far as the inferior aspect of the sacrum.
- Repeat this technique on the other side.

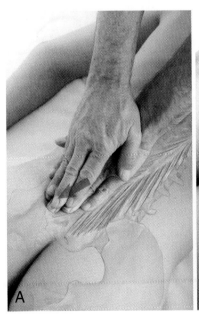
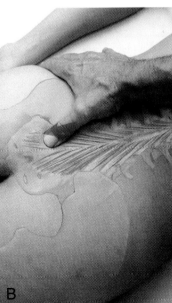

Figure 6-19 Stripping of multifidus at inferior attachments with fingertips (A) and thumb (B) (Draping option 7)

Rotatores (Fig. 6-20)

RO-ta-TOR-ace

Etymology Latin *rotatores*, rotators

Comment

Rotatores are the deepest of the three layers of transversospinalis muscles, chiefly developed in the thoracic region. Because they have a very high density of muscle spindles, they probably function as organs of proprioception. Their motor function appears to be in fine adjustments rather than gross movements of the spine.

Attachments

■ Inferiorly, from the transverse process of one vertebra
■ Superiorly, into the root of the spinous process of the next two or three vertebrae above

Action

■ Bilaterally, extension of the spine
■ Unilaterally, rotation of the vertebrae
■ Proprioception

Referral Area

Along the midline of the spine

Other Muscles to Examine

Other superficial and deep paraspinal muscles

Manual Therapy for Multifidi and Rotatores

CROSS-FIBER STROKING
■ The client lies prone.
■ The therapist stands at the client's side, beginning at the waist.

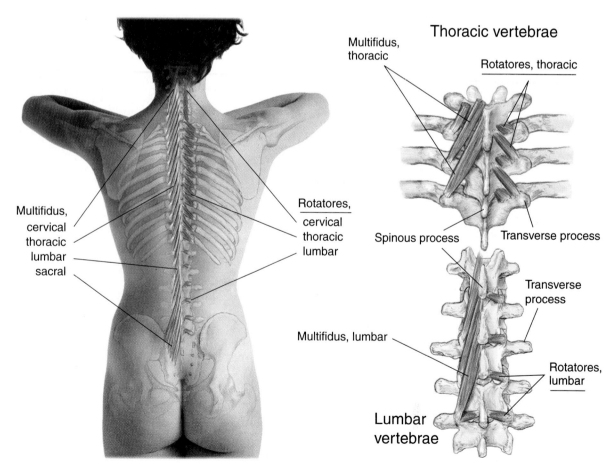

Figure 6-20 Anatomy of rotatores

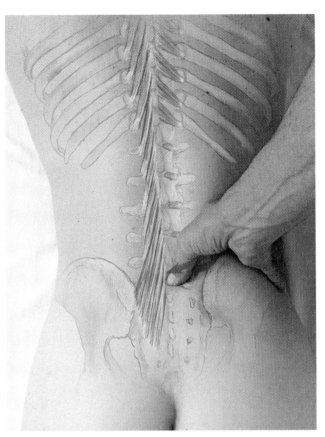

Figure 6-21 Cross-fiber stroking of rotatores in lumbar region using thumb (Draping option 7)

Caution

■ Use this technique with great care in the cervical region, and only after other work has been performed in that area as described in Chapter 3 to release the more superficial posterior neck muscles.

■ This technique is contraindicated in any area of the spine where there is diagnosed or suspected spinal pathology.

■ When using this technique, get regular feedback from the client regarding any local or referred pain or other sensation.

■ Place the thumb or fingertip (supported or unsupported) on the space between the spinous process of L5 and the sacrum (Fig. 6-21).

■ Press laterally (away from yourself) and diagonally caudad, pushing the superficial muscles out of the way to reach the intrinsic muscles.

■ If the client reports tenderness, hold for release.

■ Shifting cephalad, repeat this technique between each two spinous processes as far as the space between T12 and L1.

■ Beginning with the space between T11 and T12, perform the same technique gliding the thumb into the space between the ribs.

■ Repeat this technique (Fig. 6-22) as far as C7.

■ From C7 to the cranial base, use your unsupported thumb.

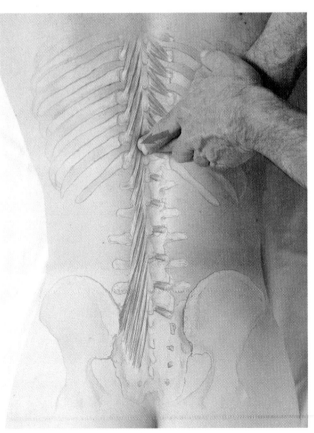

Figure 6-22 Cross-fiber stroking of rotatores in thoracic region using support fingertips (Draping option 7)

REFERENCES

1 Simons DG, Travell JG, Simons LS: Travell & Simons' Myofascial Pain and Dysfunction: The Trigger Point Manual, Vol. 1, Ed. 2. Williams & Wilkins, Baltimore, 1999, pages 261-263, 354, 436, 809-812

2 Simons, David G., MD, private communication, September 25, 2001

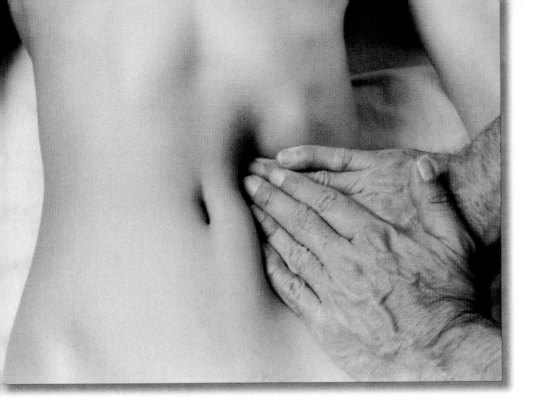

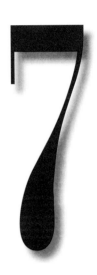

CHAPTER

7

The Low Back and Abdomen

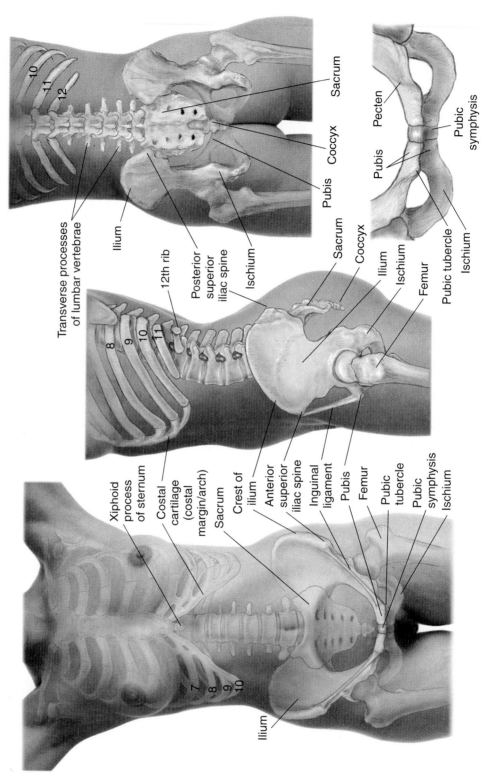

Plate 7-1 Skeletal features of the abdominal region and lower back

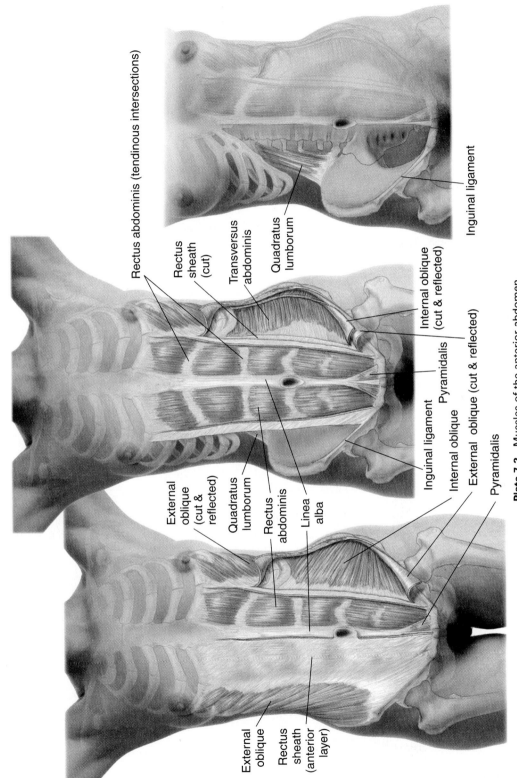

Rectus abdominis (tendinous intersections)

Rectus sheath (cut)

Transversus abdominis

Quadratus lumborum

Inguinal ligament

Internal oblique (cut & reflected)

Internal oblique (cut & reflected)

Pyramidalis

External oblique (cut & reflected)

Pyramidalis

Inguinal ligament

Internal oblique

External oblique (cut & reflected)

Quadratus lumborum

Rectus abdominis

Linea alba

External oblique

Rectus sheath (anterior layer)

Plate 7-2 Muscles of the anterior abdomen

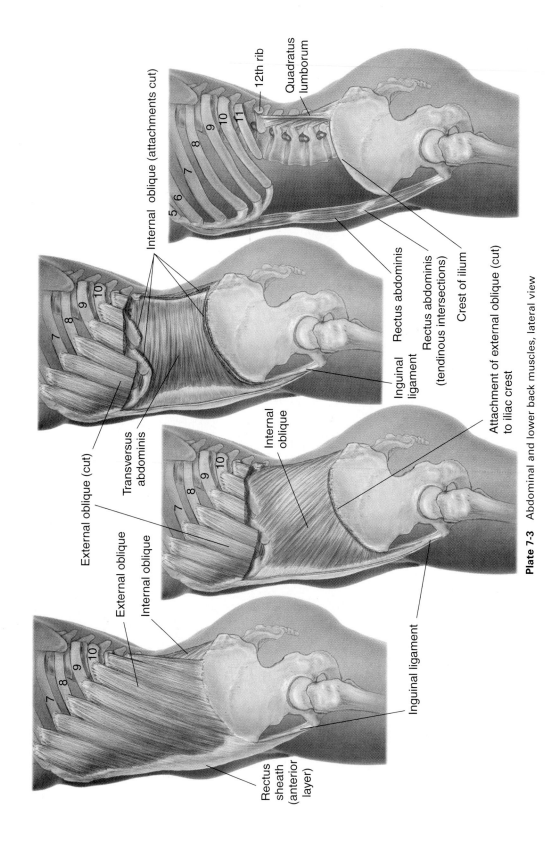

Plate 7-3 Abdominal and lower back muscles, lateral view

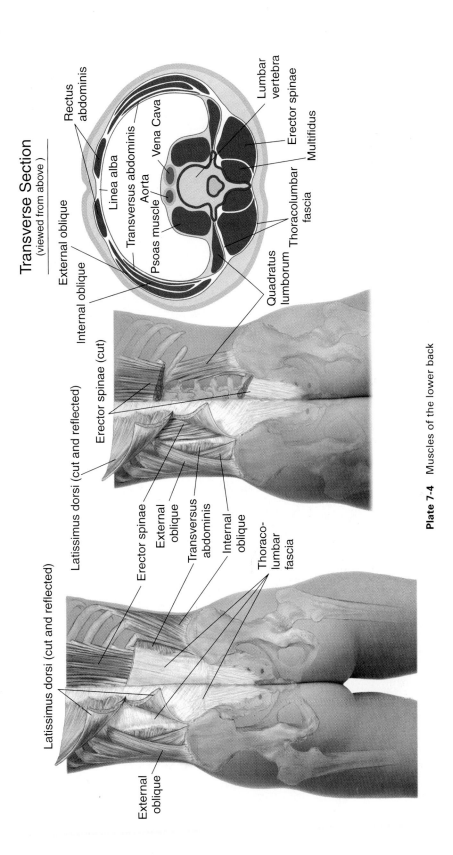

Transverse Section
(viewed from above)

- Rectus abdominis
- External oblique
- Linea alba
- Internal oblique
- Transversus abdominis
- Vena Cava
- Aorta
- Psoas muscle
- Lumbar vertebra
- Erector spinae
- Multifidus
- Thoracolumbar fascia
- Quadratus lumborum

- Latissimus dorsi (cut and reflected)
- Erector spinae (cut)
- Latissimus dorsi (cut and reflected)
- Erector spinae
- External oblique
- Transversus abdominis
- Internal oblique
- Thoraco-lumbar fascia
- External oblique

Plate 7-4 Muscles of the lower back

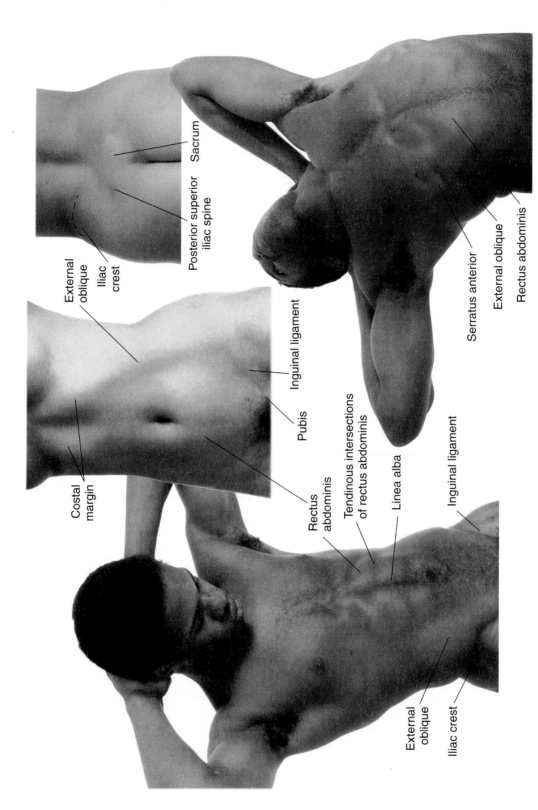

Plate 7-5 Surface anatomy of the abdomen and lower back

OVERVIEW OF THE REGION

The waist, which includes the low back (lumbar region) and middle abdomen, is a very vulnerable area because of its lack of bony armor and support. Above, the torso and spine are stabilized and the internal organs protected by the rib cage. Below, the pelvis provides stability and protection. In between, however, our need for flexibility and mobility require a space with very little support or protection. The muscles of this region, therefore, have a lot of work to do and are easily stressed or injured. Their primary actions are movement of the upper body in relation to the lower and vice versa: anterior flexion, lateral flexion, and rotation of the torso. Trigger points in these muscles refer to an extensive territory: upward into the back and chest; inward into the viscera; and downward into the buttocks, lower abdomen, groin, genitals, and legs.

The lower back region is characterized by several layers of thick, strong tendinous and fascial tissue, including the thoracolumbar fascia and tendinous portions of the erector spinae and latissimus dorsi. These connective tissues may themselves become tight, congested, and tender, and they should be treated along with the muscles.

The lumbar/abdominal muscles constitute one of the muscle groups chiefly implicated in complaints of low back pain. The others are the buttock muscles, pelvic floor muscles, and iliopsoas, all of which are addressed in the next chapter.

MUSCLES OF THE ABDOMEN

Comment

These muscles form the wall of the abdomen, and include **rectus abdominis, transversus abdominis,** and the **external** and **internal oblique muscles.** Aside from their various primary functions, all of these muscles assist in forced exhalation through compression of the abdominal cavity. They are extremely important clinically, as trigger points in these muscles can refer pain into the viscera and even cause visceral problems (somatovisceral disease). Likewise, visceral disorders can cause pain in the abdominal musculature that can persist even after the disorder is resolved. They can also refer pain into the low back.

It is helpful to do some preparatory work on the abdomen prior to deeper manual therapy on specific muscles in order to stimulate local blood flow and relax the superficial musculature. This work may include general massage techniques such as effleurage as well as myofascial stretching.

 Manual Therapy for the Abdomen

MYOFASCIAL STRETCHING
- The client lies supine.
- The therapist stands beside the client at the hips.
- Place one hand flat on the upper abdomen on the near side of the client, the fingers resting just inferior to the rib cage
- Cross the other hand over the first and place it on the lower abdomen on the far side of the client, the fingers over the ASIS (anterior superior iliac spine) (Fig. 7-1).
- Let the hands sink into the tissue until they engage the superficial fascia of the abdomen.

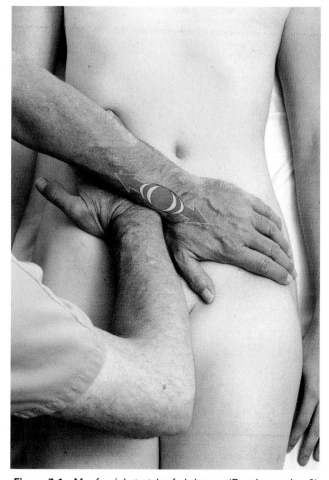

Figure 7-1   Myofascial stretch of abdomen (Draping option 2)

- Press the hands apart without allowing them to glide on the skin. Hold for release.
- Repeat on the opposite side.

Rectus Abdominis (Fig. 7-2)

REK-tus ab-DAHM-in-iss

Etymology   Latin *rectus,* straight, upright + *abdominis,* of the abdomen

Comment

Rectus abdominis is composed of a series of muscle bodies separated by tendinous intersections and divided in the center by the **linea alba** (Latin *linea,* line + *alba,* white). This muscle connects the anterior thorax (rib cage) to the anterior pelvis (pubis). It flexes the spine, and resists extension of the spine.

Attachments

- Inferiorly, to the crest and symphysis of the pubis
- Superiorly, to the xiphoid process and fifth to seventh costal cartilages

Action

- Flexes the lumbar vertebral column
- Draws the thorax inferiorly toward the pubis

Referral Area

- Over the abdomen from the xiphoid process to the pubis
- Across the back just below the scapulae; the region around the xiphoid process (epigastrium, precordium)
- Across the top of the buttocks (iliac crest) and sacrum
- Into the lower lateral quadrant of the abdomen
- Mid-abdomen just inferior to umbilicus
- (Also abdominal fullness, dysmenorrhea)

Other Muscles to Examine

- Pyramidalis
- Serratus posterior inferior
- Iliopsoas
- Abdominal obliques
- Transversus abdominis
- Gluteal muscles
- Quadratus lumborum

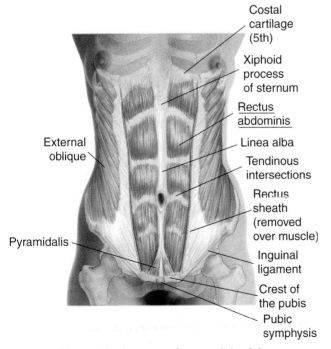

Costal cartilage (5th)
Xiphoid process of sternum
Rectus abdominis
Linea alba
Tendinous intersections
Rectus sheath (removed over muscle)
Inguinal ligament
Crest of the pubis
Pubic symphysis
External oblique
Pyramidalis

Figure 7-2 Anatomy of rectus abdominis

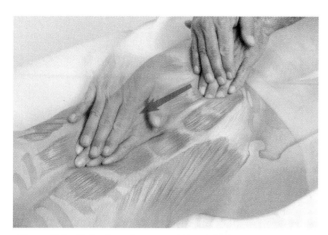

Figure 7-3 Stripping of rectus abdominis (Draping option 2)

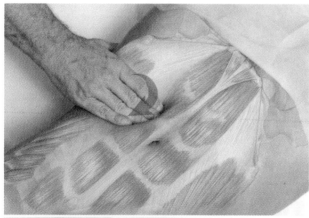

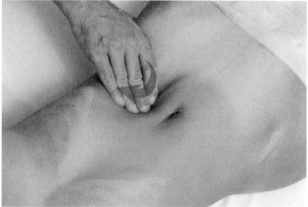

Figure 7-4 Stripping of lateral border of rectus abdominis (Draping option 2)

Manual Therapy

STRIPPING (1)

- The client lies supine.
- The therapist stands beside the client at the hip.
- Place the fingertips on one side of the rectus just superior to the pubis.
- Pressing firmly into the tissue, slide the fingertips superiorly along the muscle to its attachments on the ribs (Fig. 7-3).
- Repeat the same procedure on the other side.

STRIPPING (2)

- The client lies supine.
- The therapist stands beside the client at the waist.
- Place the fingertips on the lateral border of the rectus just above the pubis.
- Pressing firmly into the tissue, rotate the hand so that the fingertips move superiorly along the edge of the muscle (Fig. 7-4).
- Beginning just superior to the previous spot, repeat this procedure all the way along the muscle to the rib cage.
- Repeat the same procedure on the other side.

STRIPPING (3)

- The client lies supine.
- The therapist stands beside the client at the hip.
- Place the fingertips (Fig. 7-5A) or supported thumb (Fig. 7-5B) on the lateral border of the rectus just above the pubis.
- Pressing firmly into the tissue, slide the fingertips or thumb along the muscle to its attachments on the rib cage.
- Repeat the same procedure on the other side.

COMPRESSION

- The client lies supine.
- The therapist stands beside the client at the chest.
- Place the supported thumb at the attachment of the rectus to the pubis at the side nearest you.
- Press the muscle firmly against the bone, looking for tender spots. Hold for release.

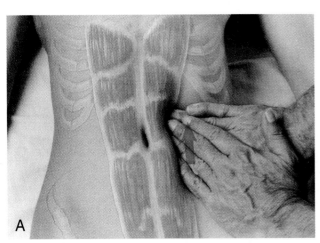
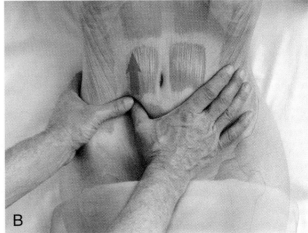

Figure 7-5 Stripping of lateral border of rectus abdominis with fingertips (A) or supported thumb (B) (Draping option 2)

- Move the hand medially to the next spot and repeat until you reach the linea alba at the center (Fig. 7-6).
- Repeat this procedure on the other side.

CROSS-FIBER STROKING

- The client lies supine.
- The therapist stands beside the client at the waist.
- Place the tip of the thumb on rectus abdominis at the linea alba (center line) just superior to the pubic symphysis, with the fingertips resting on the abdomen laterally.
- Pressing firmly into the tissue, slide the tip of the thumb laterally toward the fingertips.
- Beginning just superior to the previous point, repeat this procedure.
- Repeat the same procedure (Fig. 7-7), continuing along the rectus until you reach the rib cage.
- Repeat this procedure on the other side.

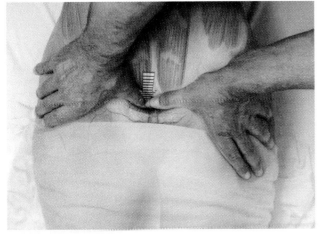

Figure 7-6 Compression of rectus abdominis attachments at the pubis (Draping option 2)

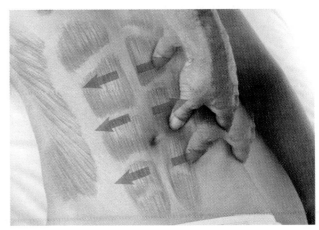

Figure 7-7 Cross-fiber stroking of rectus abdominis (Draping option 2)

Pyramidalis (Fig. 7-8)

pi-RAM-I-DAL-iss

Etymology Latin *pyramidalis,* shaped like a pyramid

Comment

Pyramidalis very commonly occurs on one side only, and may be absent in many people. It may harbor a trigger point at its attachment to the pubis.

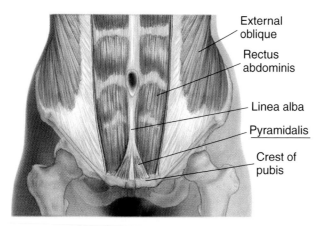

Figure 7-8 Anatomy of pyramidalis

External oblique
Rectus abdominis
Linea alba
Pyramidalis
Crest of pubis

Attachments

- Inferiorly, to the crest of the pubis
- Superiorly, to the lower portion of the linea alba

Action

Tenses the linea alba

Referral Area

- To its attachment to the pubis
- Along the midline to the umbilicus

Other Muscles to Examine

- Rectus abdominis
- Iliopsoas
- Abdominal obliques

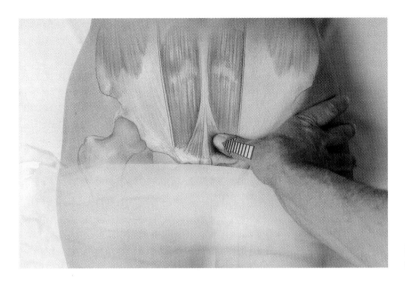

Figure 7-9 Compression of pyramidalis (Draping option 2)

Manual Therapy

COMPRESSION
- The client lies supine.
- The therapist stands beside the client at the hip.

- Place the thumb on pyramidalis, just superior and lateral to the symphysis pubis (Fig. 7-9).
- Press firmly into the tissue, examining for tenderness. Hold for release.
- Repeat this procedure on the other side.

Abdominal Obliques (Fig. 7-10, 7-11)

oh-BLEEKS

Etymology   Latin *obliquus,* slanting, diagonal

Comment

The external and internal abdominal obliques run in the same respective directions as the external and internal intercostals. A good way to remember their directions is to place one hand on the opposite side of the abdomen with your fingers pointing diagonally downward, then place the other hand on top of it pointing perpendicularly. The top hand represents the externals, the bottom hand the internals (Fig. 7-12).

Attachments

External

- Superiorly, to the fifth to twelfth ribs
- Inferiorly, to the anterior half of the lateral lip of the iliac crest, the inguinal ligament, and the anterior layer of the rectus sheath

Internal

- Inferiorly, to the iliac fascia deep to the lateral part of inguinal ligament, to the anterior half of the crest of the ilium, and to the lumbar fascia
- Superiorly, to the tenth to twelfth ribs and the sheath of the rectus abdominis

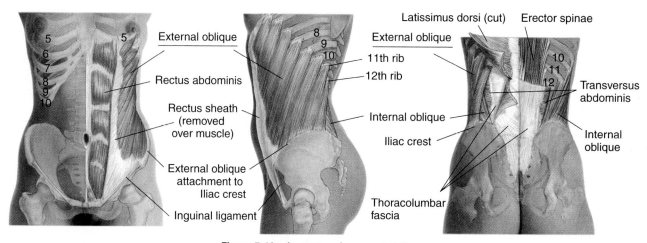

Figure 7-10   Anatomy of external oblique

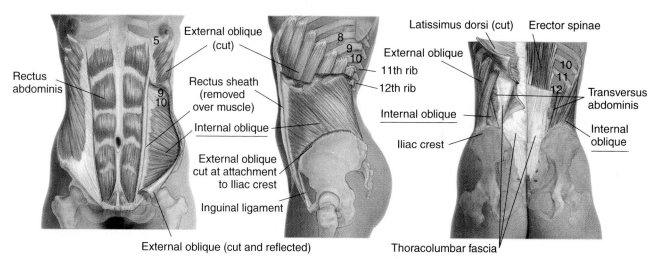

Figure 7-11   Anatomy of internal oblique

Action

Bilaterally, increase intra-abdominal pressure and flexes the spine.
Unilaterally, assist in lateral flexion and rotation of the spine.

Referral Area

- To the epigastric region (below the xiphoid process between the costal arches), over the lower chest, and diagonally below the costal arch
- The lower lateral quadrant of the abdomen, into the groin and the testicle, up over the abdomen to the pubis, the umbilicus, and the costal arch

Other Muscles to Examine

- Rectus abdominis
- Iliopsoas
- Quadratus lumborum

Manual Therapy

STRIPPING
- The client lies prone.
- The therapist stands beside the client at the chest.

- Place the hand between the client's abdomen and the table (Fig. 7-13A) with the palm on the abdomen and the fingertips just superior to the pubis at the attachment of the inguinal ligament.
- Pressing firmly upward into the tissue, slide the fingertips superolaterally along the muscle to the rib cage (Fig. 7-13B). (NOTE: the client is shown standing in the photograph for illustration of the procedure.)
- Beginning at the same spot, repeat this procedure at a more oblique angle until the whole surface of the abdomen has been treated.
- Repeat the same procedure on the other side.

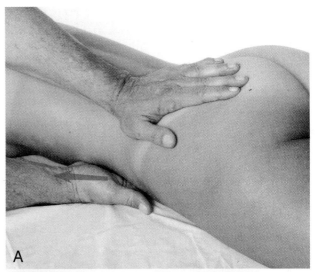

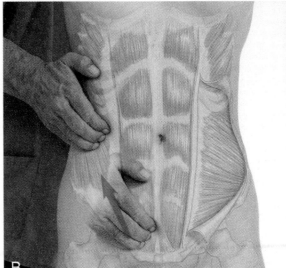

Figure 7-13 Client prone (A) for stripping of obliques (B) with fingertips (Draping option 7)

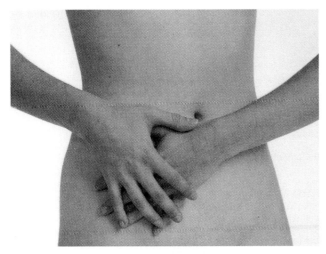

Figure 7-12 Mnemonic hand position for direction of external and internal obliques (top hand, external; bottom hand, internal)

Transversus Abdominis (Fig. 7-14)

trans-VERS-us ab-DOM-in-iss

Etymology   Latin *trans,* across + *versus,* turned

Comment

Transversus abdominis lies deep to the other abdominal muscles. There is no separate manual treatment for it that is appropriate to this text.

 Attachments

- Laterally, to the seventh to twelfth costal cartilages (interdigitating with fibers of the diaphragm), lumbar fascia, iliac crest, and inguinal ligament
- Medially, to the xiphoid cartilage and linea alba and, through the conjoint tendon, to the pubic tubercle and pecten

 Action

Compresses the abdomen

 Referral Area

Along and between the anterior costal margins

 Other Muscles to Examine

- Rectus abdominis
- Abdominal obliques

 Manual Therapy

Not applicable

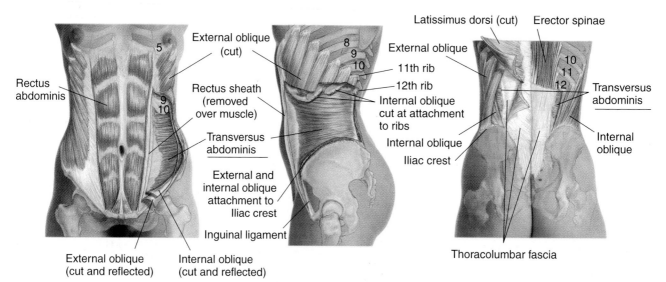

Figure 7-14   Anatomy of transversus abdominis

MUSCLES OF THE LOWER BACK

Comment

Shoulder muscles in the lower back are covered in Chapter 4. Vertebral muscles in the lower back are covered in Chapter 6.

Quadratus Lumborum (Fig. 7-15)

kwa-DRAY-tus lum-BOR-um

Etymology Latin *quadratus,* four-sided + *lumborum,* of the loins

Comment

When cinematographers have to shoot a scene in which the camera is moving around, either on someone's back or on a truck, they use a device called Steadicam™—to prevent the movement of the carrier being transferred to the camera. The same coordination between our upper and lower bodies is needed when we perform complex actions with our eyes and hands while running or riding on horseback, or keep our feet and legs steady while performing actions with our arms. In addition to its responsibility for side-bending, **quadratus lumborum** performs this service. For this reason, you will often find quadratus lumbo-rum problems in horseback riders, kayakers, golfers, and anyone whose activities involve separation of movement between the upper and lower body.

Quadratus lumborum is not an easy muscle to access manually, as it lies deep to the lumbar paraspinal muscles (erector spinae) and the thick layers of fascia and aponeurotic tissue of the lumbar region. It can be approached obliquely with the elbow just adjacent to the lumbar paraspinal muscles or laterally with the fingers or thumbs.

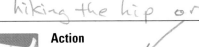

Attachments

- Inferiorly, to the iliac crest, iliolumbar ligament, and transverse processes of the lower lumbar vertebrae
- Superiorly, to the twelfth rib and transverse processes of the upper lumbar vertebrae

hiking the hip or

Action

- Lateral flexion of the spine (unilaterally)
- Extension of the spine (bilaterally)
- Stabilization of the lumbar spine

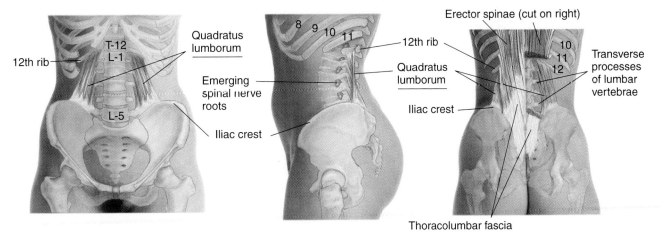

Figure 7-15 Anatomy of quadratus lumborum

Referral Area

- Into the buttock
- Over the hip
- Down the back of the leg
- Over the iliac crest
- Into the groin and sometimes the testicle
- Into the lower lateral quadrant of the abdomen

Other Muscles to Examine

- Iliopsoas
- Lumbar paraspinal muscles
- Gluteal muscles
- Piriformis and other deep lateral rotators
- Rectus abdominis and pyramidalis

Caution

In working in a superior direction on quadratus lumborum, do not place excessive pressure on the last rib. It is joined only to T12, and can be broken with pressure.

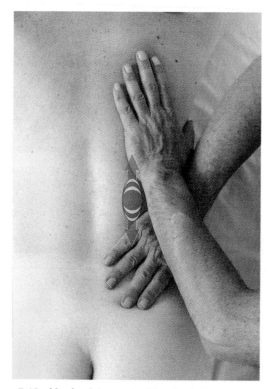

Figure 7-16 Myofascial stretch of low back (Draping option 7)

Manual Therapy

MYOFASCIAL STRETCH

- The client lies prone.
- The therapist stands beside the client at the waist.
- Place the hand nearest the client's head flat on the lumbar area lateral to the vertebrae with the fingers over the iliac crest just lateral to the sacrum.
- Crossing the other hand over or under the first, place it flat on the thoracic area over the lowest three or four ribs.
- Let your hands sink into the tissue until you feel contact with the superficial fascia.
- Press the hands in opposite directions, with enough downward pressure to engage and stretch the superficial fascia (Fig. 7-16).
- Hold until you feel significant release in the fascia.
- Shift both hands laterally (toward yourself) by one hand's width and repeat the technique.

COMPRESSION

- The client lies prone or on one side.
- The therapist stands beside the client at the waist.
- Grasp the client's waist laterally, with either the thumb (Fig. 7-17, 7-18A) or the fingertips (Fig. 7-18B) pressing under the erector spinae bundle into quadratus lumborum.
- Press firmly into the muscle, looking for tender spots, which may range from the attachments to the ilium to the attachments to the last rib. Hold for release.

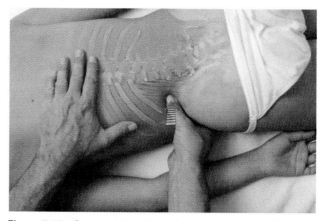

Figure 7-17 Compression of quadratus lumborum with the thumb, client prone (Draping option 7)

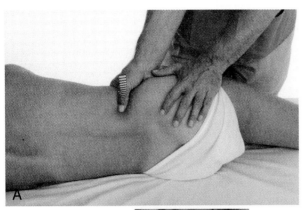

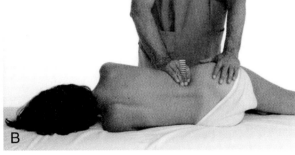

Figure 7-18 Compression of quadratus lumborum with the client side-lying, using the thumb (A) or fingertips (B) (Draping options 11,15)

COMPRESSION
- The client lies prone.
- The therapist stands beside the client at the waist.
- Place the elbow just lateral to the erector spinae bundle.
- Press firmly into the tissue, obliquely in a deep and medial direction. Hold for release.
- Repeat this procedure, first pressing superiorly toward the muscle's attachment to the last rib (Fig. 7-19A), then inferiorly toward the muscle's attachment to the ilium (Fig. 7-19B).

STRETCH
- The client lies prone.
- The therapist stands beside the client at the waist.
- Place the heel of the hand just lateral to the erector spinae bundle on the opposite side of the client's body, between the ilium and the last rib.
- Pressing deeply toward the table, let the heel of your hand slide slowly away from you (Fig. 7-20), compressing all the muscles between the pelvis and the last rib, until your hand comes off the client's side.

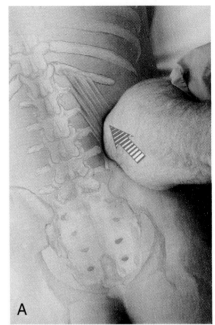

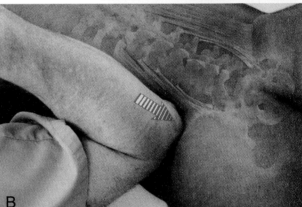

Figure 7-19 Compression of quadratus lumborum with the elbow superiorly (A) and inferiorly (B), client side-lying (Draping option 7)

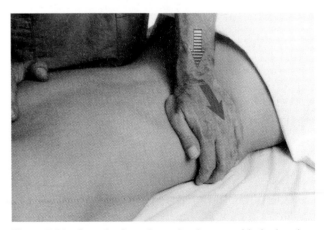

Figure 7-20 Stretch of quadratus lumborum with the hand (Draping option 7)

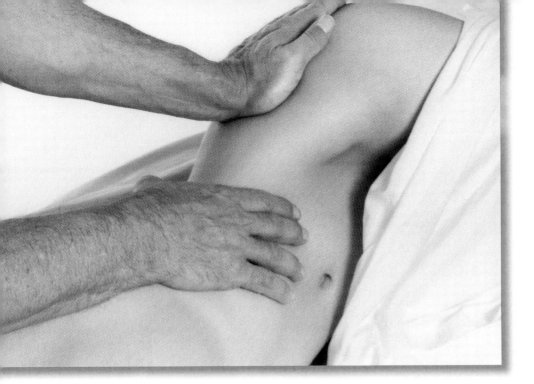

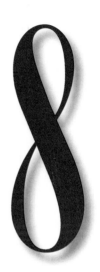

The Pelvis

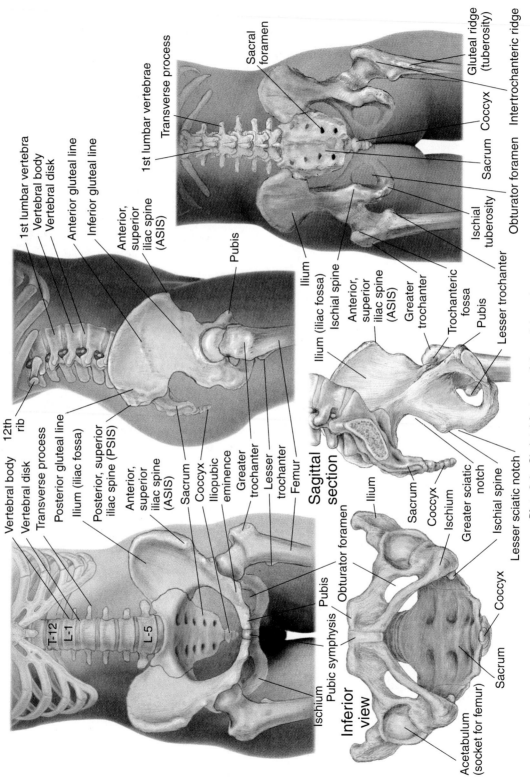

Plate 8-1 Skeletal features of the pelvic region

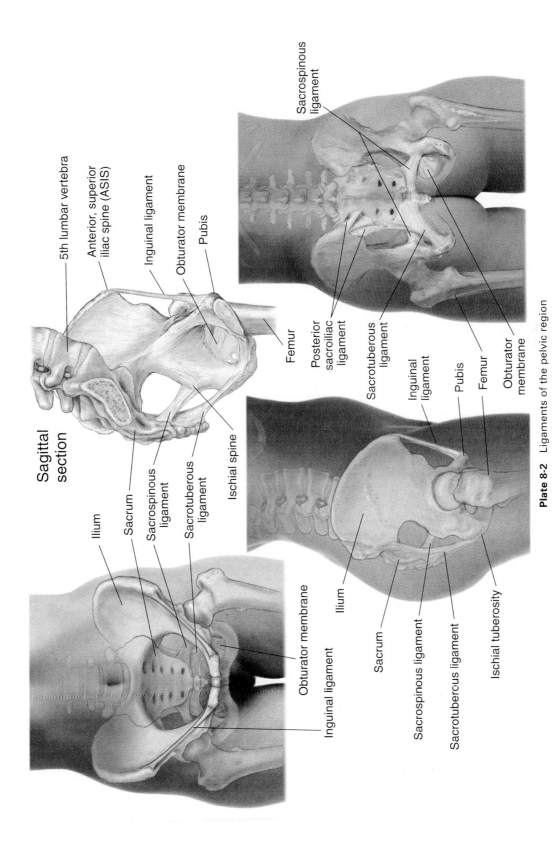

5th lumbar vertebra

Anterior, superior iliac spine (ASIS)

Inguinal ligament

Obturator membrane

Pubis

Sagittal section

Ilium

Sacrum

Sacrospinous ligament

Sacrotuberous ligament

Ischial spine

Femur

Posterior sacroiliac ligament

Sacrotuberous ligament

Inguinal ligament

Pubis

Femur

Obturator membrane

Sacrospinous ligament

Obturator membrane

Inguinal ligament

Ilium

Sacrum

Sacrospinous ligament

Sacrotuberous ligament

Ischial tuberosity

Plate 8-2 Ligaments of the pelvic region

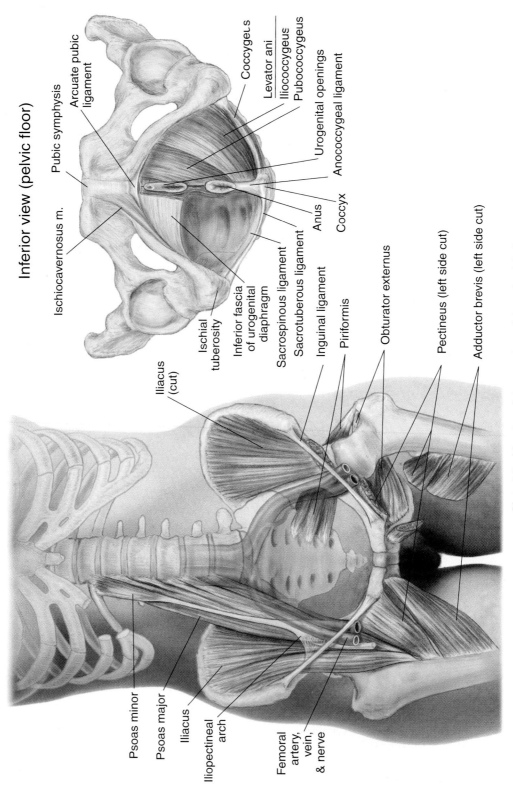

Inferior view (pelvic floor)

Arcuate pubic ligament
Pubic symphysis
Coccygeus
Levator ani
Iliococcygeus
Pubococcygeus
Urogenital openings
Anococcygeal ligament
Anus
Coccyx
Ischiocavernosus m.
Ischial tuberosity
Inferior fascia of urogenital diaphragm
Sacrospinous ligament
Sacrotuberous ligament
Inguinal ligament
Piriformis
Obturator externus
Pectineus (left side cut)
Adductor brevis (left side cut)
Iliacus (cut)
Psoas minor
Psoas major
Iliacus
Iliopectineal arch
Femoral artery, vein, & nerve

Plate 8-3 Muscles of the anterior pelvis and pelvic floor

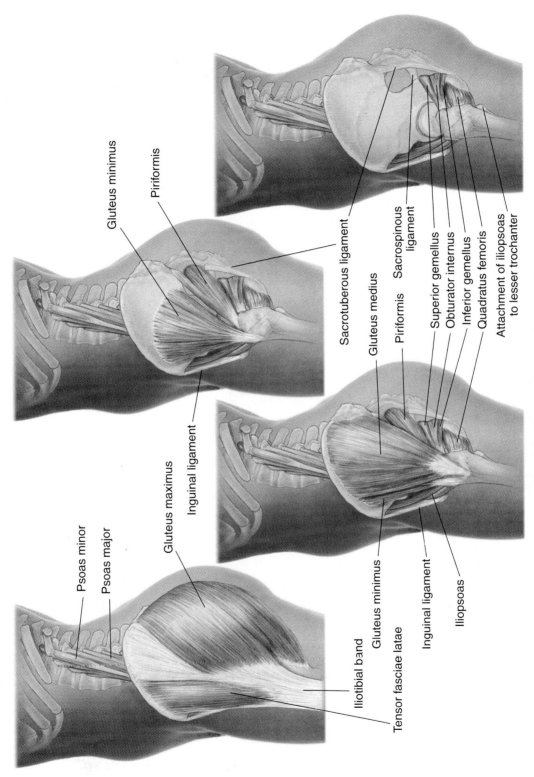

Gluteus minimus

Piriformis

Sacrotuberous ligament

Gluteus medius

Piriformis

Sacrospinous ligament

Superior gemellus

Obturator internus

Inferior gemellus

Quadratus femoris

Attachment of iliopsoas to lesser trochanter

Gluteus maximus

Inguinal ligament

Psoas minor

Psoas major

Iliotibial band

Gluteus minimus

Tensor fasciae latae

Inguinal ligament

Iliopsoas

Plate 8-4 Muscles of the pelvis, lateral view

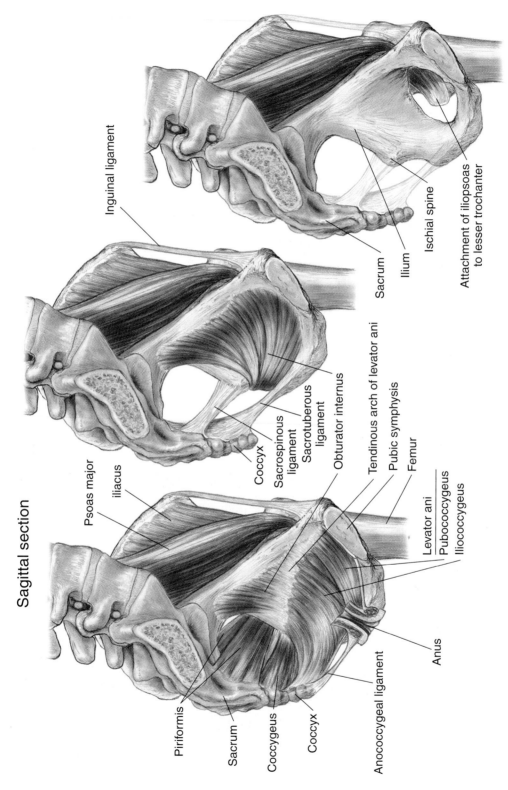

Sagittal section

Inguinal ligament

Sacrum
Ilium
Ischial spine
Attachment of iliopsoas
to lesser trochanter

Psoas major
iliacus

Coccyx
Sacrospinous
ligament
Sacrotuberous
ligament
Obturator internus

Tendinous arch of levator ani
Pubic symphysis
Femur

Levator ani
Pubococcygeus
Iliococcygeus

Anus

Piriformis
Sacrum
Coccygeus
Coccyx
Anococcygeal ligament

Plate 8-5 Muscles of the pelvis, sagittal section

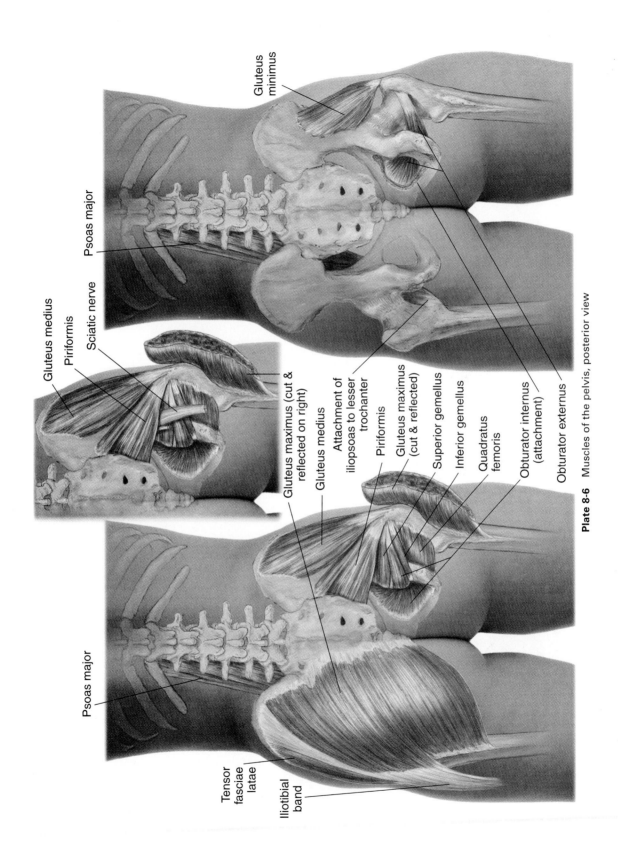

Gluteus minimus

Psoas major

Gluteus medius
Piriformis
Sciatic nerve

Gluteus maximus (cut & reflected on right)
Gluteus medius
Attachment of iliopsoas to lesser trochanter
Piriformis
Gluteus maximus (cut & reflected)
Superior gemellus
Inferior gemellus
Quadratus femoris
Obturator internus (attachment)
Obturator externus

Psoas major

Tensor fasciae latae
Iliotibial band

Plate 8-6 Muscles of the pelvis, posterior view

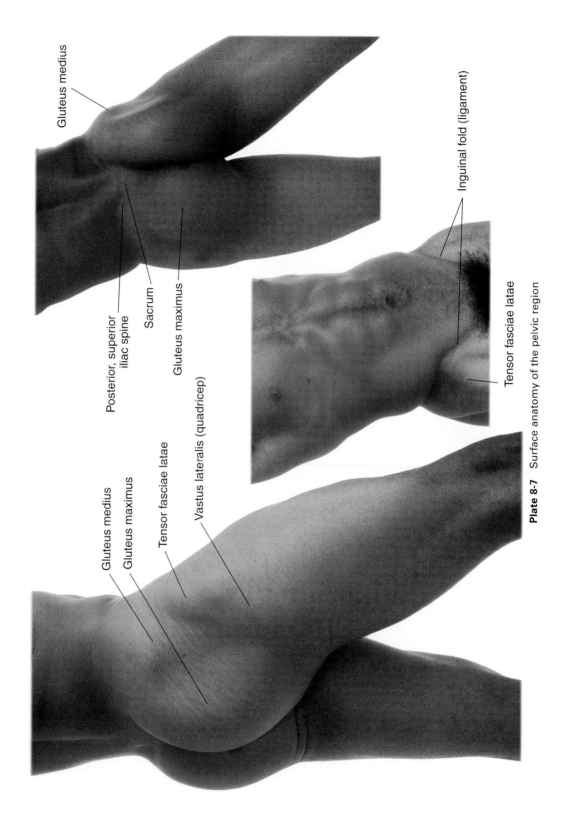

Gluteus medius

Posterior, superior iliac spine

Sacrum

Gluteus maximus

Gluteus medius

Gluteus maximus

Tensor fasciae latae

Vastus lateralis (quadricep)

Inguinal fold (ligament)

Tensor fasciae latae

Plate 8-7 Surface anatomy of the pelvic region

OVERVIEW OF THE REGION

The structural, functional, and emotional importance of the human pelvis cannot be overemphasized. The pelvis balances the torso and its appendages on the legs. It is the container, support, and protector of the abdominal and pelvic organs, especially the organs of reproduction and elimination. It is therefore a very personal and intimate area. Its position and freedom of movement are of principal importance in postural alignment.

Although we tend to think of the pelvis as a single entity, it is actually composed of two halves, or hemipelves, connected posteriorly at the sacroiliac joints and anteriorly at the symphysis pubis. The pelvis as a whole can be rotated forward or backward, or tilted to either side. Each hemipelvis, however, can have a greater or lesser anterior or posterior rotation in relation to the other, resulting in what is called a torqued pelvis. Since each hemipelvis is the site of one acetabulum, in which the head of the femur rests, the position of the hemipelvis will affect the position of the hip joint and its corresponding leg. The anterior or posterior rotation of the pelvis as a whole will also affect the normal curve of the lumbar spine, which in turn will affect the carriage of the entire upper body.

A lateral tilt in the pelvis, determined by the relative positions of the two sacroiliac joints, will result in an uneven distribution of the body weight on the legs, and will require a compensatory shifting of the rib cage and its attached structures. Any combination of tilt or rotation in the frontal or sagittal planes and torque of the hemipelves will result in a postural misalignment that is likely to cause a wide variety of myofascial problems in both the lower extremities and the entire upper body. In addition to postural issues, tightness or trigger points in the muscles of the pelvis can interfere with reproductive or eliminatory functions and can refer pain into the viscera.

The muscles of the pelvis should always be considered and addressed in any interview and examination. Because of the intimate nature of the pelvic region, it is necessary to approach examination and treatment with a great deal of sensitivity to the client's feelings and concerns with regard to privacy and modesty and should be carried out only with informed consent.

Psoas Major (Iliopsoas) (Fig. 8-1)

SO-az MAY-jer

Etymology   Greek *psoa*, the muscles of the loins + Latin *major*, larger

Overview

Psoas major, which joins **iliacus** at the groin to form **iliopsoas,** is one of the most important muscles in the body, not only for its primary function as hip flexor, but also for its postural and clinical significance.

In four-legged domestic animals, iliopsoas has little challenging work to do, since it has no real postural function and acts only to swing the hind leg forward in walking. For this reason, it tends to be a tender cut of meat: it is the tenderloin or filet, the source of the filet mignon. In humans, the story is altogether different: since we walk upright, much greater muscular effort is required to flex the hip and lift the leg. In addition, psoas plays a major role in determining the positioning of the pelvis and low back in relation to each other.

During gestation, the hips of the fetus remain fully flexed most of the time. If you observe human babies, you will notice that they do not lie flat–the hips tend to stay partially flexed. In fact, a baby does not usually attain full extension of the hips until she begins to walk. This full extension is necessary for a relaxed and comfortable upright posture. Children spend a great deal of time sitting, either in class at school, or at home studying or watching television. Most adults spend even more time in this position at desks or computers or, again, in front of the television. Iliopsoas, therefore, spends a lot of time shortened and very little time stretched.

Psoas attaches to the lumbar vertebrae and passes downward through the abdominal cavity to

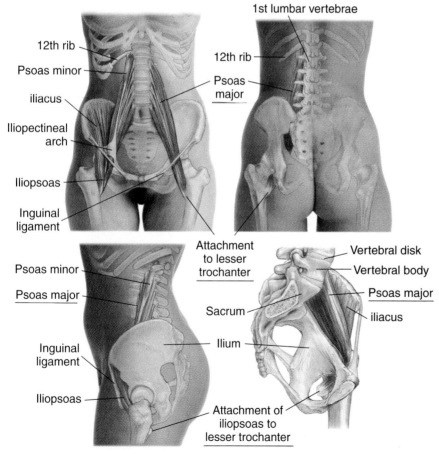

Sagittal section

Figure 8-1   Anatomy of psoas major

the groin, where it merges with iliacus and passes over the anterior rim of the ilium, then obliquely in a posterior and inferior direction to attach to the **lesser trochanter** of the femur. In this way, it uses the anterior rim of the ilium as a pulley, exerting an inferior and posterior force against it. Thus, by pulling forward on the lumbar spine and pressing downward and backward on the anterior inferior ilium, it tilts the pelvis forward and draws the lumbar curve into lordosis (Fig. 8-2). This effect can easily be seen in children, who tend to have this tilt and lordosis to a pronounced degree, and it is quite common for this postural tendency to persist into adulthood to a lesser, but still measurable, extent. One result of an anterior pelvic tilt is to shift the weight of the contents of the abdominal cavity forward, causing the abdomen to protrude. In addition, this tilt moves the hip joint posteriorly, placing strain on the muscles controlling the knees and ankles. An exaggerated lumbar lordosis requires compensatory positioning of all the structures superior to it.

The clinical significance of psoas is both indirect and direct: indirect, in the postural influences described above, and direct, by referring pain into the low back, abdomen, groin, and upper thigh. The pain referral patterns of psoas can include the viscera. In this way, psoas problems can mimic pain from visceral causes.

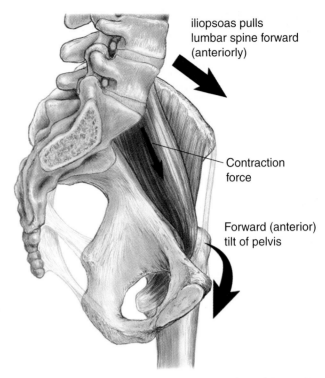

iliopsoas pulls lumbar spine forward (anteriorly)

Contraction force

Forward (anterior) tilt of pelvis

Figure 8-2   Influence of psoas major on anterior pelvic rotation

Attachments

- Superiorly, to the vertebral bodies and intervertebral disks of the twelfth thoracic to the fifth lumbar, and to the transverse processes of the lumbar vertebrae
- Inferiorly, with the iliacus muscle to the lesser trochanter of the femur

Action

Flexes the hip; is a major postural muscle

Referral Area

- To the medial lumbar region
- To the abdomen from the epigastrium to the groin
- To the anterior thigh from the groin halfway to the knee

Other Muscles to Examine

- Iliacus
- Rectus abdominis
- Abdominal obliques
- Diaphragm
- Hip adductors
- Quadratus lumborum
- Lumbar erector spinae muscles

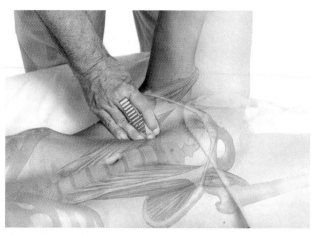

Figure 8-3 Position of hand for work on psoas major (Draping option 5)

Manual Therapy

COMPRESSION

■ The client lies supine, with the hip and knee on the side to be to be treated flexed about 45°.
■ The therapist stands beside the client, at the client's hip.

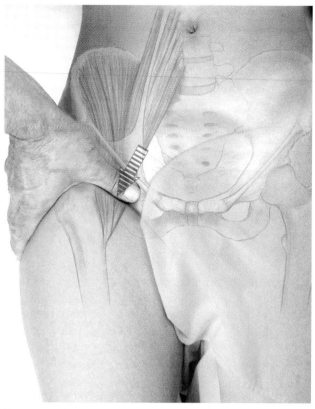

Figure 8-5 Compression of iliopsoas below the inguinal ligament (Draping option 5)

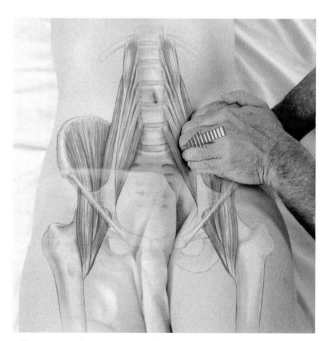

Figure 8-4 Compression of psoas major (Draping option 5)

■ Place the fingertips of the hand nearest the client on the near side of the abdomen, a few inches inferior and lateral to the navel (Fig. 8-3).
■ Press firmly and slowly into the abdomen, moving the fingertips in a circular fashion to nudge the viscera out of the way.
■ When you encounter the psoas, press into the muscle searching for tender areas (Fig. 8-4). Hold for release.
■ Move the hand caudally so that the fingertips are just inferior to the previous spot.
■ Repeat this procedure until you reach the inguinal ligament.
■ Repeat at the groin below the inguinal ligament (the circular motion is not necessary here) (Fig. 8-5).
■ This work on psoas may also be done from the opposite side of the client (Fig. 8-6), with the client in a sitting position (Fig. 8-7), or standing bent over the table (Fig. 8-8).

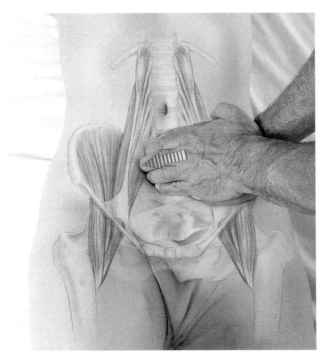

Figure 8-6 Compression of psoas major from opposite side of client (Draping option 5)

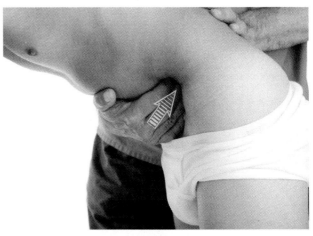

Figure 8-8 Compression of psoas major with client standing bent forward (Draping: underwear or swimsuit)

COMPRESSION OF THE INFERIOR ATTACHMENT
- The client lies supine.
- The therapist stands beside the client at the client's knees.
- Place the supported thumb on the anterior thigh, about two inches below the groin, medial to the rectus femoris.
- Press firmly into the tissue, looking for the attachment to the lesser trochanter (Fig. 8-9). If tender, hold for release.

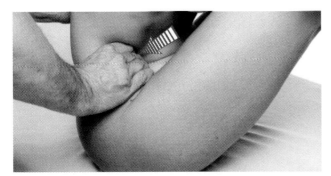

Figure 8-7 Compression of psoas major with client in sitting position (Draping: underwear, swimsuit, or exam gown)

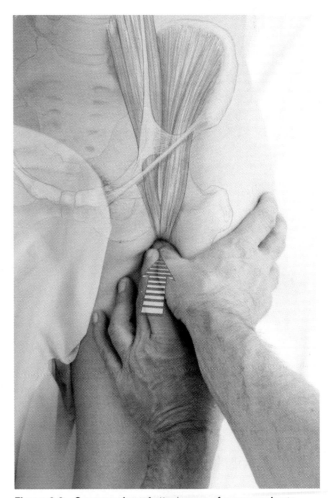

Figure 8-9 Compression of attachment of psoas major to lesser trochanter (Draping option 5)

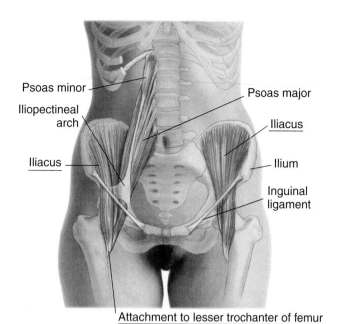

Psoas minor

Iliopectineal arch

Iliacus

Psoas major

Iliacus

Ilium

Inguinal ligament

Attachment to lesser trochanter of femur

Figure 8-10　Anatomy of iliacus

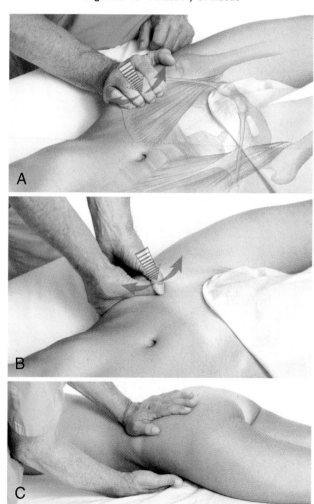

A

B

C

Figure 8-11　Stripping and cross-fiber stroking of iliacus with fingertips (A), supported thumb (B), and from underneath the client (C) (Draping options 7, 2)

Iliacus (Fig. 8-10)

il-lee-ACK-us, il-EYE-a-cus

Etymology　Relating to the ilium: Latin *ilium*, flank, groin

Overview

See discussion of psoas, above.

 Attachments

- Superiorly, to the iliac fossa
- Inferiorly, to the tendon of psoas, the anterior surface of lesser trochanter, and the capsule of the hip joint

 Action

Flexes the hip

 Referral Area

See psoas, above.

 Other Muscles to Examine

See psoas, above.

 Manual Therapy

STRIPPING AND CROSS-FIBER STROKING

- The client lies supine.
- The therapist stands beside the client at the hip.
- Place the fingertips just medial to the ilium.
- Pressing firmly into the tissue, move the fingertips back and forth and rotate the hand from side to side to slide the fingertips across the muscle (Fig. 8-11A).
- This procedure may also be carried out with the supported thumb (8-11B), or with the client prone and the hand underneath the pelvis (Fig. 8-11C).

Psoas Minor (Fig. 8-12)

SO-az MY-ner

Etymology

Greek *psoa,* the muscles of the loins + Latin *minor,* smaller

Overview

Psoas minor is absent in approximately 40% of the population, and in some people may be present on one side only. It has no recorded clinical significance.

Attachments

- Superiorly to the bodies of the twelfth thoracic and first lumbar vertebrae and the disk between them
- Inferiorly, to the iliopubic eminence via the iliopectineal arch (iliac fascia)

Action

Assists in flexion of the lumbar spine

Referral Area

Not applicable

Other Muscles to Examine

Not applicable

Manual Therapy

Not applicable

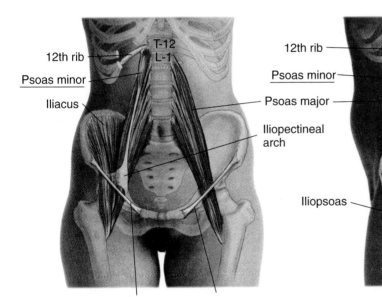

12th rib
T-12
L-1
Psoas minor
Iliacus

12th rib
Psoas minor
Psoas major
Iliopectineal arch

Iliopsoas

Attachment to iliopubic eminence
Inguinal ligament

Figure 8-12 Anatomy of psoas minor

MUSCLES OF THE PELVIC FLOOR

Overview

The pelvic floor might more usefully be called the pelvic hammock, both for psychological reasons (a hammock sounds softer than a floor) and descriptive reasons. These muscles form a supportive hammock for the pelvic organs, secured to the coccyx behind, the pubis in front, the ischial tuberosities on either side, as well as to various connective tissue structures in between.

The muscle group has openings to admit the rectum, the vagina, and the urethra, and parts of it serve as sphincters for these passages. It is common for people to hold tension in the pelvic floor muscles along with the buttock muscles, and this tension can affect the pelvic organs and cause discomfort in such activities as bowel movements and sexual intercourse.

Some examination and treatment of these muscles can be carried out externally, working between the buttocks and on the perineum, but a thorough and effective treatment will often require internal work through the rectum. Internal examination and treatment of the pelvic floor muscles is an advanced, specialized technique that is beyond the scope of this book.

For external work between the buttocks or on the perineum, the client may lie prone, preferably with a pillow or bolster under the hips.

Coccygeus (Fig. 8-13)

cock-SIDGE-us

Etymology   Latin, relating to the coccyx, from Greek *kokkyx,* cuckoo, coccyx

Attachments

- Inferiorly, to the spine of the ischium and the sacrospinous ligament
- Superiorly, to the sides of the lower part of the sacrum and the upper part of the coccyx

Action

Assists in the support of the pelvic floor, especially when intra-abdominal pressures increase. Wagging of tail (flexion of coccyx).

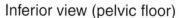

Inferior view (pelvic floor)

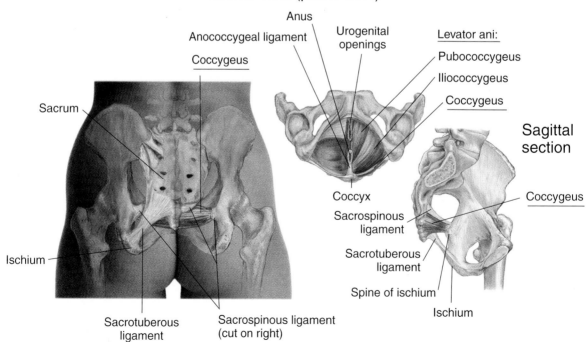

Figure 8-13   Anatomy of coccygeus

Referral Area

To the lower sacrum, the coccyx, and the surrounding area (medial aspect of the buttocks)

Other Muscles to Examine

- Gluteus maximus
- Obturator internus
- Quadratus lumborum

Manual Therapy

See Manual Therapy for the Pelvic Floor Muscles and Obturator Internus, below.

Levator ani (Fig. 8-14)

le-VAY-ter AYN-eye

Etymology Latin *levator*, raiser + *ani*, of the anus

Overview

Levator ani is comprised of the pubococcygeus, iliococcygeus, and puborectalis muscles, forming the pelvic diaphragm.

Attachments

- Anteriorly, to the posterior body of the pubis, the tendinous arch of the obturator fascia, and the spine of the ischium
- Posteriorly, to the anococcygeal ligament, the sides of the lower part of the sacrum and of the coccyx

Action

Resists prolapsing forces and draws the anus upward following defecation; helps support the pelvic viscera.

Referral Area

To the lower sacrum, the coccyx, and the surrounding area (medial aspect of the buttocks)

Other Muscles to Examine

- Gluteus maximus
- Obturator internus
- Quadratus lumborum

Sagittal section   Inferior view (pelvic floor)

Figure 8-14 Anatomy of levator ani

Manual Therapy

Levator ani cannot be externally treated effectively.

Manual Therapy for the Pelvic Floor Muscles and Obturator Internus

COMPRESSION

- The client lies prone. A pillow may be placed under the client's pelvis.
- The therapist stands beside the client at the hip.
- Place the palm of the gloved hand nearest the client on the opposite but-

tock, inserting the thumb between the buttocks to rest on the inferior end of the coccyx externally.

- Press firmly under the coccyx (Fig. 8-15), then into the tissue on either side of the coccyx, looking for tender spots. Hold for release.
- Repeat this procedure, shifting the thumb in an inferior direction, exploring the pelvic floor muscles and the inner aspect of gluteus maximus (Fig. 8-16).
- At the level of the obturator foramen, press into the foramen to explore obturator internus, holding for release as necessary (Fig. 8-17).

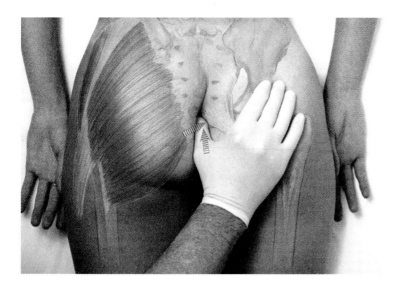

Figure 8-15 External examination under the coccyx (Draping option 8)

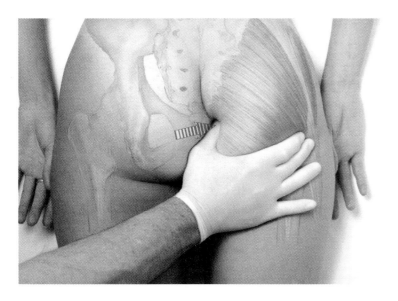

Figure 8-16 External examination and treatment between the buttocks (Draping option 8)

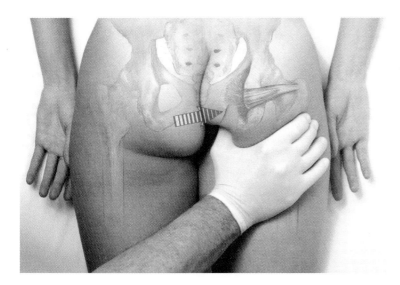

Figure 8-17 Compression of obturator internus (Draping option 8)

GLUTEAL MUSCLES

Overview

Since gluteus maximus covers gluteus medius and much of gluteus minimus, much of the work on the buttock applies to all three muscles, especially over the lateral aspect. The only distinction lies in the intention and depth of the work. Therapy of the gluteal muscles will be found after descriptions of all the individual muscles.

Gluteus maximus (Fig. 8-18)

GLUE-tee-us MAX-im-us

Etymology   Latin *gluteus*, buttock muscle + *maximus*, largest

Overview

Gluteus maximus is the powerful climbing muscle, antagonist to iliopsoas. It is very commonly involved in low back pain.

Attachments

- Superiorly, to the ilium behind the posterior gluteal line, to the posterior surface of the sacrum and coccyx, and to the sacrotuberous ligament

- Inferiorly, to the iliotibial band of the fascia lata (superficial three-quarters) and to the gluteal tuberosity (postero-lateral proximal one-quarter) of the femur

Action

Extends the thigh, especially from a flexed position, as in climbing stairs or rising from a sitting position

Referral Area

To the entire buttock and into the upper posterior thigh

Other Muscles to Examine

- Other gluteal muscles
- Deep lateral rotators of the hip
- Quadratus lumborum
- Pelvic floor muscle

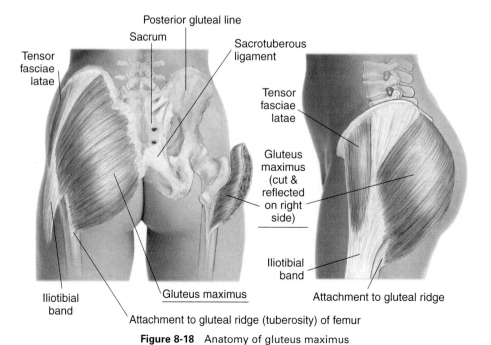

Figure 8-18   Anatomy of gluteus maximus

Manual Therapy

See Manual Therapy for the Gluteal Muscles below.

Note: For working the medial aspect of gluteus maximus, use the technique for external work between the buttocks described under Pelvic Floor Muscles and Obturator Internus above (Fig. 8-16).

Gluteus medius (Fig. 8-19)

GLUE-tee-us ME-dee-us

Etymology   Latin *gluteus,* buttock muscle + *medius,* middle

Overview

Gluteus medius, with gluteus minimus, is a powerful abductor of the hip. It is very commonly involved in low back pain.

 Attachments

- Superiorly, to the ilium between the anterior and posterior gluteal lines
- Inferiorly, to the lateral surface of the greater trochanter

 Action

Abducts and contributes to rotation of the thigh; stabilizes the pelvis in walking

 Referral Area

- Over the buttock
- Over the sacrum
- Into the medial lumbar region
- Into the upper posterior thigh

 Other Muscles to Examine

- Quadratus lumborum
- Lumbar erector spinae muscles
- Other gluteal muscles
- Deep lateral rotators of the hip
- Pelvic floor muscles

 Manual Therapy

See Manual Therapy for the Gluteal Muscles, below.

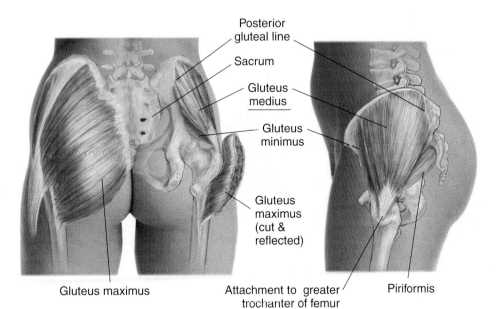

Figure 8-19   Anatomy of gluteus medius

Gluteus minimus (Fig. 8-20)

GLUE-tee-us MIN-im-us

Etymology Latin *gluteus*, buttock muscle + *minimus*, smallest

Overview

Gluteus minimus, with gluteus medius, is a powerful abductor of the hip. It has a far-ranging pain referral pattern, and is commonly involved in hip and leg pain.

Attachments

- Superiorly, to the ilium between the anterior and inferior gluteal lines
- Inferiorly, to the greater trochanter of the femur

Action

Abducts and medially rotates the thigh

Referral Area

- Over the buttock and lateral hip
- Over the posterior thigh
- Over the posterior calf
- Over the lateral thigh
- Over the lateral calf to the ankle

Other Muscles to Examine

- Other gluteal muscles
- Deep lateral rotators of the hip
- Tensor fascia latae
- Iliotibial band
- Vastus lateralis
- Hamstrings
- Calf muscles

Manual Therapy for the Gluteal Muscles

MYOFASCIAL STRETCH
- The client lies prone.
- The therapist stands beside the client at the waist, facing the client.
- Place the palm of your cephalad hand on the upper aspect of the client's near buttock, the fingers pointing inferiorly.
- Cross the caudad hand over, placing it on the client's waist at the iliac crest.

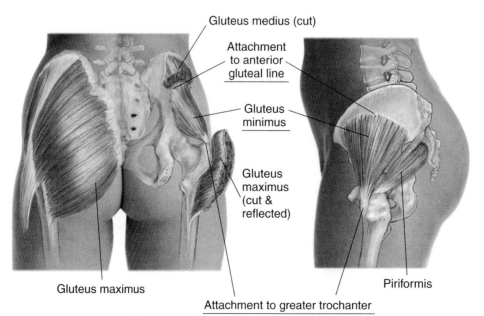

Figure 8-20 Anatomy of gluteus minimus

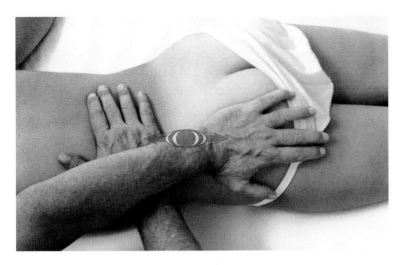

Figure 8-21 Myofascial release on gluteal region (Draping options 6, 8, 10, underwear or swimsuit)

■ Lean into the hands to push them apart, pressing firmly into the tissue (Fig. 8-21).

■ Hold this stretch until you feel the underlying fascia release.

STRIPPING
■ The client lies prone.

■ The therapist stands beside the client at the level of the chest.

■ Place the palm of the hand on the buttock just above the iliac crest and lateral to the sacrum, the thumb pointing inferiorly (Fig. 8-22A).

■ Pressing firmly into the tissue with the heel of the hand, slide the hand along the muscle to its most inferior aspect.

■ Beginning just lateral to the previous spot, repeat this procedure until the entire buttock has been covered, including the attachment of gluteus maximus to the iliotibial band, and gluteus minimus along the side of the hip (Fig. 8-22B).

■ The same procedure may be carried out with the knuckles (Fig. 8-23), the fingertips (Fig. 8-24), or the supported thumb (Fig. 8-25).

STRIPPING
■ The client lies on her side, with the lower leg straight and the upper leg flexed at the hip and knee.

■ The therapist stands beside the client at the waist.

■ Place the supported thumb on the superior lateral aspect of the buttock at the iliac crest.

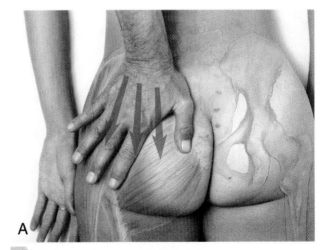

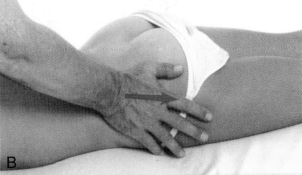

Figure 8-22 Stripping of gluteal muscles with the heel of the hand: A, beginning stroke; B, ending stroke (Draping options 6, 8, 10, underwear or swimsuit)

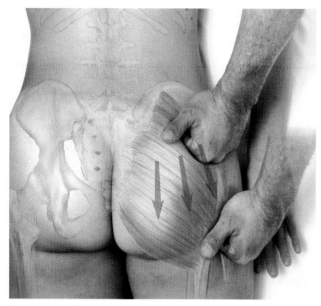

Figure 8-23 Stripping of gluteal muscles with the knuckles (Draping options 6, 8, 10, underwear or swimsuit)

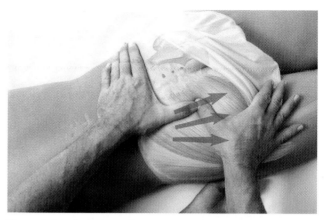

Figure 8-25 Stripping of gluteal muscles with the thumb (Draping options 6, 8, 10, underwear or swimsuit)

- Pressing firmly into the tissue, slide the thumbs inferiorly along the muscle to its attachments on the greater trochanter (Fig. 8-26).

COMPRESSION
- The client lies prone.
- The therapist stands beside the client at the client's waist.
- Place the supported thumb on the lateral aspect of the buttock just inferior to the iliac crest.

- Press firmly into the tissue, moving your thumb back and forth, to search for tender areas. Hold for release (Fig. 8-27).
- Explore the gluteal muscles in this way over the entire buttock.

Reversing Anterior Pelvic Rotation

These procedures should be performed after working all the muscles affecting anterior pelvic rotation (quadratus lumborum, gluteal muscles, latissimus dorsi, iliopsoas, rectus femoris, hip adductors).

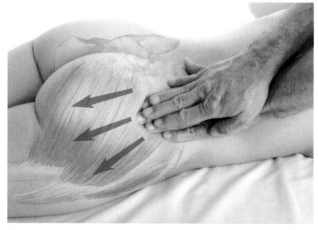

Figure 8-24 Stripping of gluteal muscles with the fingertips (Draping options 6, 8, 10, underwear or swimsuit)

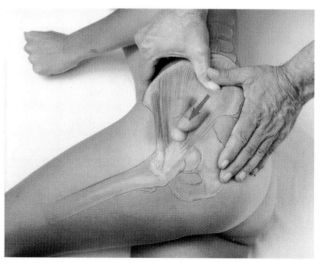

Figure 8-26 Stripping of gluteal muscles in side-lying position (Draping option 13, underwear or swimsuit)

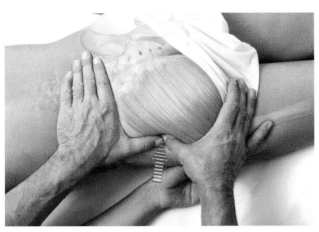

Figure 8-27 Examination and compression of gluteal muscles (Draping options 6, 8, 10, underwear or swimsuit)

SUPINE POSITION
- The client lies supine, with the leg flexed at the hip and the knee.
- The therapist stands beside the client's leg, facing the head.
- Wrapping the arm nearest the client around the client's leg, place your shoulder firmly just below the knee and the heel of your hand on the ASIS.
- Place your far hand underneath the client's buttock, with the fingertips resting on the iliac crest.
- Ask the client to resist you with 20% of her/his strength as you simultaneously press the leg to the client's chest, push superiorly against the ASIS, and pull inferiorly on the buttock and iliac crest (Fig. 8-29).

PRONE POSITION
- The client lies prone.
- The therapist stands beside the client at the client's waist.
- Place one hand on the buttock at the iliac crest, the fingers pointing inferiorly. Place the other hand under the ilium with the fingertips on the anterior superior iliac spine (ASIS).
- Simultaneously pull the ASIS in a superior direction while pushing the iliac crest in an inferior direction (Fig. 8-28).

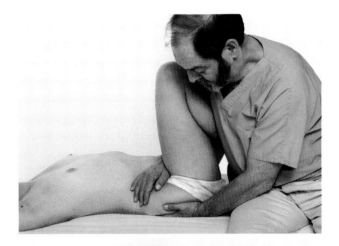

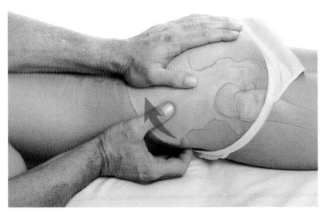

Figure 8-28 Reversing anterior pelvic rotation in prone position (Draping option 8, 10, underwear or swimsuit)

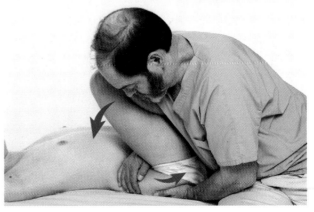

Figure 8-29 Reversing anterior pelvic rotation in supine position (Draping option 5, underwear or swimsuit)

DEEP LATERAL ROTATORS OF THE HIP

Piriformis (Fig. 8-30)

PEER-re-FORM-is

Etymology   Latin *pirum*, pear + *forma*, form

Overview

Piriformis is a primary lateral rotator of the hip, as well as a principal stabilizer of the hip joint. It has profound clinical significance.

The sciatic nerve may pass under, over, or even through (or partially through) piriformis, depending on the individual. Therefore, a tightened piriformis may cause pain not only through its own referral patterns, but also by entrapment of the sciatic nerve. This entrapment is called *piriformis syndrome*. Piriformis problems are common in ballet dancers because of the constant demand for "turnout" (lateral rotation of the hip) in ballet. It is also very common in general because of its role in stabilizing the hip.

Attachments

■ Medially and superiorly, to the margins of the anterior pelvic sacral foramina and the greater sciatic notch of the ilium
■ Laterally and inferiorly, to the upper border of greater trochanter

Action

Rotates thigh laterally; assists in abduction of flexed hip; stabilizes hip joint

Referral Area

■ Over the buttock (especially the lateral border of the sacrum and the inferolateral aspect of the buttock)
■ Into the posterior thigh
■ By entrapment of the sciatic nerve, over the entire posterior leg to the foot, and into the low back, hip, groin, perineum, and rectum

Other Muscles to Examine

■ Gluteal muscles
■ Other deep lateral rotators of the hip
■ Quadratus lumborum

Manual Therapy

COMPRESSION
■ The client lies prone.
■ The therapist stands beside the client's hip.
■ Place the thumb (Fig. 8-31) or supported thumb (Fig. 8-32) on the midpoint between the greater trochanter and the sacrum.

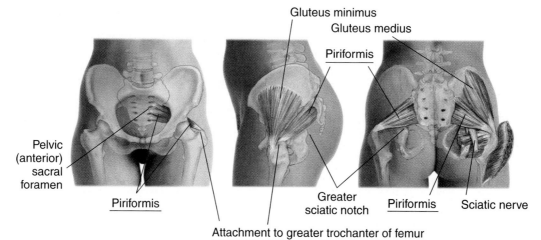

Figure 8-30   Anatomy of piriformis

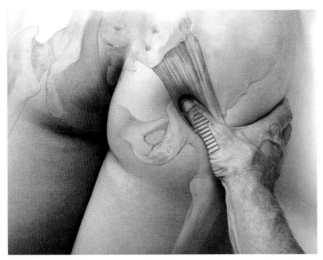

Figure 8-31   Compression of piriformis with thumb (Draping option 10)

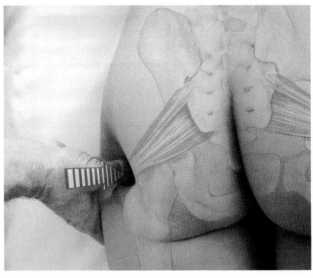

Figure 8-33   Compression of piriformis attachment at greater trochanter (Draping option 10)

- Press firmly into the tissue, looking for tender areas. Hold for release.
- Explore the entire muscle in this manner, from the sacral border to the attachment on the greater trochanter (Fig. 8-33).

COMPRESSION WITH STRETCH
- The client lies prone.
- The therapist stands at the client's hip
- Place the knuckles of one hand on the buttock just medial to the greater trochanter, pressing firmly in a medial and anterior direction.

- With the other hand, grasp the client's ankle and flex the knee to 90°.
- Still holding the knuckles firmly against piriformis, pull the client's foot toward yourself, rotating the hip medially (Fig. 8-34).

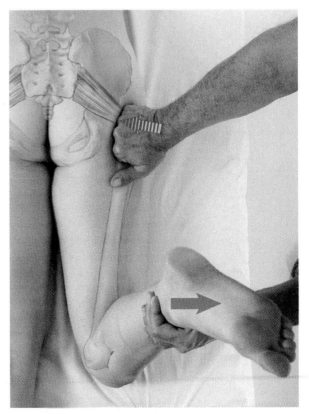

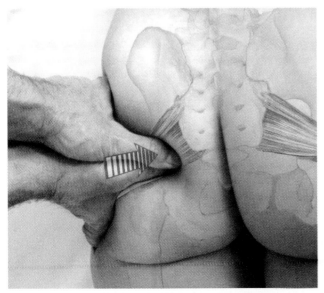

Figure 8-32   Compression of piriformis with supported thumb (Draping option 10)

Figure 8-34   Passive stretch of piriformis (Draping option 10)

Superior Gemellus (Fig. 8-35)

sue-PEER-ee-or je-MELL-us

Etymology   Latin *superior,* higher + *gemellus,* diminutive of *geminus,* twin

Overview

This muscle has no clinical significance separate from piriformis.

Attachments

- Medially, to the ischial spine and margin of the lesser sciatic notch
- Laterally, to the medial surface of the greater trochanter via the tendon of obturator internus

Action

Rotates thigh laterally; stabilizes the hip joint

Referral Area

Not applicable

Other Muscles to Examine

Not applicable

Manual Therapy

Not applicable

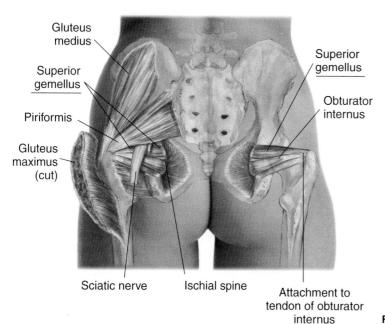

Gluteus medius
Superior gemellus
Piriformis
Gluteus maximus (cut)
Superior gemellus
Obturator internus
Sciatic nerve   Ischial spine
Attachment to tendon of obturator internus

Figure 8-35   Anatomy of superior gemellus

Inferior Gemellus (Fig. 8-36)

in-FEER-ee-or je-MELL-us

Etymology Latin *inferior,* lower + *gemellus,* diminutive of *geminus,* twin

Overview

This muscle has no clinical significance separate from piriformis.

Attachments

- Medially, to the ischial tuberosity
- Laterally, to the medial surface of the greater trochanter via the tendon of obturator internus

Action

Rotates thigh laterally

Referral Area

Not applicable

Other Muscles to Examine

Not applicable

Manual Therapy

Not appicable

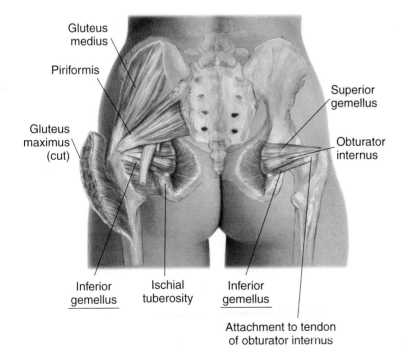

Gluteus medius

Piriformis

Gluteus maximus (cut)

Superior gemellus

Obturator internus

Inferior gemellus

Ischial tuberosity

Inferior gemellus

Attachment to tendon of obturator internus

Figure 8-36 Anatomy of inferior gemellus

Obturator Internus (Fig. 8-37)

AHB-tu-ray-ter in-TURN-us

Etymology Latin *obturator,* that which occludes or stops up + *internus,* internal

Overview

Obturator internus has much the same referral pattern as levator ani and coccygeus, discussed above.

Attachments

■ Medially, to the pelvic surface of the obturator membrane and margin of obturator foramen
■ Laterally, through the lesser sciatic notch, turning 90° to insert into the medial surface of the greater trochanter

Action

Rotates thigh laterally; stabilizes the hip joint

Referral Area

■ To the lower sacrum and coccyx
■ Into the posterior upper thigh

Other Muscles to Examine

■ Pelvic floor muscles
■ Piriformis
■ Gluteus maximus

Manual Therapy

See Manual Therapy for the Pelvic Floor Muscles and Obturator Internus, above (see page 284)

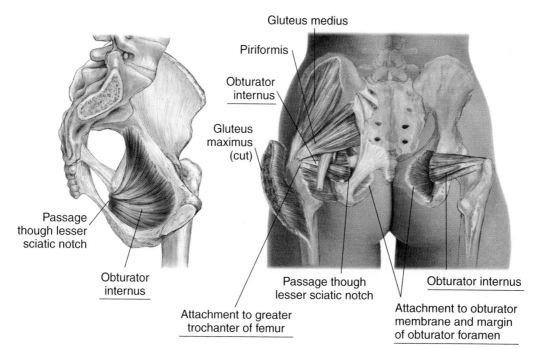

Figure 8-37 Anatomy of obturator internus

Obturator Externus (Fig. 8-38)

AHB-tu-ray-ter ex-TURN-us

Etymology   Latin *obturator,* that which occludes or stops up + *externus,* external

Overview

Obturator externus may, with quadratus femoris, cause tenderness just medial to the lower aspect of the greater trochanter. This muscle may be palpated deeply in the groin between pectineus and adductor brevis.

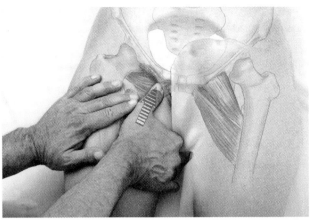

Figure 8-39   Compression of obturator externus through the groin (Draping option 5)

Attachments

■ Medially, to the lower half of margin of obturator foramen and adjacent part of external surface of obturator membrane
■ Laterally, to the trochanteric fossa of greater trochanter

Action

Rotates thigh laterally; stabilizes the hip joint

Referral Area

Just medial to the lower aspect of the greater trochanter

Other Muscles to Examine

■ Quadratus femoris and other deep lateral rotators of the hip
■ Pectineus
■ Adductor brevis

Manual Therapy

COMPRESSION
■ The client lies supine.
■ The therapist stands at the client's knee.
■ Using the thumb, locate pectineus and adductor brevis.
■ Press firmly and deeply into the tissue between pectineus and adductor brevis exploring for tenderness (Fig. 8-39). Hold for release.

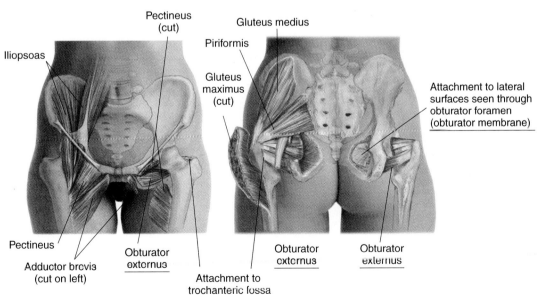

Figure 8-38   Anatomy of obturator externus

Quadratus Femoris (Fig. 8-40)

kwa-DRAY-tus FEM-or-is

Etymology Latin *quadratus,* four-sided + *femoris,* of the femur (thigh bone)

Overview

Quadratus femoris may, with obturator externus, cause tenderness just medial to the lower aspect of the greater trochanter.

Attachments

- Medially, to the lateral border of tuberosity of ischium
- Laterally, to the intertrochanteric crest

Action

Rotates thigh laterally

Referral Area

With obturator externus, just medial to the lower aspect of the greater trochanter

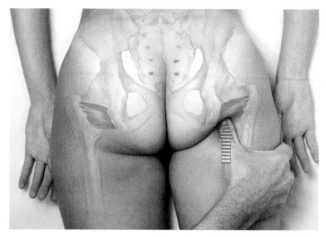

Figure 8-41 Compression of quadratus femoris (Draping option 10)

Other Muscles to Examine

- Obturator externus
- Other deep lateral rotators of the hip

Manual Therapy

COMPRESSION
- The client lies prone.
- The therapist stands at the client's knee.
- Place the thumb at the crease of the buttock between the ischial tuberosity and the greater trochanter.
- Press firmly in a superior direction, exploring for tender areas (Fig. 8-41). Hold for release.

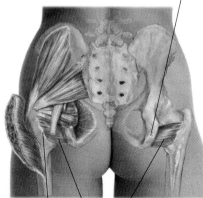
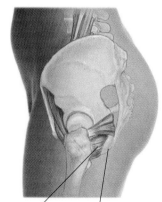

Ischial tuberosity

Quadratus femoris

Attachment to intertrochanteric ridge of femur

Quadratus femoris   Ischial tuberosity

Figure 8-40 Anatomy of quadratus femoris

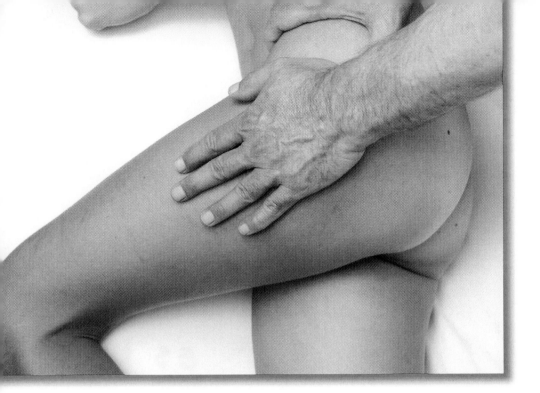

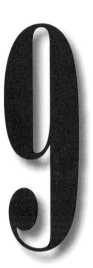

The Thigh

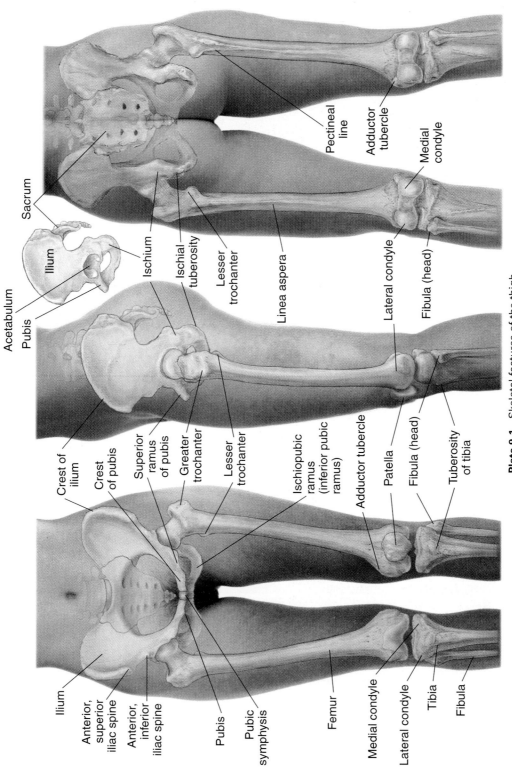

Plate 9-1 Skeletal features of the thigh

Sacrum

Acetabulum

Ilium

Pubis

Ischium

Ischial tuberosity

Lesser trochanter

Linea aspera

Lateral condyle

Fibula (head)

Pectineal line

Adductor tubercle

Medial condyle

Crest of ilium

Crest of pubis

Superior ramus of pubis

Greater trochanter

Lesser trochanter

Ischiopubic ramus (inferior pubic ramus)

Adductor tubercle

Patella

Fibula (head)

Tuberosity of tibia

Ilium

Anterior, superior iliac spine

Anterior, inferior iliac spine

Pubis

Pubic symphysis

Femur

Medial condyle

Lateral condyle

Tibia

Fibula

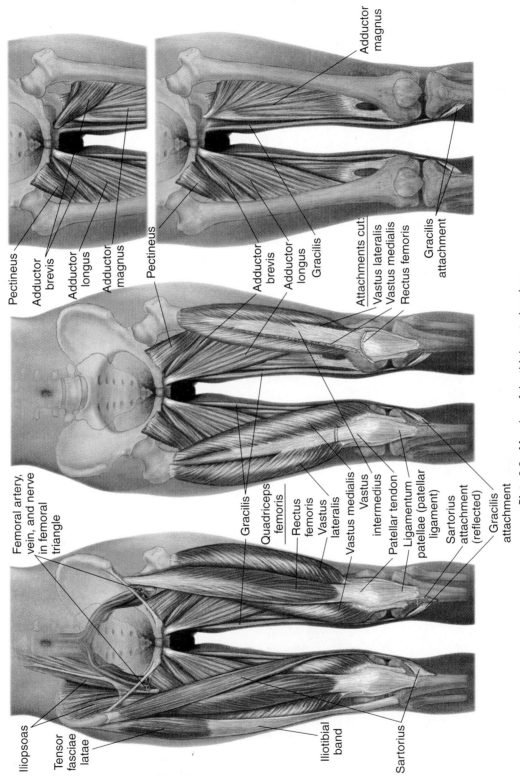

Pectineus

Adductor brevis

Adductor longus

Adductor magnus

Pectineus

Adductor brevis

Adductor longus

Gracilis

Adductor magnus

Attachments cut:
Vastus lateralis
Vastus medialis
Rectus femoris

Gracilis attachment

Femoral artery, vein, and nerve in femoral triangle

Gracilis

Quadriceps femoris

Rectus femoris
Vastus lateralis
Vastus medialis
Vastus intermedius

Patellar tendon

Ligamentum patellae (patellar ligament)

Sartorius attachment (reflected)

Gracilis attachment

Iliopsoas

Tensor fasciae latae

Iliotibial band

Sartorius

Plate 9-2 Muscles of the thigh, anterior view

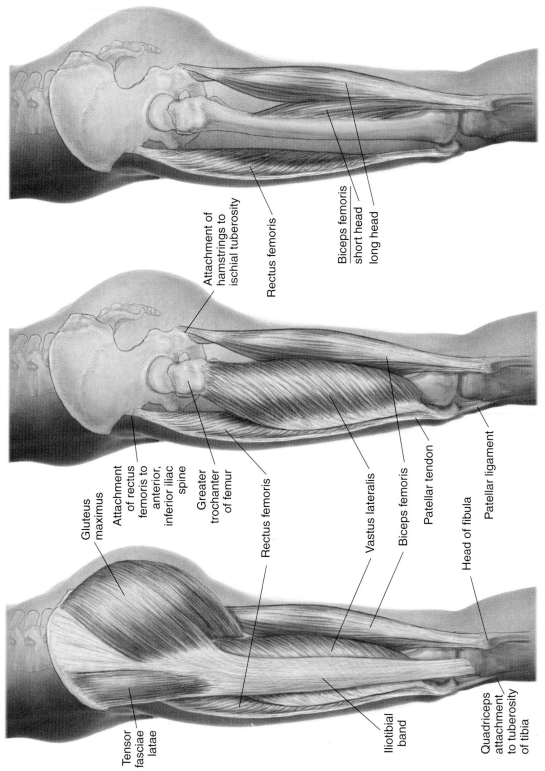

Gluteus
maximus

Attachment
of rectus
femoris to
anterior,
inferior iliac
spine

Greater
trochanter
of femur

Rectus femoris

Tensor
fasciae
latae

Iliotibial
band

Vastus lateralis

Biceps femoris

Patellar tendon

Head of fibula

Patellar ligament

Quadriceps
attachment
to tuberosity
of tibia

Attachment of
hamstrings to
ischial tuberosity

Rectus femoris

Biceps femoris
short head
long head

Plate 9-3   Muscles of the thigh, lateral view

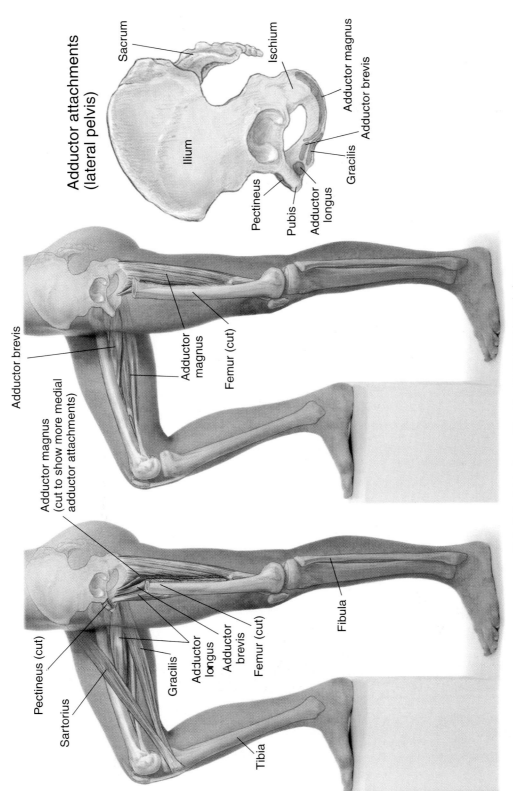

Adductor attachments
(lateral pelvis)

Sacrum

Ischium

Adductor magnus

Adductor brevis

Ilium

Gracilis

Pectineus

Pubis

Adductor longus

Adductor brevis

Adductor magnus
(cut to show more medial
adductor attachments)

Adductor magnus

Femur (cut)

Pectineus (cut)

Sartorius

Gracilis

Adductor longus

Adductor brevis

Femur (cut)

Fibula

Tibia

Plate 9-4 Adductors of the hip, medial and lateral views

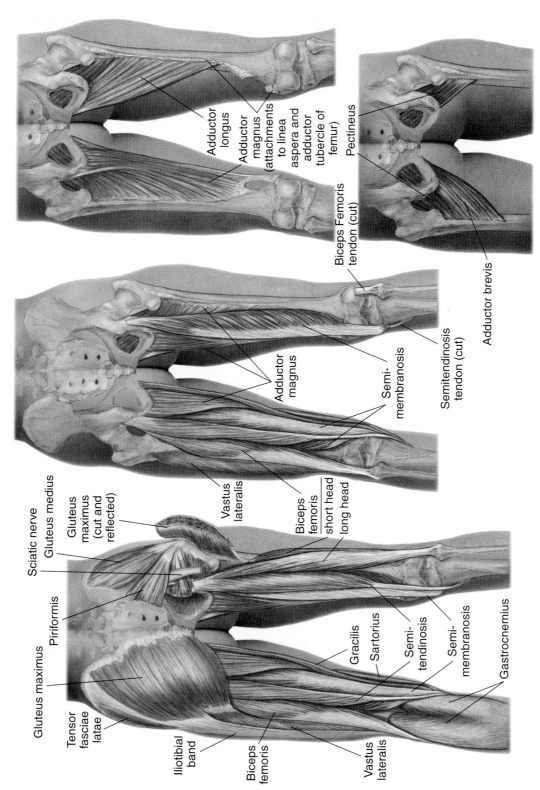

Plate 9-5 Muscles of the thigh, posterior view

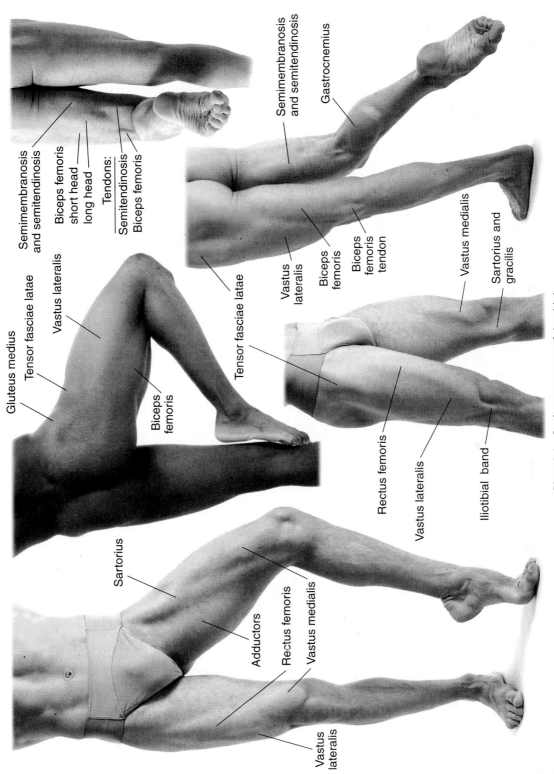

Plate 9-6 Surface anatomy of the thigh

OVERVIEW OF THE REGION

The powerful muscles of the thigh can be divided into four basic groups: anterior **(quadriceps and sartorius)**, posterior **(hamstrings)**, lateral **(tensor fasciae latae** and **iliotibial band)**, and medial **(hip adductors)**. Although some pain in the thigh is referred from superior muscles in and around the pelvis and from the lower leg, pain may also originate in the thigh muscles themselves.

The muscles of the thigh are one of the principal contributors to knee pain, as their primary function is to move and stabilize the knee joint. Their importance in maintaining posture is considerable, both in their control of the knee and in the influence of **rectus femoris** and the hip adductors on the position of the pelvis. Rectus femoris attaches at the **ASIS**, and **adductor longus, adductor brevis, pectineus,** and **gracilis** all have attachments to various anterior aspects of the **pubis**. Therefore, all these muscles can contribute to an anterior pelvic rotation. The hamstrings, on the other hand, attach to the ischial tuberosity and can pull the pelvis into posterior rotation. When we say that quadriceps and hamstrings are antagonists, we usually think of their opposing functions in flexing and extending the knee, but they are also antagonists in the positioning of the pelvis.

The relative tension of the muscles of the thigh also determines the position of the **head of the femur** in the **acetabulum**, and thus the position and movement of the femur in standing and walking. In addition, since the muscles of the **quadriceps** group attach to the **tibia** via a common tendon enclosing the **patella**, these muscles determine the position of the patella. Together, the quadriceps and hamstrings dictate the position and balance of stress in the knee joint.

Careful observation of the gait of the client in the initial examination will reveal much information about the muscles of the thigh, because they affect the position and movement of the hips and knees throughout the gait cycle.

Note that the connective tissue structure attaching quadriceps to the tibia and enclosing the patella is generally referred to as the *patellar tendon* above the patella and as the *patellar ligament* below the patella.

 Caution

Be familiar with the femoral triangle, a triangular space at the upper part of the thigh, bounded by sartorius laterally, adductor longus medially, and the inguinal ligament superiorly (see Plate 9-2). Deep to these muscles it is bounded laterally by iliopsoas and medially by pectineus. The femoral triangle contains the femoral vessels and the branches of the femoral nerve. When working on the anterior and medial thigh, take care not to exert pressure on these structures.

MUSCLES OF THE ANTERIOR THIGH

Quadriceps Femoris (Fig. 9-1)

KWAD-ris-seps fe-MOR-is, FEM-or-is

Etymology Latin *quadri,* four + *caput,* head, therefore, four-headed

Comment

Three of the muscles (the vasti) of the quadriceps group cross only the knee joint, while one (rectus femoris) crosses both the hip and the knee joint.

All have a common inferior attachment via the patellar tendon.

Attachments

- Inferiorly, by four heads: rectus femoris, vastus lateralis, vastus intermedius, and vastus medialis to the patella, and thence by ligamentum patellae (patellar ligament) to the tibial tuberosity; vastus medialis also to the medial condyle of the tibia
- Superiorly, as follows:
    - Rectus Femoris: to the anterior inferior spine of ilium and upper margin of acetabulum
    - Vastus lateralis: to the lateral lip of the linea aspera as far as the greater trochanter
    - Vastus medialis: to the medial lip of the linea aspera
    - Vastus intermedius: to the upper three-fourths of the anterior surface of the shaft of the femur

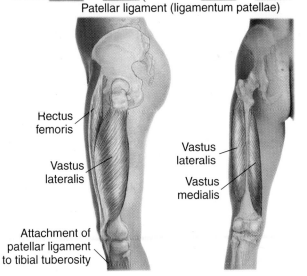

Anterior view

Vastus lateralis

Anterior, inferior iliac spine

Vastus lateralis
Rectus femoris
Vastus medialis
Patellar tendon
Medial condyle of tibia

Vastus inter-medius

Cut attach-ments of superficial quadriceps heads

Patellar ligament (ligamentum patellae)

Hectus femoris

Vastus lateralis

Vastus lateralis

Vastus medialis

Attachment of patellar ligament to tibial tuberosity

Lateral view   Posterior attachment

Figure 9-1 Anatomy of quadriceps femoris

Action

Extends the knee; flexes the hip by the action of rectus femoris

Referral area

- Vastus medialis and intermedius: to the anterior thigh and the knee
- Vastus lateralis: to the lateral thigh and the knee

Other muscles to examine

- Hip adductors
- Tensor fasciae latae and iliotibial band
- Obturator internus (may cause pain in the anterior thigh through entrapment of the obturator nerve)

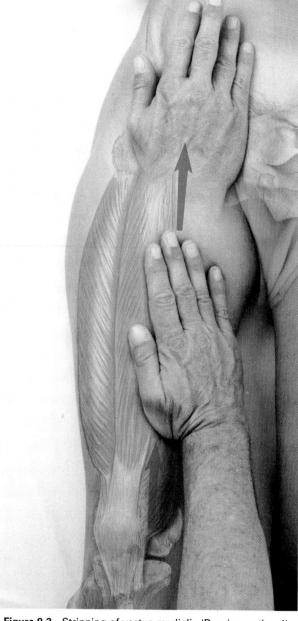

Figure 9-3 Stripping of vastus medialis (Draping option 4)

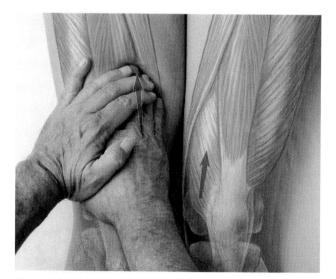

Figure 9-2 Stripping of vastus medialis with the fingertips (Draping option 4)

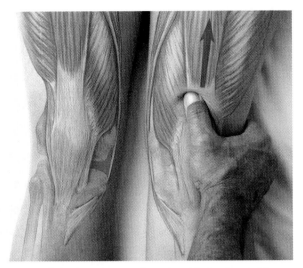

Figure 9-4 Stripping of rectus femoris with the thumb (Draping option 5)

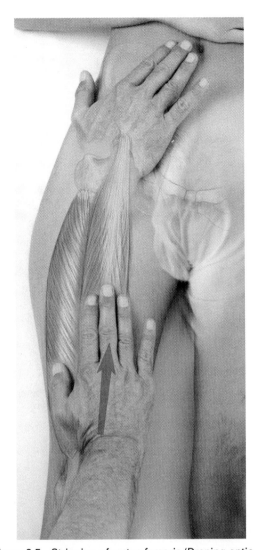

Figure 9-5 Stripping of rectus femoris (Draping option 5)

Manual Therapy

STRIPPING

- The client lies supine.
- The therapist stands beside the client at the lower legs.
- Place the heel of the hand, the thumb, or the fingertips (Fig. 9-2) on the quadriceps tendon where it attaches to the patella on the medial side.
- Pressing firmly into the tissue, slide along vastus medialis to its attachment on the upper femur (Fig. 9-3).
- Beginning again at the kneecap in the center, repeat this procedure, continuing the stroke along rectus femoris to its attachment at the ASIS (Fig. 9-4–9-5).
- Repeat the same procedure laterally on vastus lateralis (Fig. 9-6–9-7).
- Note: Vastus intermedius lies deep to the other quadriceps muscles, and is therefore treated through them.

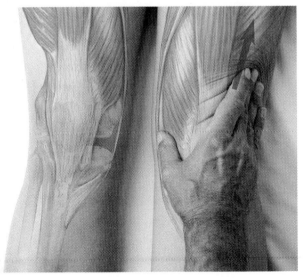

Figure 9-6 Stripping of vastus lateralis with the fingertips (Draping option 4)

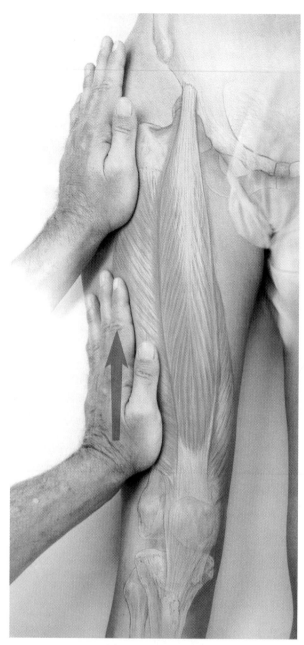

Figure 9-7 Stripping of vastus lateralis (Draping option 4)

CROSS-FIBER FRICTION FOR THE PATELLAR TENDON AND LIGAMENT

- The client lies supine.
- The therapist stands beside the client at the legs.
- Place the thumb on the patellar tendon (superior to the patella).
- Press firmly into the tissue, and move the thumb back and forth across the tendon until you feel a softening and relaxation in the tissue (Fig. 9-8A).
- Repeat this procedure on the patellar ligament (inferior to the patella) (Fig. 9-8B).

CROSS-FIBER FRICTION ON DEEP SURFACE OF PATELLA

- With one hand, displace the patella away from yourself.
- Place the fingertips of the other hand under the patella.
- Pressing upward into the patella, move your fingertips back and forth until you feel a softening and relaxation in the tissue (Fig. 9-9A).
- Repeat the procedure medially (Fig. 9-9B).

Caution

The above procedure should not be performed on a client who has had recent knee surgery, or is scheduled for such surgery. If a client has had knee surgery in the past, or complains of knee pain, question the client thoroughly before proceeding. When in doubt, have the client obtain permission from her or his physician before proceeding.

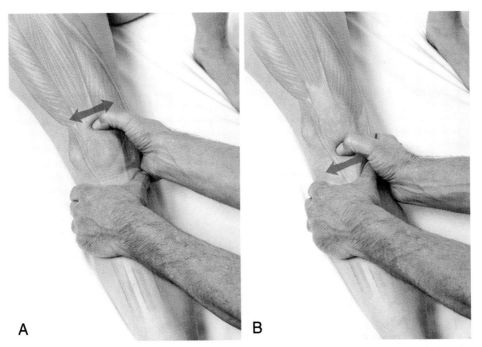

Figure 9-8 Cross-fiber friction of the patellar tendon (A) and ligament (B) (Draping option 4)

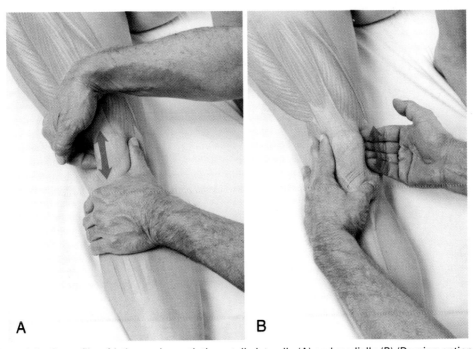

Figure 9-9 Cross-fiber friction underneath the patella laterally (A) and medially (B) (Draping option 4)

Sartorius (Fig. 9-10)

sar-TORE-ee-us

Etymology Latin *sartor,* tailor (from the cross-legged position in which a tailor sits)

Overview

A tight sartorius muscle will often interfere with the stretching of piriformis. If you attempt to stretch piriformis and the client reports feeling the stretch in the anterior thigh, release sartorius before proceeding.

Attachments

- Superiorly, to the anterior superior iliac spine
- Inferiorly, to the medial border of the tuberosity of the tibia

Action

Flexes hip and knee, rotates knee medially and hip laterally

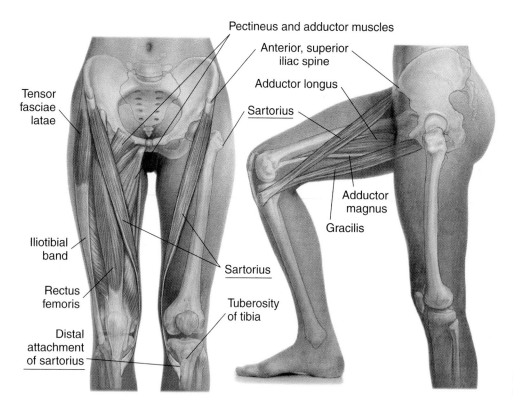

Figure 9-10 Anatomy of sartorius

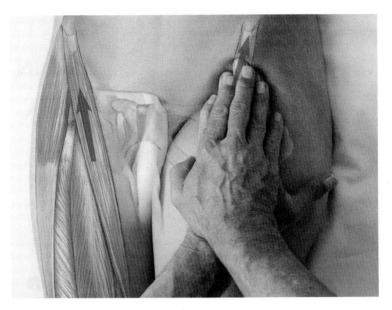

Figure 9-11 Stripping of sartorius with the fingertips (Draping option 5)

Referral Area

To the anterior and medial aspects of the thigh

Other Muscles to Examine

■ Quadriceps
■ Hip adductors

Manual Therapy

STRIPPING
■ The client lies supine.
■ The therapist stands beside the client at the legs.
■ Place the heel of the hand, thumb, or fingertips on the medial thigh just superior to the patella.
■ Pressing firmly into the tissue, slide the fingertips diagonally along the muscle across the quadriceps to its attachment on the ASIS (Fig. 9-11).

MUSCLES OF THE POSTERIOR THIGH (HAMSTRINGS)

Overview

From the word "ham," denoting the buttock and back of the thigh, "hamstrings" is an old term for the muscles of the posterior thigh, comprising the long head of biceps, the semitendinosus, and the semimembranosus muscles. Note that these muscles cross both the hip and knee joints, and are therefore important in both movement and stabilization of these joints.

Semitendinosus (Fig. 9-12)

SEM-i-ten-di-NO-sus

Etymology   Latin *semi,* half + *tendinosus,* tendinous

Attachments

- Superiorly, to the ischial tuberosity
- Inferiorly, to the medial surface of the superior fourth of the shaft of the tibia

Action

Extends hip, flexes knee and rotates it medially when flexed

Referral Area

Over the back of the leg from the buttock to the mid-calf

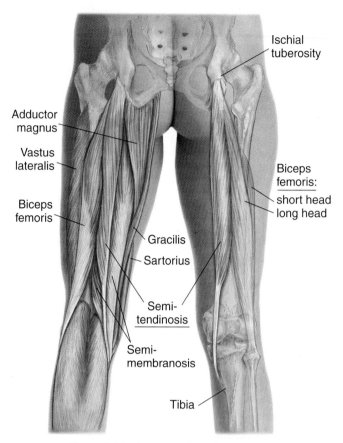

Figure 9-12   Anatomy of semitendinosus

Other Muscles to Examine

- Quadratus lumborum
- Piriformis
- Gluteal muscles
- Hip adductors

Semimembranosus (Fig. 9-13)

SEM-i-mem-bra-NO-sus

Etymology   Latin *semi*, half + *membranosus*, membranous

Attachments

- Superiorly, to the ischial tuberosity
- Inferiorly, to the posterior aspect of the medial condyle of the tibia

Action

Flexes knee and rotates knee medially when flexed; contributes to the stability of extended knee by making capsule of knee joint tense; extends hip

Referral Area

Over the back of the leg from the buttock to the mid-calf

Other Muscles to Examine

- Quadratus lumborum
- Piriformis
- Gluteal muscles
- Hip adductors

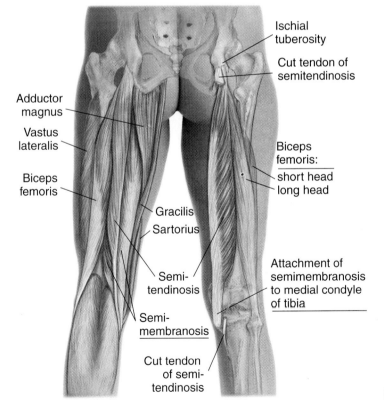

Figure 9-13   Anatomy of semimembranosus

Biceps Femoris (Fig. 9-14)

BUY-seps fe-MORE-is

Etymology Latin *biceps*, two-headed + *femoris*, of the femur

Attachments

- Superiorly, the long head to the ischial tuberosity, the short head to the lower half of the lateral lip of linea aspera
- Inferiorly, to the head of the fibula

Action

Flexes knee and rotates flexed knee laterally; long head extends hip

Referral Area

Over the back of the leg from the buttock to the mid-calf

Other Muscles to Examine

- Quadratus lumborum
- Piriformis
- Gluteal muscles
- Hip adductors

Manual Therapy for Hamstrings

STRIPPING
- The client lies prone.
- The therapist stands beside the client at the calves.
- Place the fingertips, heel of the hand, forearm, or knuckles on the medial aspect of the hamstrings just superior to the knee.
- Pressing firmly into the tissue, slide along the muscle to its attachment on the ischial tuberosity (Fig. 9-15).
- Beginning in the center, repeat this procedure (Fig. 9-16).
- Repeat the same procedure on the lateral aspect (Fig. 9-17).

Caution

At the beginning of the above procedure, avoid pressure into the popliteal space behind the knee.

COMPRESSION AND CROSS-FIBER FRICTION
- Place the thumbs on the attachment of the hamstrings to the ischial tuberosity (Fig. 9-18).
- Press superiorly into the tissue and hold for release.
- Alternatively, move the thumbs from side to side until you feel a softening and relaxation in the tissue.

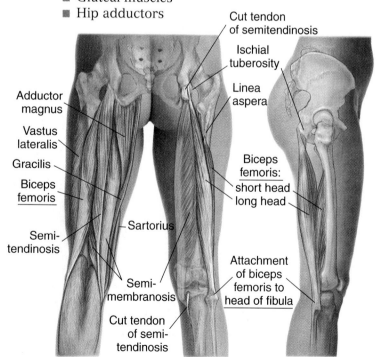

Figure 9-14 Anatomy of biceps femoris

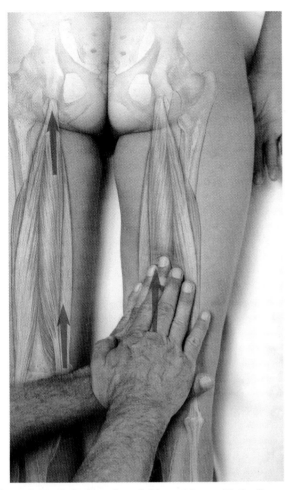

Figure 9-15 Stripping of medial hamstrings with the fingertips (Draping option 10)

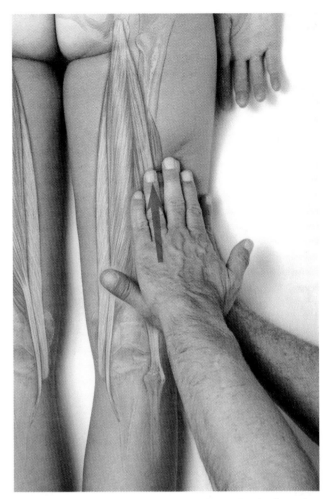

Figure 9-17 Stripping of lateral hamstrings with the fingertips (Draping option 10)

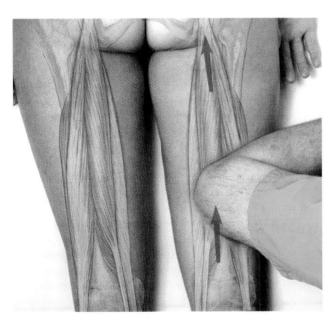

Figure 9-16 Stripping of hamstrings with the forearm (Draping option 10)

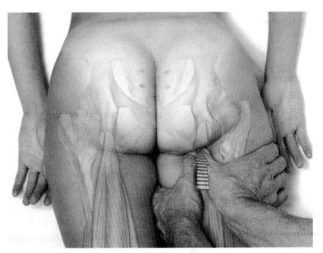

Figure 9-18 Compression of hamstring attachments against the ischial tuberosity (Draping option 10)

THE LATERAL THIGH: TENSOR FASCIAE LATAE AND THE ILIOTIBIAL BAND (ILIOTIBIAL TRACT, ITB)

Overview

The iliotibial band is a fibrous reinforcement (thickening) of the fascia lata (the deep fascia of the thigh) on the lateral surface of the thigh, extending from the crest of the ilium to the lateral condyle of the tibia. Tensor fasciae latae attaches to it and tenses the deep fascia. Together they serve as a flexor, abductor, and medial rotator of the hip. Tensor fasciae latae and gluteus maximus are the two muscles that insert on and control the iliotibial band.

Tensor Fasciae Latae and the Iliotibial Band (Fig. 9-19)

TEN-ser FASH-a LAT-a
ILL-ee-o-TIB-ee-al band

Etymology Latin *tensor*, tightener + *fasciae*, of the bandage + *latae*, wide

Attachments

- Superiorly, (tensor fasciae latae) to the anterior superior iliac spine and the adjacent lateral and posterior surface of the ilium
- Inferiorly, to the iliotibial band of fascia lata, which attaches to the lateral condyle of the tibia

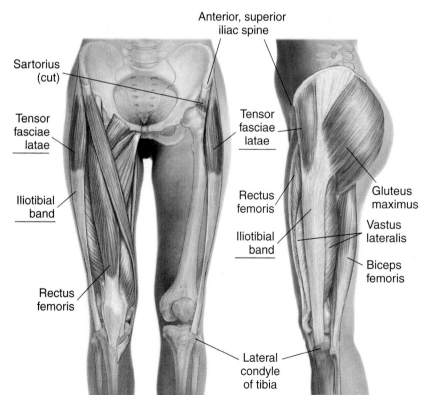

Anterior, superior iliac spine

Sartorius (cut)

Tensor fasciae latae

Iliotibial band

Rectus femoris

Tensor fasciae latae

Rectus femoris

Iliotibial band

Gluteus maximus

Vastus lateralis

Biceps femoris

Lateral condyle of tibia

Figure 9-19 Anatomy of tensor fasciae latae and the iliotibial band

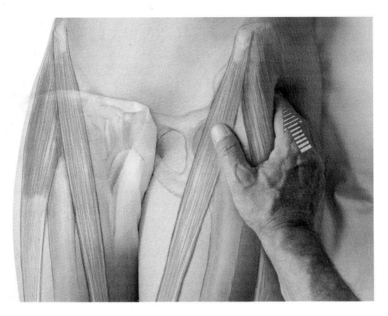

Figure 9-20 Compression of tensor fasciae latae with the fingertips (Draping option 5)

Action

Tenses fascia lata; flexes, abducts and medially rotates hip; also contributes to the lateral stability of the knee

Referral Area

To the lateral aspect of the thigh

Other Muscles to Examine

Vastus lateralis

Manual Therapy for Tensor Fasciae Latae

COMPRESSION
- The client lies supine.
- The therapist stands beside the client at the knee.
- Place the fingertips on the tensor fasciae latae between the greater trochanter and the crest of the ilium.
- Press firmly into the tissue, searching for tender areas. Hold for release (Fig. 9-20).

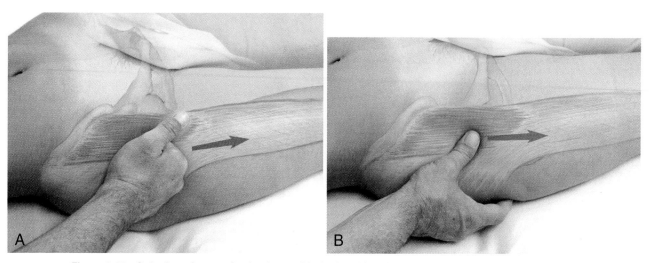

Figure 9-21 Stripping of tensor fasciae latae with the knuckles (A) and the thumb (B) (Draping option 5)

STRIPPING
- The client lies supine.
- The therapist stands beside the client at the chest.
- Place the fingertips, thumb, or knuckles on the tensor fasciae latae just below the iliac crest.

- Pressing firmly into the tissue, glide along the muscle past the greater trochanter (Fig. 9-21, Fig. 9-22).
- Continue the stroke with the next technique for the ITB.

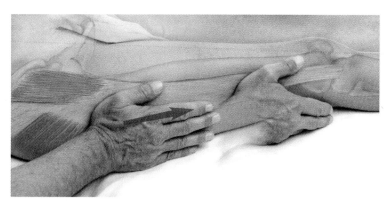

Figure 9-22 Stripping of iliotibial band with client supine (Draping option 5)

Manual Therapy for the Iliotibial Band (ITB)

STRIPPING
- The client lies supine.
- The therapist stands beside the client at the waist.
- Place the heel of the hand or knuckles on the ITB just below the greater trochanter.
- Pressing firmly into the tissue, glide along the muscle to the lateral condyle of the tibia (Fig. 9-22).

STRIPPING
- The client lies on her or his side, with the lower leg straight, and the upper leg flexed at the hip and the knee.
- The therapist stands behind the client at the pelvis.
- Place the heel of the hand or knuckles on the ITB just below the greater trochanter.
- Pressing firmly into the tissue, slide along the muscle to the lateral condyle of the tibia (Fig. 9-23).

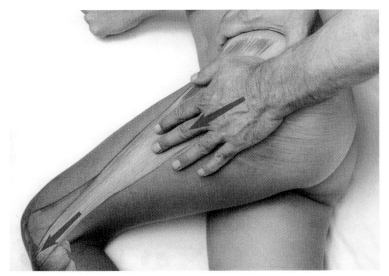

Figure 9-23 Stripping of iliotibial band with client side-lying (Draping option 12)

MUSCLES OF THE MEDIAL THIGH (HIP ADDUCTORS)

Overview

Although we associate the hip adductors chiefly with adduction of the hip, they contribute to flexion, extension, rotation, and stability of the hip in complex ways in standing, walking, climbing stairs, and other activities involving the legs. In your assessment of the client's gait, observe the medial thigh closely for any anomalies such as twitches or catches in the motion of the thigh.

Adductor Magnus (Fig. 9-24)

ad-DUCK-ter MAG-nus

Etymology Latin *ad*, toward + *ducere*, pull + *magnus*, large

Overview

The superior part of adductor magnus is called adductor minimus.

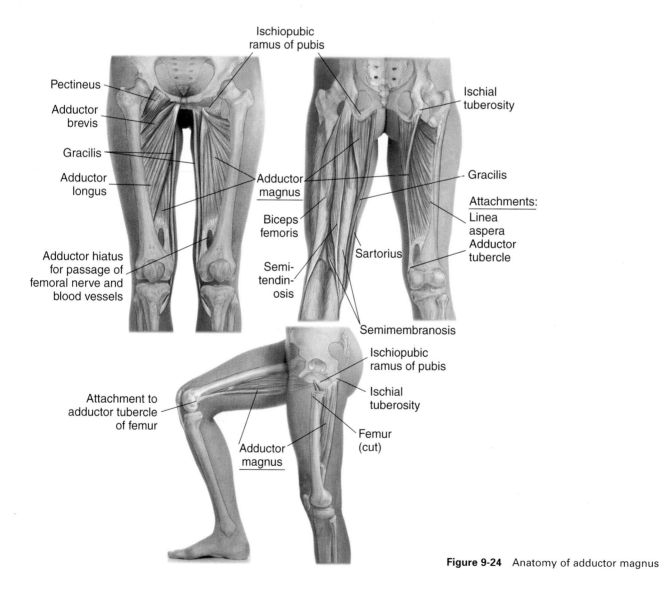

Figure 9-24 Anatomy of adductor magnus

Attachments

■ Superiorly, to the ischial tuberosity and ischiopubic ramus
■ Inferiorly, to the linea aspera and adductor tubercle of the femur

Action

Adducts and extends hip

Referral Area

To the medial aspect of the thigh

Other Muscles to Examine

Other hip adductors

Adductor Longus (Fig. 9-25)

ad-DUCK-ter LONG-gus

Etymology   Latin *ad,* toward + *ducere,* pull + *longus,* long

Attachments

■ Superiorly, symphysis and crest of pubis
■ Inferiorly, to the middle third of medial lip of linea aspera

Action

Adducts hip

Referral Area

To the medial aspect of the thigh

Other Muscles to Examine

Other hip adductors

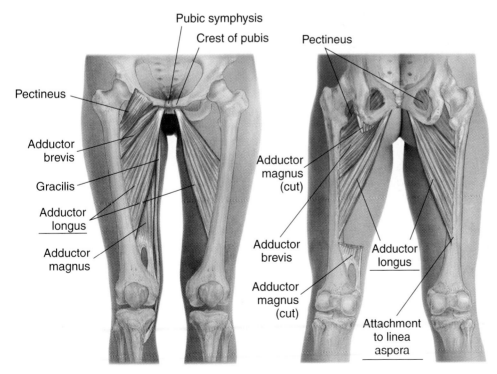

Figure 9-25   Anatomy of adductor longus

Adductor Brevis (Fig. 9-26)

ad-DUCK-ter BREV-is

Etymology   Latin *ad,* toward + *ducere,* pull + *brevis,* short

Attachments

- Superiorly, to the inferior ramus of the pubis
- Inferiorly, to the upper third of medial lip of linea aspera

Action

Adducts hip

Referral Area

To the medial aspect of the thigh

Other Muscles to Examine

Other hip adductors

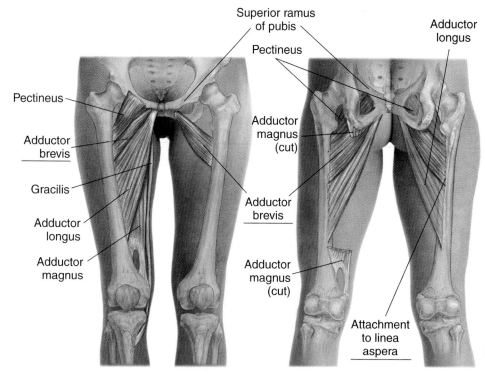

Figure 9-26   Anatomy of adductor brevis

Pectineus (Fig. 9-27)

peck-TIN-ee-us

Etymology Latin *pecten,* comb

Overview

Pectineus is named for its attachment to the pecten, a sharp ridge on the superior pubic ramus.

Attachments

- Superiorly, to the crest of the pubis
- Inferiorly, to the pectineal line of femur between the lesser trochanter and the linea aspera

Action

Adducts and assists in flexion of hip

Referral Area

To the medial aspect of the thigh

Other Muscles to Examine

Other hip adductors

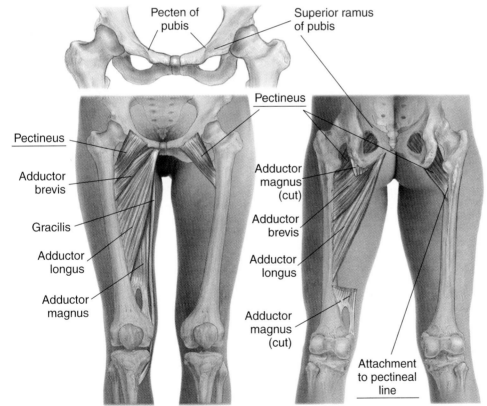

Pecten of pubis

Superior ramus of pubis

Pectineus

Pectineus

Adductor brevis

Gracilis

Adductor longus

Adductor magnus

Adductor magnus (cut)

Adductor brevis

Adductor longus

Adductor magnus (cut)

Attachment to pectineal line

Figure 9-27 Anatomy of pectineus

Gracilis (Fig. 9-28)

GRASS-ill-iss, gra-SILL-iss

Etymology Latin *gracilis,* slender

Attachments

- Superiorly, to the body and inferior ramus of the pubis near the symphysis
- Inferiorly, to the medial shaft of the tibia below the tibial tuberosity

Action

Adducts the hip, flexes the knee, rotates the flexed knee medially

Referral Area

To the medial aspect of the thigh

Other Muscles to Examine

Other hip adductors

Manual Therapy for the Hip Adductors

Note: Some clients may be more comfortable keeping underwear on for work on the hip adductors.

COMPRESSION OF THE ADDUCTOR ATTACHMENTS
- The client lies supine.
- The therapist stands beside the client at the knee.
- Place your thumb on the lateral edge of the pubic crest on the attachment of pectineus (Fig. 9-29).
- Press firmly into the tissue, looking for tender spots. Hold for release.
- Shift the thumb inferiorly and posteriorly along the pubic crest, compressing each adductor attachment (Fig. 9-30).
- Repeat this procedure until you reach the attachment of adductor magnus (Fig. 9-31).
- This technique may also be performed with the hip abducted and externally rotated and the knee partially flexed, and may also be performed with the fingertips (Fig. 9-32).

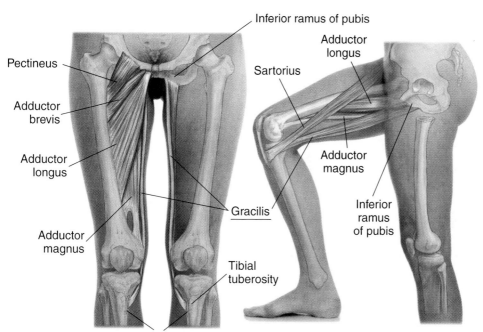

Figure 9-28 Anatomy of gracilis

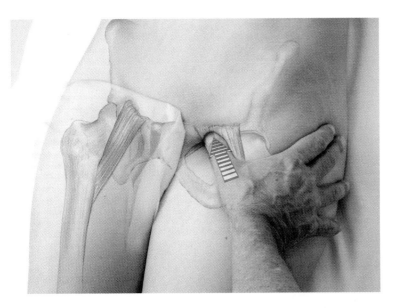

Figure 9-29   Compression of attachment of pectineus (Draping option 5)

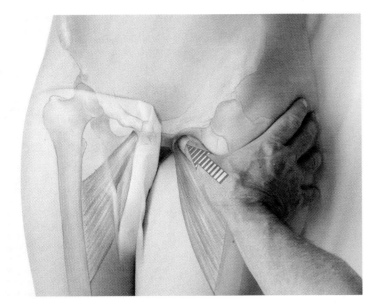

Figure 9-30   Compression of attachment of adductor brevis (Draping option 5)

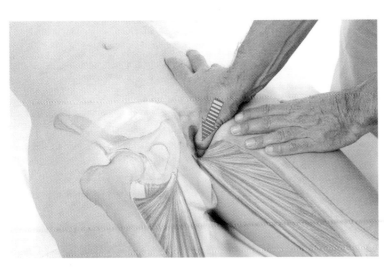

Figure 9-31   Compression of attachment of adductor magnus with thumb (Draping option 5)

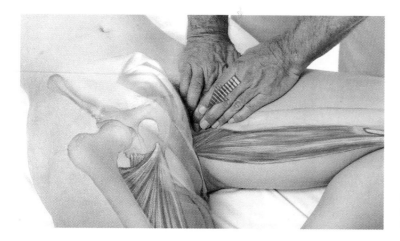

Figure 9-32 Compression of attachment of adductor magnus with fingertips, hip adducted and rotated (Draping option 5)

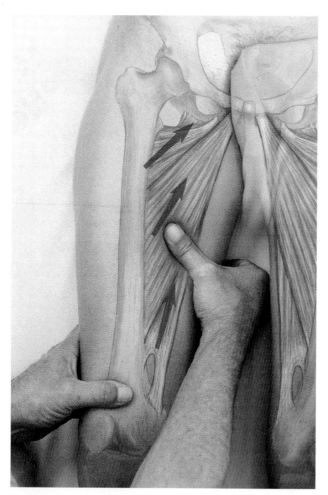

Figure 9-33 Stripping of adductor magnus and longus with thumb, client supine, leg straight, hip slightly abducted (Draping option 5)

STRIPPING AND COMPRESSION OF THE HIP ADDUCTORS

- The client lies supine, either with the leg straight and the hip slightly abducted, or with the hip abducted and externally rotated and the knee partially flexed.
- The therapist stands beside the client at the knees.
- Place the fingertips or thumb(s) just above the medial epicondyle of the femur.
- Pressing firmly into the tissue, glide the fingertips along the adductors to the anterior aspect of the pubic arch.
- Beginning at the same spot, repeat this procedure, ending each time more posteriorly along the pubis (Fig. 9-33, Fig. 9-34, Fig. 9-35).
- You may also perform compression against the femur along each hip adductor in the same position, using the thumbs (Fig. 9-36).
- Both of these procedures may also be performed with the client lying on her side, with either the lower leg straight and the upper leg flexed at the hip and the knee (Fig. 9-37), or with the upper leg straight and the lower leg flexed at the hip and the knee (Fig. 9-38). However, in these positions it is not possible to work close to the attachments without contacting the genitals.

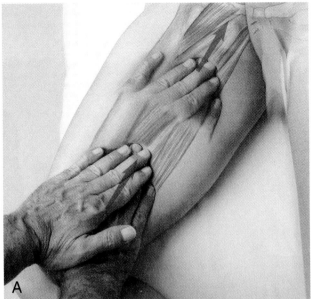

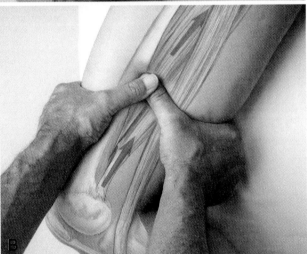

Figure 9-34 Stripping of adductor magnus and gracilis, client supine, hip adducted and externally rotated, hip and knee flexed: (A) with fingertips, (B) with thumb (Draping option 5)

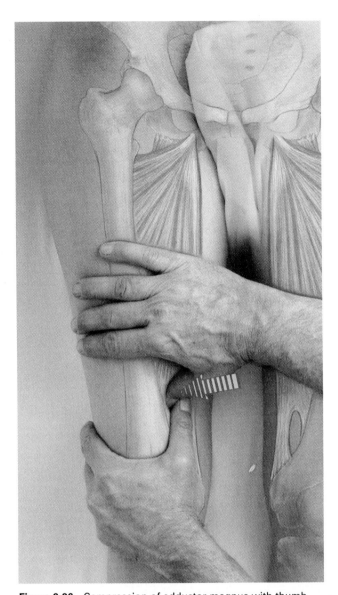

Figure 9-36 Compression of adductor magnus with thumb, leg straight (Draping option 5)

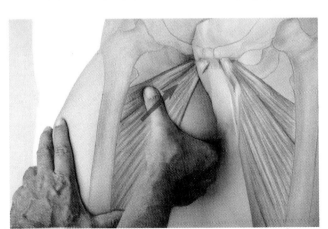

Figure 9-35 Stripping of adductor brevis and longus with thumb, client supine, hip adducted and externally rotated, hip and knee flexed (Draping option 5)

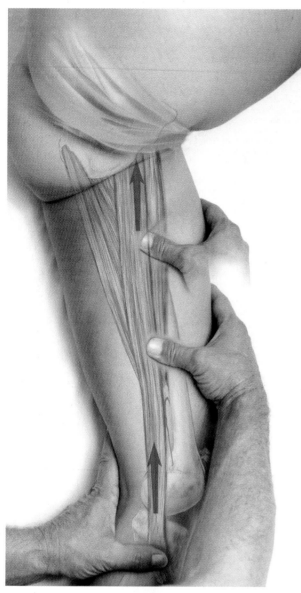

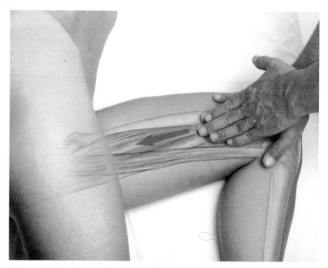

Figure 9-38   Stripping of adductors with client side-lying, upper leg straight (Draping option 12 or underwear)

Figure 9-37   Stripping of adductors with client side-lying, lower leg straight (Draping option 12 or underwear)

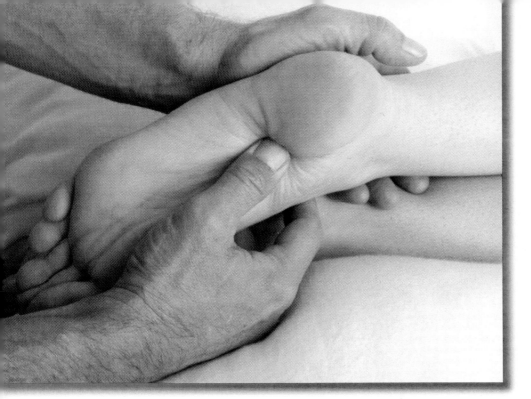

Muscles of the Leg, Ankle, and Foot

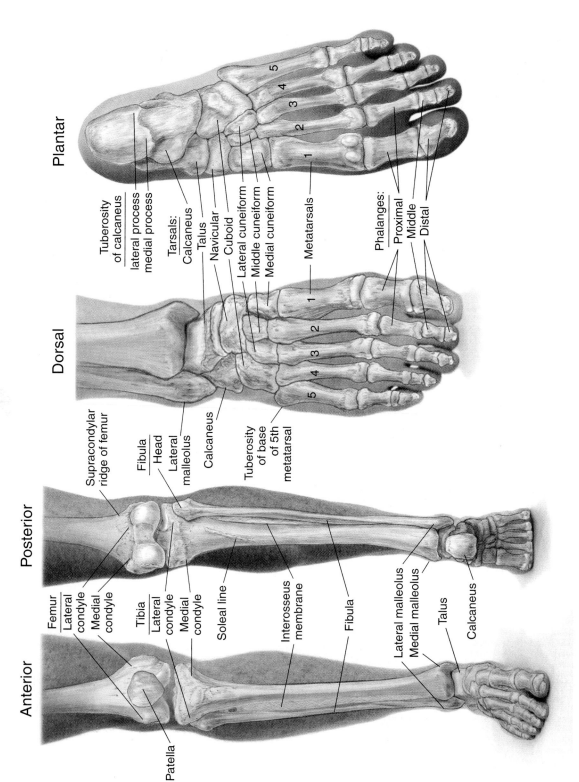

Plantar

Tuberosity
of calcaneus
lateral process
medial process

Tarsals:
Calcaneus
Talus
Navicular
Cuboid
Lateral cuneiform
Middle cuneiform
Medial cuneiform

Metatarsals

Phalanges:
Proximal
Middle
Distal

Dorsal

Supracondylar
ridge of femur

Fibula
Head
Lateral
malleolus

Calcaneus

Tuberosity
of base
of 5th
metatarsal

Posterior

Femur
Lateral
condyle
Medial
condyle

Tibia
Lateral
condyle
Medial
condyle

Soleal line

Interosseus
membrane

Fibula

Lateral malleolus
Medial malleolus

Talus

Calcaneus

Anterior

Patella

Plate 10-1 Skeletal features of the leg and foot

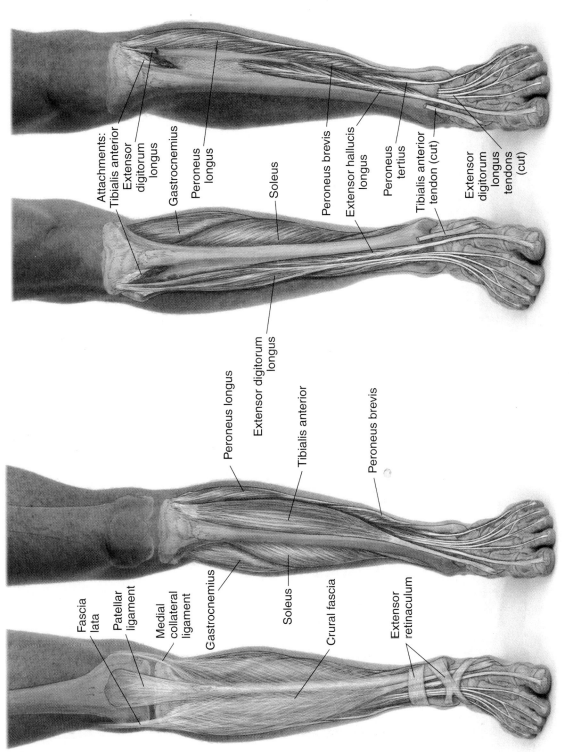

Attachments:
Tibialis anterior
Extensor digitorum longus
Gastrocnemius
Peroneus longus
Soleus
Peroneus brevis
Extensor hallucis longus
Peroneus tertius
Tibialis anterior tendon (cut)
Extensor digitorum longus tendons (cut)

Peroneus longus
Extensor digitorum longus
Tibialis anterior
Peroneus brevis

Fascia lata
Patellar ligament
Medial collateral ligament
Gastrocnemius
Soleus
Crural fascia
Extensor retinaculum

Plate 10-2   Muscles of the leg, anterior view

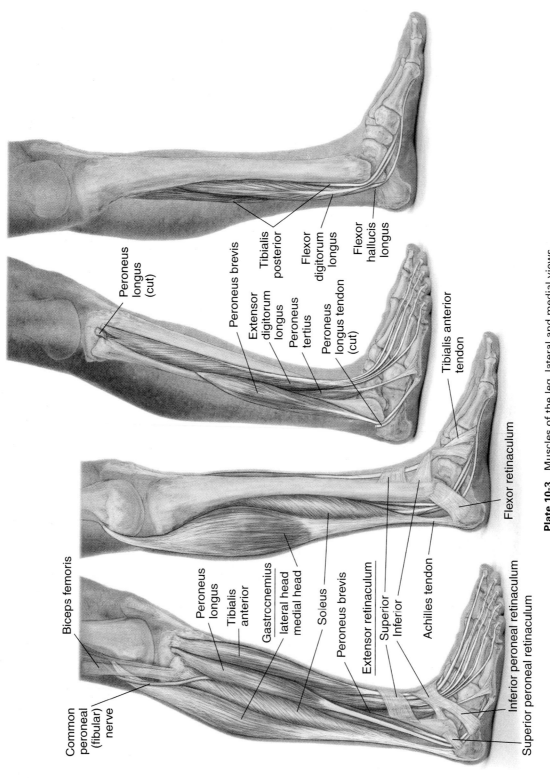

Biceps femoris

Common peroneal (fibular) nerve

Peroneus longus

Tibialis anterior

Gastrocnemius
lateral head
medial head

Soleus

Peroneus brevis

Extensor retinaculum
Superior
Inferior

Achilles tendon

Inferior peroneal retinaculum

Superior peroneal retinaculum

Peroneus longus (cut)

Peroneus brevis   Tibialis posterior

Extensor digitorum longus

Peroneus tertius

Peroneus longus tendon (cut)

Flexor digitorum longus

Flexor hallucis longus

Tibialis anterior tendon

Flexor retinaculum

Plate 10-3   Muscles of the leg, lateral and medial views

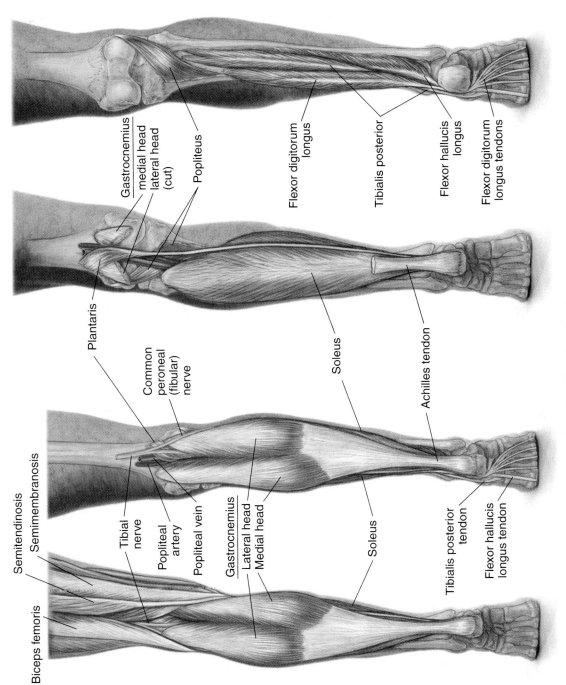

Plate 10-4   Muscles of the leg, posterior view

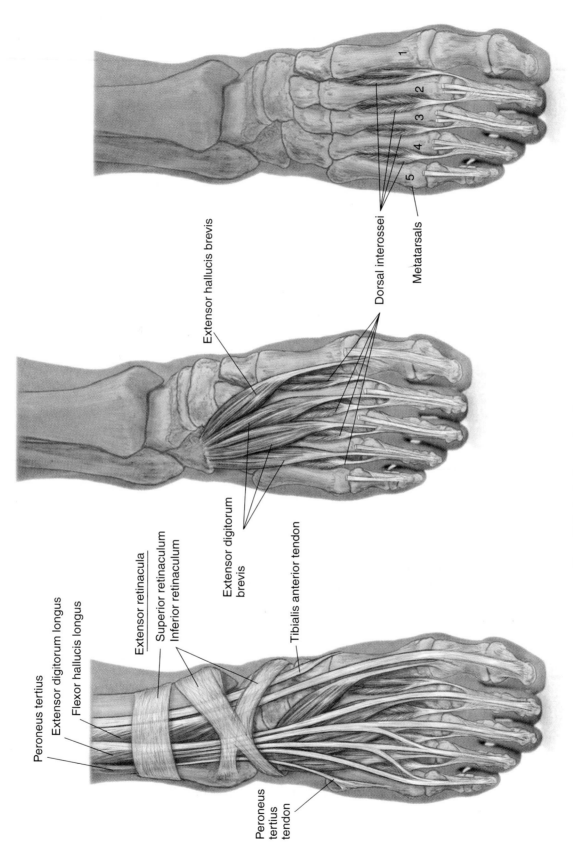

Peroneus tertius

Extensor digitorum longus

Flexor hallucis longus

Extensor retinacula
Superior retinaculum
Inferior retinaculum

Extensor digitorum brevis

Tibialis anterior tendon

Peroneus tertius tendon

Extensor hallucis brevis

Dorsal interossei

Metatarsals

1
2
3
4
5

Plate 10-5   Intrinsic muscles of the foot, dorsal view

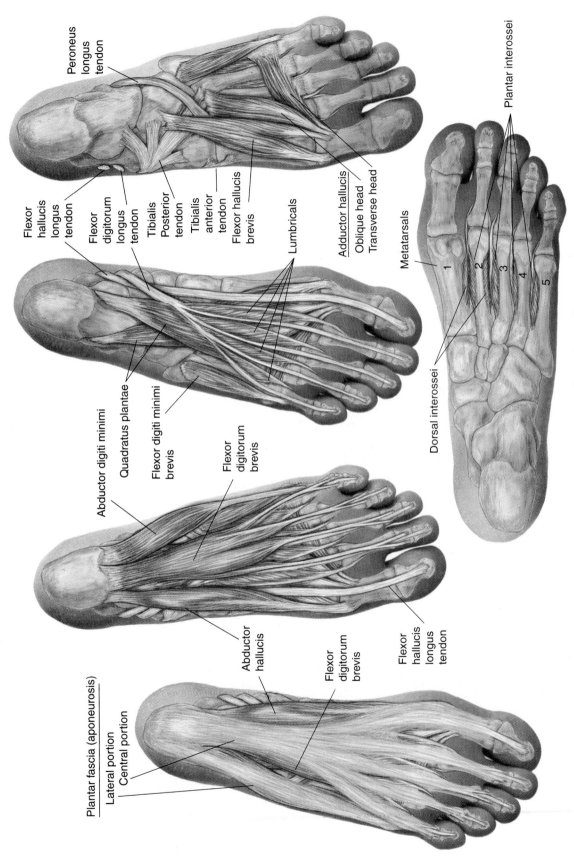

Peroneus
longus
tendon

Plantar interossei

Flexor
hallucis
longus
tendon

Flexor
digitorum
longus
tendon

Tibialis
Posterior
tendon

Tibialis
anterior
tendon

Flexor hallucis
brevis

Lumbricals

Adductor hallucis
Oblique head
Transverse head

Metatarsals

1
2
3
4
5

Abductor digiti minimi

Quadratus plantae

Flexor digiti minimi
brevis

Flexor
digitorum
brevis

Dorsal interossei

Abductor
hallucis

Flexor
digitorum
brevis

Flexor
hallucis
longus
tendon

Plantar fascia (aponeurosis)
Lateral portion
Central portion

Plate 10-6 Intrinsic muscles of the foot, plantar view

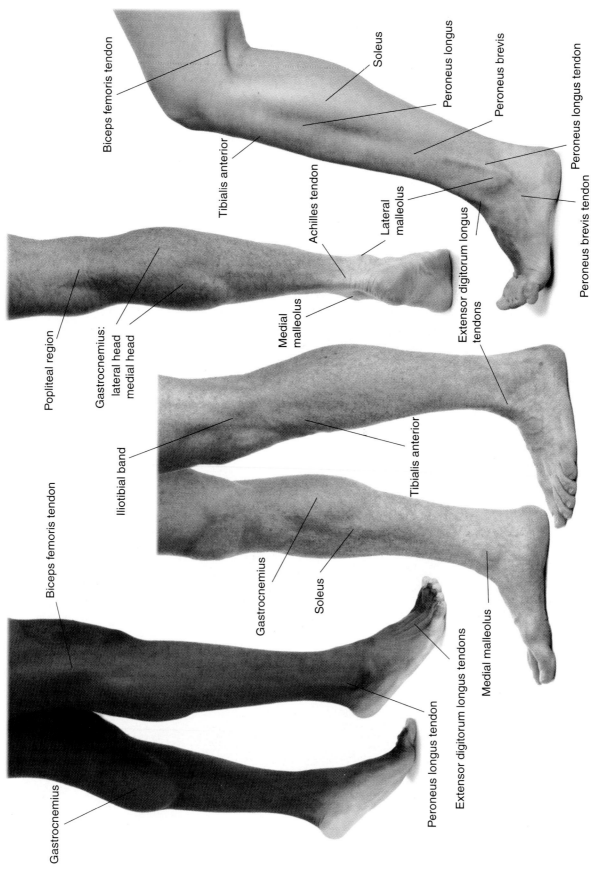

Plate 10-7 Surface Anatomy of the leg and foot

Biceps femoris tendon

Tibialis anterior

Soleus

Peroneus longus

Peroneus brevis

Peroneus longus tendon

Achilles tendon

Lateral malleolus

Extensor digitorum longus tendons

Peroneus brevis tendon

Popliteal region

Gastrocnemius: lateral head medial head

Medial malleolus

Biceps femoris tendon

Iliotibial band

Tibialis anterior

Gastrocnemius

Soleus

Peroneus longus tendon

Extensor digitorum longus tendons

Medial malleolus

Gastrocnemius

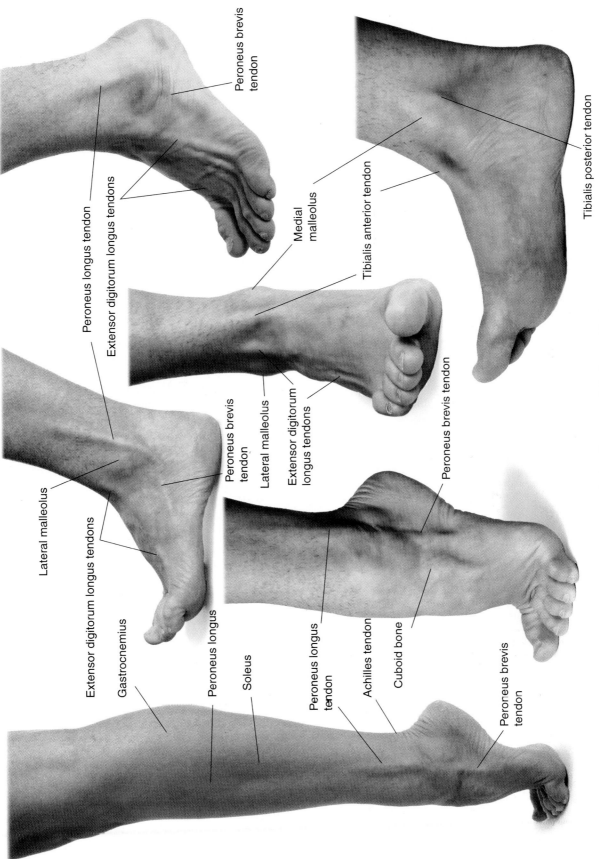

Peroneus brevis tendon

Peroneus longus tendon

Extensor digitorum longus tendons

Medial malleolus

Tibialis posterior tendon

Tibialis anterior tendon

Peroneus brevis tendon

Lateral malleolus

Extensor digitorum longus tendons

Peroneus brevis tendon

Lateral malleolus

Extensor digitorum longus tendons

Gastrocnemius

Peroneus longus

Soleus

Peroneus longus tendon

Achilles tendon

Cuboid bone

Peroreus brevis tendon

Plate 10-8 Surface Anatomy of the leg and foot

OVERVIEW OF THE REGION

The feet are the foundation of the human body and the pivot points for its locomotion. The principal muscles controlling the feet are found in the leg. Tendons of these muscles reach various points in the foot via the ankle, usually making right-angle turns and covering long distances to do so. The complex structure of the leg, ankle, and foot, along with its massive weight-bearing requirements, makes it vulnerable to a wide variety of injuries and chronic myofascial problems.

Because they serve as the foundation, the feet, ankles, and legs affect and are profoundly affected by posture. For balanced posture, the weight of the body should rest at a point just forward of the ankle. The body will compensate in a variety of ways to ensure that the weight does not fall behind this point. If the weight falls in front of this point, the calf and foot muscles must work constantly to keep the body from falling forward. Chronic tightness and trigger points in the calf muscle are usually attributable to this imbalance and are very common.

Note that the bones and joints in the leg, ankle, and foot are similar in number to those in the forearm, wrist, and hand, but their functions and the demands placed on them are quite different.

The ankle joint itself allows for virtually no lateral or medial movement. External and internal rotation of the feet are accomplished primarily at the hip. The foot is capable of external and internal rotation, inversion, eversion, supination, and pronation. Chronic supination or pronation of the foot are dysfunctions requiring correction appropriate to their cause.

The principal movements of the foot at the ankle are plantar and dorsal flexion. These are the primary movements of locomotion, and they are accompanied by complex activity in both the muscles of the foot that reside one the leg and the intrinsic muscles of the foot. In locomotion, weight is transferred successively from the back to the front, as the action proceeds from the heel strike to the function of the toes in pushing off. Many other movements involve intricate coordination of these muscles: running, climbing, diving, dancing, to name but a few. The healthy foot and leg are well-equipped to carry out these activities with impressive dexterity.

Aside from traumatic injuries, the most stressful activity for the legs, ankles, and feet is simply standing for long periods of time. If the posture is out of balance, standing places tremendous stress on these structures, as already described. But even if the posture is good, muscles function best either in motion or at rest—not under constant stress.

CONNECTIVE TISSUE OF THE LEG AND FOOT

Crural Fascia (Fig. 10-1)

Comment

The crural fascia is the deep fascia of the entire lower limb. It is continuous with the fascia lata, attaches to the ligaments of the patella, and thickens at the ankle to form the retinacula. Treatment of the crural fascia, including the fascia over the tibia, frees the structures of the leg.

Manual Therapy

FASCIAL STRIPPING
- The client lies supine.
- The therapist stands at the client's feet.
- Place the heel of the hand on the medial side of the leg just superior to the ankle.
- Pressing firmly into the tissue, slide the heel of the hand in a cephalad and posterior direction (Fig. 10-2A).

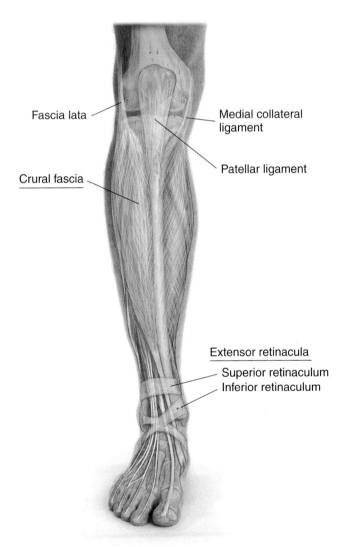

Figure 10-1   Anatomy of the crural fascia

Fascia lata

Crural fascia

Medial collateral ligament

Patellar ligament

Extensor retinacula
Superior retinaculum
Inferior retinaculum

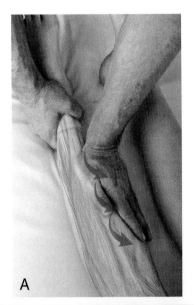

A

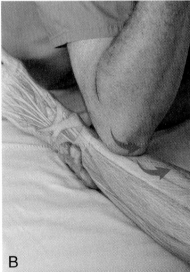

B

Figure 10-2   Deep stroking of the crural fascia with the heel of the hand (A) and the elbow (B)

- Repeat this procedure, with the hand just above the previous starting position.
- Repeat the same procedure, proceeding up the leg as far as the medial condyle.
- You may also use the elbow (Fig. 10-2B) or supported thumb (Fig. 10-3) for this procedure.

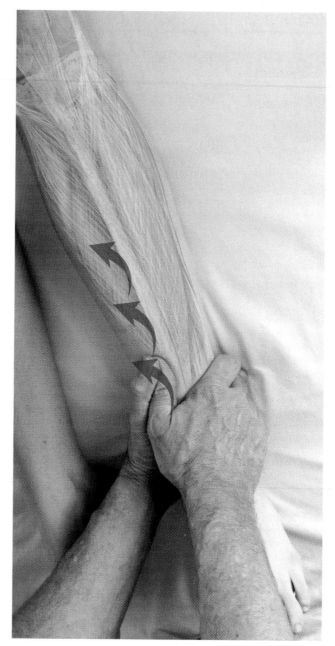

Figure 10-3 Deep stroking of the crural fascia with supported thumb

FLEXOR, EXTENSOR, AND PERONEAL RETINACULA (FIG. 10-4)

Flexor Retinaculum

Overview

The flexor retinaculum is a wide band passing from the medial malleolus to the medial and upper border of the calcaneus and to the plantar surface as far as the navicular bone. It holds in place the tendons of the tibialis posterior, flexor digitorum longus, and flexor hallucis longus.

Inferior Extensor Retinaculum

Overview

The inferior extensor retinaculum is a Y-shaped ligament restraining the extensor tendons of the foot distal to the ankle joint.

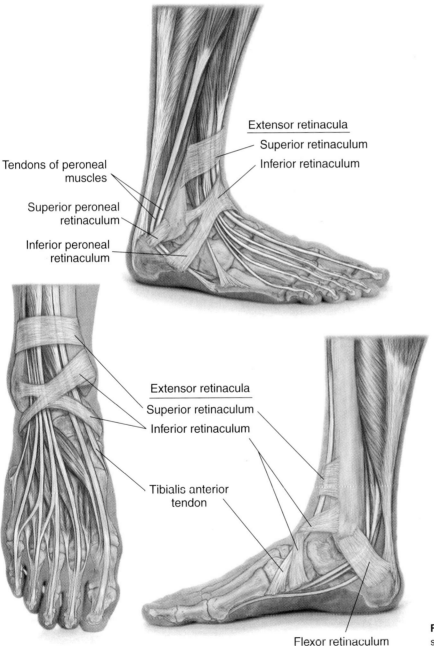

Extensor retinacula
- Superior retinaculum
- Inferior retinaculum

Tendons of peroneal muscles

Superior peroneal retinaculum

Inferior peroneal retinaculum

Extensor retinacula
- Superior retinaculum
- Inferior retinaculum

Tibialis anterior tendon

Flexor retinaculum

Figure 10-4 Anatomy of the flexor, extensor, and peroneal retinacula

Superior Extensor Retinaculum

Overview

The superior extensor retinaculum is a ligament that binds the extensor tendons proximal to the ankle joint; it is continuous with (a thickening of) the deep fascia of the leg.

Peroneal Retinaculum

Overview

The peroneal retinaculum consists of superior and inferior fibrous bands that retain the tendons of the peroneus longus and brevis in position as they cross the lateral side of the ankle.

Manual Therapy for the Retinacula

Comment

Although there are distinct retinacula of the ankle, they are treated together.

CROSS-FIBER STROKING
- The client lies supine.
- The therapist stands at the client's feet.
- Place the thumb on the dorsum of the foot just below the ankle, over the navicular bone.
- Pressing firmly into the tissue, slide the thumb up the ankle about three inches (Fig. 10-5A).
- Repeat this procedure (Fig. 10-5B), moving laterally around the ankle all the way to the Achilles tendon (Fig. 10-5C).
- Repeat this procedure, moving around the ankle medially (Fig. 10-6A) all the way to the Achilles tendon (Fig. 10-6B).
- Note that the distal aspect of the retinaculum lies more distal on the foot on the lateral side.

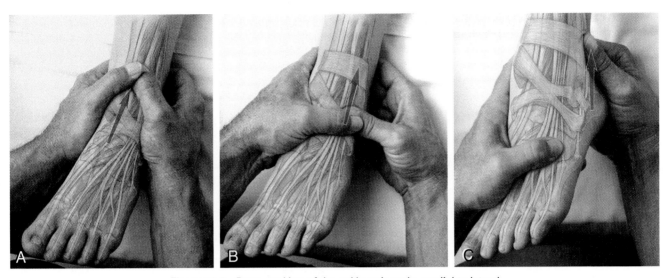

Figure 10-5   Deep stroking of the ankle retinacula, medial to lateral

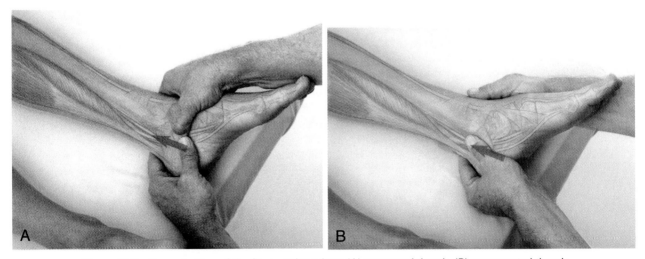

Figure 10-6   Deep stroking of the flexor retinaculum: (A) supported thumb, (B) unsupported thumb

PLANTAR FASCIA (PLANTAR APONEUROSIS) (FIG. 10-7)

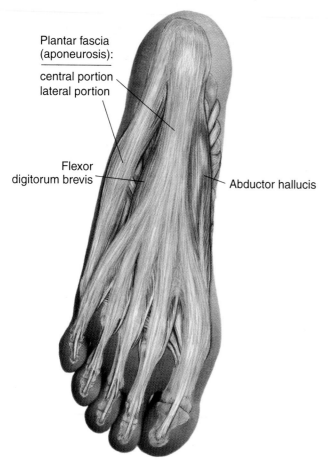

Plantar fascia (aponeurosis):

central portion
lateral portion

Flexor digitorum brevis

Abductor hallucis

Figure 10-7 Anatomy of the plantar fascia

Overview

The plantar fascia is the very thick, central portion of the fascia investing the plantar muscles; it radiates toward the toes from the medial process of the calcaneal tuberosity and provides attachment to the short flexor muscle of the toes.

Manual Therapy

- The client lies prone, the feet on a pillow or bolster.
- The therapist stands or sits at the client's feet.
- Place the thumb or supported thumb on the plantar aspect of the foot on the medial side, just proximal to the base of the big toe.
- Pressing firmly into the tissue, glide the thumb to the heel (Fig. 10-8).
- Repeat this procedure, starting just lateral to the previous starting position.
- Repeat the same procedure until the entire plantar surface has been treated.
- This procedure can be carried out for the entire plantar surface with the knuckles (Fig. 10-9).

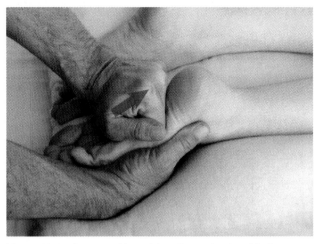

Figure 10-9   Deep stroking of the plantar fascia with the knuckles

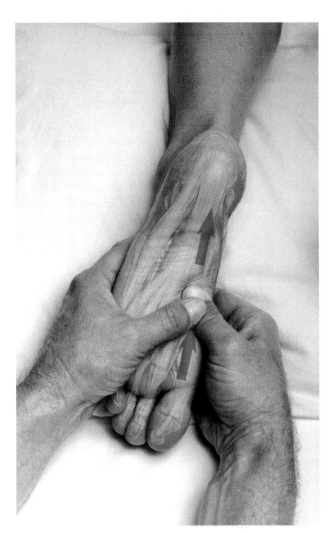

Figure 10-8   Deep stroking of the plantar fascia with the thumbs

ANTERIOR MUSCLES OF THE LEG

Tibialis Anterior

tib-ee-AL-is an-TEER-ee-or
(Fig. 10-10)

Etymology Latin *tibialis,* of the tibia + *anterior,* front

Comment

Be aware that tibialis anterior crosses from the anterolateral side of the leg to the medial side of the foot.

Attachments

- Proximally, to the superior two-thirds of the lateral surface of tibia, and to the interosseous membrane
- Distally, to the medial cuneiform and the base of the first metatarsal

Action

Dorsiflexion and inversion of foot

Referral Area

- To the anterior aspect of the ankle
- Over the dorsal aspect of the phalanx of the great toe

Other Muscles to Examine

Extensor hallucis longus

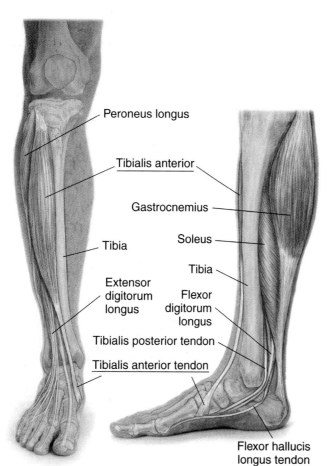

Peroneus longus

Tibialis anterior

Gastrocnemius

Soleus

Tibia

Tibia

Extensor digitorum longus

Flexor digitorum longus

Tibialis posterior tendon

Tibialis anterior tendon

Flexor hallucis longus tendon

Figure 10-10 Anatomy of tibialis anterior

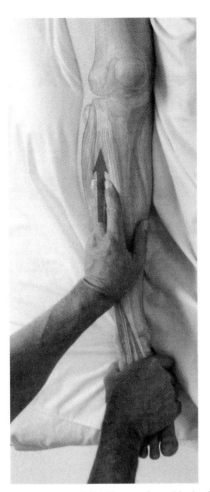

Figure 10-11   Stripping of tibialis anterior with the fingertips

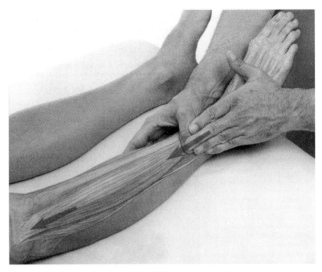

Figure 10-12   Stripping of tibialis anterior with supported thumb

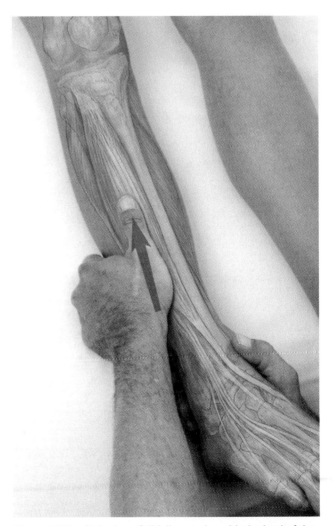

Figure 10.13   Stripping of tibialis anterior with the heel of the hand

Manual Therapy

STRIPPING

- The client lies supine.
- The therapist stands at the client's feet.
- Stabilize the foot with the non-treating hand.
- Place the fingertips on the distal end of the tibialis anterior, just proximal to the ankle.
- Pressing firmly into the tissue, slide the fingertips along the muscle to its attachments on the tibia (Fig. 10-11).
- This procedure may also be carried out with the supported thumb (Fig. 10-12) or the heel of the hand (Fig. 10-13).

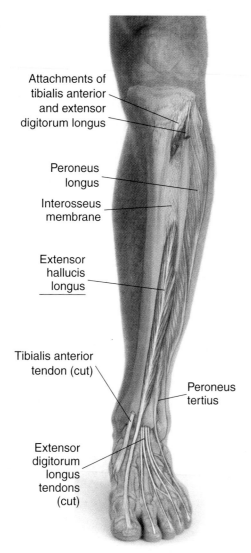

Attachments of
tibialis anterior
and extensor
digitorum longus

Peroneus
longus

Interosseus
membrane

Extensor
hallucis
longus

Tibialis anterior
tendon (cut)

Peroneus
tertius

Extensor
digitorum
longus
tendons
(cut)

Figure 10-14 Anatomy of extensor hallucis longus

Extensor Hallucis Longus (Fig. 10-14)

ex-TENSE-er hal-LOOSE-is, HALL-loose-is LONG-us

Etymology   Latin *extensor,* extender + *hallucis* (from *hallux,* great toe), of the great toe + *longus,* long

Attachments

- Proximally, to the anteromedial surface of the fibula and the interosseous membrane
- Distally, to the base of the distal phalanx of the great toe

Action

Extends the great toe

Referral Area

Over the dorsal aspect of the phalanx of the great toe

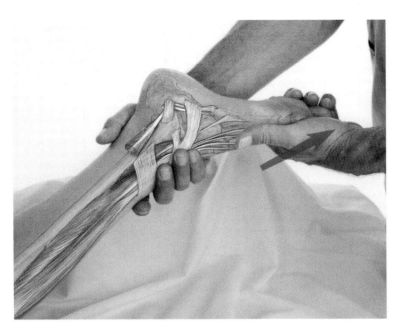

Figure 10-15   Stretch of the extensors (dorsiflexors) of the foot

Other Muscles to Examine

Tibialis anterior

Manual Therapy for Extensors (Dorsiflexors) of the Foot

STRETCH
- Client may lie prone or supine.
- Holding the leg in one hand, take the foot in the other hand and slowly extend it (Fig. 10-15).

LATERAL MUSCLES OF THE LEG

Peroneus Longus (Fig. 10-16)

pe-ROE-nee-us LONG-us

Etymology
Latin *peroneus* from Greek *perone,* fibula + *longus,* long

Comment
The name "fibularis" is sometimes used in place of "peroneus."

Attachments

- Proximally, to the superior two-thirds of the outer surface of the fibula and to the lateral condyle of tibia
- Distally, by the tendon passing posterior to the lateral malleolus and across the sole of the foot to the medial cuneiform and base of the first metatarsal

Action

Plantar flexes and everts foot

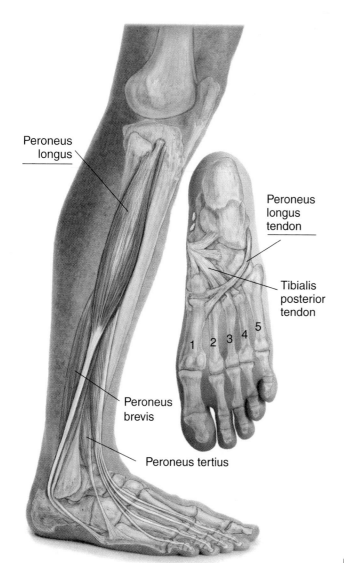

Peroneus longus

Peroneus longus tendon

Tibialis posterior tendon

1 2 3 4 5

Peroneus brevis

Peroneus tertius

Figure 10-16 Anatomy of peroneus longus

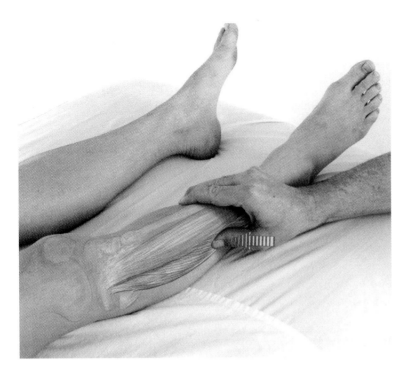

Figure 10-17 Compression of peroneus longus trigger point

Referral Area

To the lateral calf, and around the lateral malleolus

Other Muscles to Examine

Peroneus brevis

Manual Therapy

COMPRESSION
- The client lies prone.
- The therapist stands beside the client at the leg.
- Place a hand on the calf, with the thumb pressing into the lateral aspect of the leg a few inches below the knee.
- Press firmly into the tissue, searching for tender spots. Hold for release (Fig. 10-17).

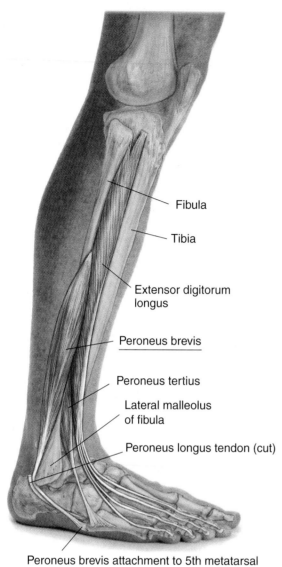

Fibula

Tibia

Extensor digitorum longus

Peroneus brevis

Peroneus tertius

Lateral malleolus of fibula

Peroneus longus tendon (cut)

Peroneus brevis attachment to 5th metatarsal

Figure 10-18   Anatomy of peroneus brevis

Peroneus Brevis (Fig. 10-18)

pe-ROE-nee-us BREV-is

Etymology   Latin *peroneus* from Greek *perone,* fibula + *brevis,* short

Comment

The name "fibularis" is sometimes used in place of "peroneus."

 Attachments

- Proximally, to the lower two-thirds of the lateral surface of the fibula
- Distally, to the base of the fifth metatarsal bone

 Action

Plantar flexes and everts the foot

 Referral Area

Around the lateral malleolus

 Other Muscles to Examine

Peroneus longus

Peroneus Tertius (Fig. 10-19)

pe-ROE-nee-us TER-shus

Etymology   Latin *peroneus* from Greek *perone*, fibula + *tertius*, third

Comment

The name "fibularis" is sometimes used in place of "peroneus."

Attachments

- Proximally, in common with musculus extensor digitorum longus
- Distally, dorsum of base of fifth metatarsal bone

Action

Assists in dorsiflexion and eversion of foot

Referral Area

- Over the anterior lateral ankle and proximal dorsal foot
- Over the lateral aspect of the heel

Other Muscles to Examine

Extensor digitorum longus

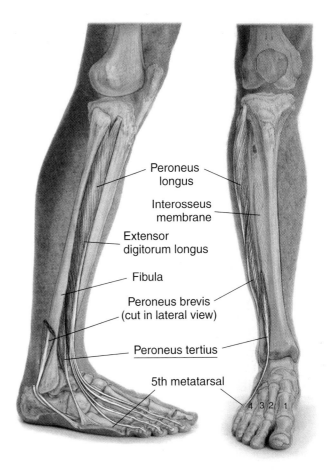

Figure 10-19   Anatomy of peroneus tertius

Labels in figure: Peroneus longus; Interosseus membrane; Extensor digitorum longus; Fibula; Peroneus brevis (cut in lateral view); Peroneus tertius; 5th metatarsal; 4 3 2 1

Extensor Digitorum Longus (Fig. 10-20)

ex-TENSE-er didge-i-TORE-um LONG-us

Etymology Latin *extensor*, extender + *digitorum*, of the digits + *longus*, long

 Attachments

- Proximally, to the lateral condyle of the tibia, and the superior two-thirds of the anterior margin of the fibula
- Distally, by four tendons to the dorsal surfaces of the bases of the proximal, middle, and distal phalanges of the second to fifth toes

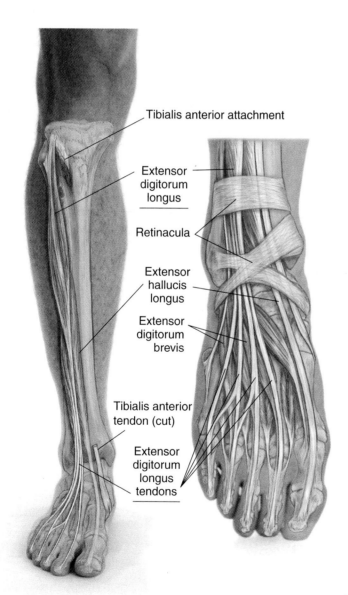

Tibialis anterior attachment

Extensor digitorum longus

Retinacula

Extensor hallucis longus

Extensor digitorum brevis

Tibialis anterior tendon (cut)

Extensor digitorum longus tendons

Figure 10-20 Anatomy of extensor digitorum longus

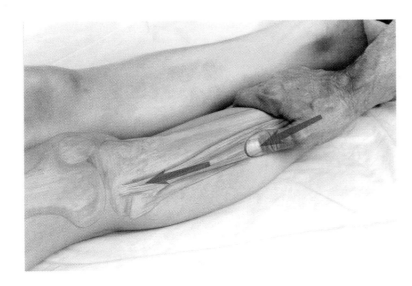

Figure 10-21   Stripping of extensor digitorum longus with thumb

Action

Extends the four lateral toes

Referral Area

Over the dorsal aspect of the second, third, and fourth digits of the foot

Other Muscles to Examine

Extensor digitorum brevis

Manual Therapy

STRIPPING
- The client lies supine.
- The therapist stands beside the client at the feet.
- Place the thumb on extensor digitorum longus at its distal end, just anterior and superior to the lateral malleolus.
- Pressing firmly into the tissue, slide the thumb along the muscle following the fibula to its head (Fig. 10-21).

POSTERIOR MUSCLES OF THE LEG

Popliteus (Fig. 10-22)

pop-LIT-ee-us

Etymology   Latin *poples, poplit-*, the ham of the knee

Attachments

- Proximally, to the lateral condyle of the femur
- Distally, to the posterior surface of the tibia above the soleal line

Action

Unlocks the knee to permit flexion

Referral Area

To the posterior knee, toward the medial side.

Other Muscles to Examine

Gastrocnemius

Manual Therapy

COMPRESSION

- The client lies on the unaffected side, with the knee to be treated flexed slightly.
- The therapist stands at the client's knees.
- Place the hand nearest the client on the posterior aspect of the knee, the thumb placed distal to the knee toward the medial side, pressing the gastrocnemius laterally to gain access to popliteus.
- Press firmly into the tissue, searching for tender spots. Hold for release (Fig. 10-23).

Caution

Avoid pressure on the popliteal artery and tibial nerve, which run along the midline of the knee.

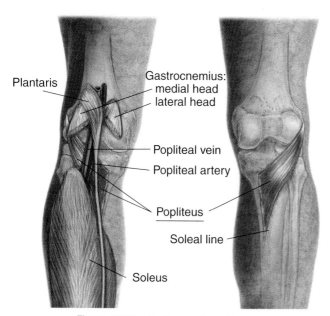

Plantaris
Gastrocnemius:
  medial head
  lateral head
Popliteal vein
Popliteal artery
Popliteus
Soleal line
Soleus

Figure 10-22   Anatomy of popliteus

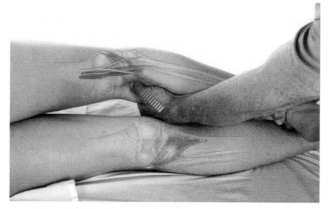

Figure 10-23   Compression of popliteus trigger point

Gastrocnemius (Fig. 10-24)

GAS-trock-NEEM-ee-us

Etymology Greek *gastroknemia,* calf of the leg, from *gaster* (*gastr-*), belly, + *kneme,* leg

Comment

Note that gastrocnemius crosses both the knee and ankle joints, while soleus crosses only the ankle joint. Therefore, while soleus can be stretched with the knee flexed, gastrocnemius can only be stretched with the knee straight.

 Attachments

- Superiorly, by two heads (lateral and medial) from the lateral and medial condyles of the femur
- Inferiorly, with soleus by the Achilles tendon into the inferior half of the posterior surface of the calcaneus

 Action

Plantar flexion of foot

 Referral Area

- Over the bellies of the muscle
- To the medial surface of the ankle
- To the longitudinal arch (medial surface of the plantar foot)

 Other Muscles to Examine

- All other muscles of the calf
- Piriformis

 Manual Therapy

See treatment of calf muscles below.

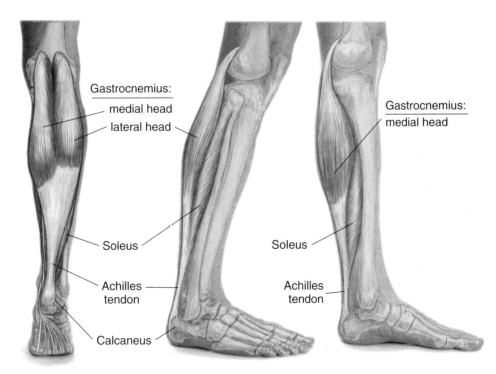

Gastrocnemius:
medial head
lateral head

Soleus

Achilles tendon

Calcaneus

Gastrocnemius:
medial head

Soleus

Achilles tendon

Figure 10-24 Anatomy of gastrocnemius

Soleus (Fig. 10-25)

SO-lee-us

Etymology Latin *solea,* a sandal, sole of the foot (of animals), from *solum,* bottom, floor, ground

Comment

A soleus trigger point is one of the most common causes of pain in the heel.

Attachments

- Superiorly, to the posterior surface of the head and superior third of the shaft of the fibula, the soleal line and middle third of the medial margin of the tibia, and a tendinous arch passing between the tibia and the fibula over the popliteal vessels
- Inferiorly, with gastrocnemius by the Achilles tendon into the tuberosity of the calcaneus

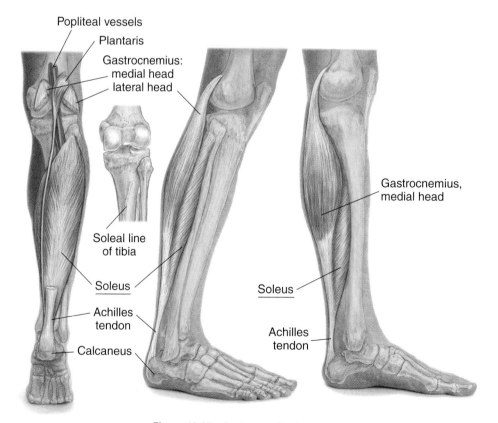

Figure 10-25 Anatomy of soleus

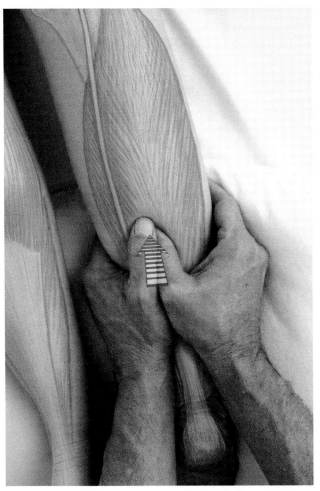

Figure 10-26 Compression of soleus trigger point

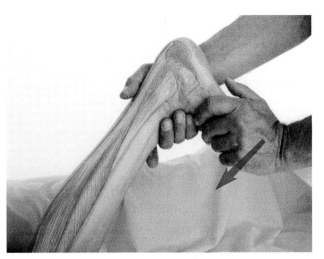

Figure 10-27 Stretch of soleus

Action

Plantar flexion of foot

Referral Area

Over the Achilles tendon to the plantar surface of the heel

Other Muscles to Examine

Quadratus plantae

Manual Therapy

COMPRESSION
- The client lies prone.
- The therapist stands at the client's feet.
- Place the hand on the soleus, the thumb pressing into the muscle proximal to the ankle about a third of the way to the knee (Fig. 10-26).
- Press firmly into the tissue, searching for tender spots. Hold for release.

Stretch of Soleus

Holding the client's leg in one hand, grasp the foot with the other hand and slowly dorsiflex it (Fig. 10-27).

Comment

See also treatment of calf muscles below.

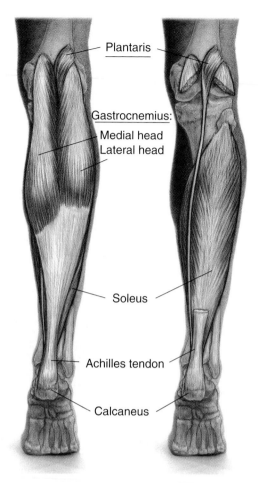

Figure 10-28 Anatomy of plantaris

Plantaris (Fig. 10-28)

plan-TARE-is

Etymology Latin *plantaris,* plantar (relating to the sole of the foot)

Attachments

- Proximally, to the lateral supracondylar ridge of the femur
- Distally, by a long tendon to the medial margin of the Achilles tendon and deep fascia of the ankle

---

Action

Assists in plantar flexion of the foot

Referral Area

To the posterior knee and the upper calf

Other Muscles to Examine

- Soleus
- Piriformis

Manual Therapy

Comment

See treatment of calf muscles below

Tibialis Posterior (Fig. 10-29)

tib-ee-AL-is pos-TEER-ee-or

Etymology   Latin *tibialis,* of the tibia + *posterior,* back

Attachments

- Proximally, to the soleal line and posterior surface of the tibia, the head and shaft of the fibula between the medial crest and interosseous border, and the posterior surface of the interosseous membrane
- Distally, to the navicular; three cuneiform; cuboid; and second, third, and fourth metatarsal bones

Action

Plantar flexion and inversion of foot

Referral Area

- Primarily, to the Achilles tendon
- Secondarily, to the surface of the calf, and the plantar surface of the heel and foot

Other Muscles to Examine

- Soleus
- Gastrocnemius
- Peroneal muscles

Manual Therapy

See treatment of calf muscles below.

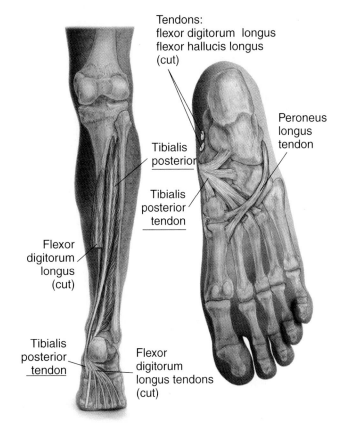

Figure 10-29   Anatomy of tibialis posterior

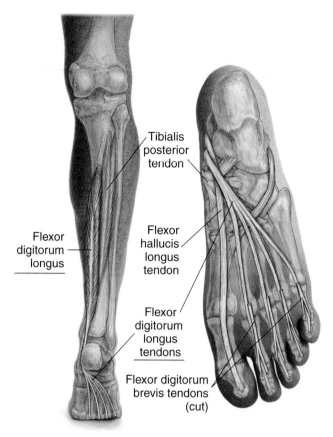

Tibialis
posterior
tendon

Flexor
digitorum
longus

Flexor
hallucis
longus
tendon

Flexor
digitorum
longus
tendons

Flexor digitorum
brevis tendons
(cut)

Figure 10-30 Anatomy of flexor digitorum longus

Flexor Digitorum Longus (Fig. 10-30)

FLEX-er DIDGE-i-TORE-um LONG-us

Etymology Latin *flexor,* flexor + *digitorum,* of the digits + *longus,* long

Attachments

- Proximally, to the middle third of the posterior surface of the tibia
- Distally, by four tendons, perforating those of the flexor brevis, into the bases of the distal phalanges of the four lateral toes

Action

Flexes second to fifth toes

Referral Area

- To the medial surface of the calf
- To the central plantar surface of the foot

Other Muscles to Examine

- Other calf muscles
- Other muscles of the plantar foot

Manual Therapy

See treatment of calf muscles, below.

Flexor Hallucis Longus (Fig. 10-31)

FLEX-er hal-LOOSE-is,
HALL-loose-is LONG-us

Etymology Latin *flexor,* flexor + *hallucis* (from *hallux,* great toe), of the great toe + *longus,* long

Attachments

- Proximally, to the lower two-thirds of the posterior surface of the fibula
- Distally, to the base of the distal phalanx of the great toe

Action

Flexes great toe

Referral Area

To the ball of the foot and the great toe

Other Muscles to Examine

Flexor hallucis brevis

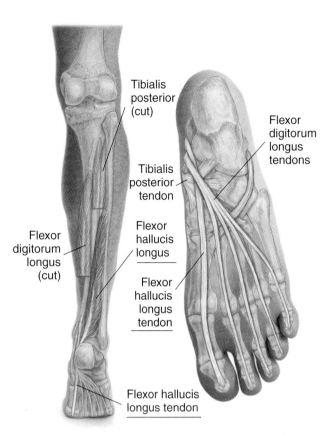

Figure 10-31 Anatomy of flexor hallucis longus

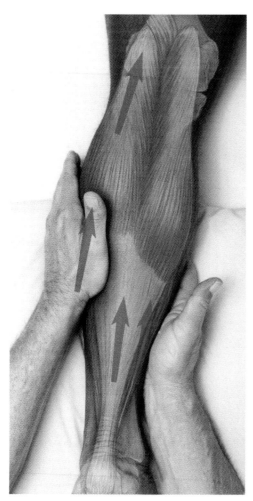

Figure 10-32   Stripping of calf muscles with the heel of the hand

Manual Therapy of the Calf Muscles

When treating the calf muscles with the client prone, avoid excessive plantar flexion of the ankle by placing the ankles on a pillow or bolster, or have the client lie with the feet off the end of the table.

STRIPPING
- The client lies prone.
- The therapist stands at the client's feet.
- Place the heel of the hand on the calf at the proximal end of the Achilles tendon, starting on the lateral side.
- Pressing firmly into the tissue (Fig. 10-32), slide the heel of the hand along the muscle to the knee.
- Repeat this procedure on the posterior calf.
- Repeat this procedure on the medial calf.
- This procedure may also be carried out using the fingertips, thumbs (Fig. 10-33), or supported thumb (Fig. 10-34).

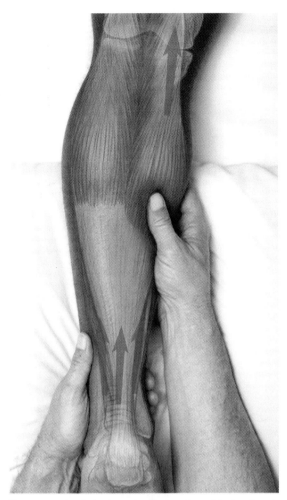

Figure 10-33 Stripping of calf muscles with the thumb

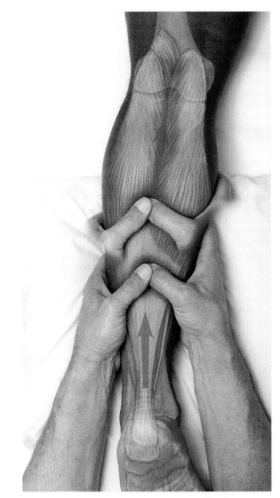

Figure 10-34 Stripping of calf muscles with the supported thumb

INTRINSIC MUSCLES OF THE FOOT

Quadratus Plantae (Fig. 10-35)

kwa-DRAY-tus PLAN-tay

Etymology Latin *quadratus,* square + *plantae,* of the sole of the foot

Comment

Quadratus plantae is sometimes called *flexor accessorius.*

Attachments

- Proximally, by two heads from the lateral and medial borders of the inferior surface of the calcaneus
- Distally, to the tendons of flexor digitorum longus

Action

Assists flexor digitorum longus

Referral Area

To the plantar aspect of the heel

Other Muscles to Examine

Soleus

Manual Therapy

COMPRESSION
- The client lies prone.
- The therapist stands at the client's feet.
- Hold the foot with both hands, the thumb resting on the plantar surface in the center, just distal to the heel (Fig. 10-36).
- Press firmly into the tissue, searching for tender spots. Hold for release.

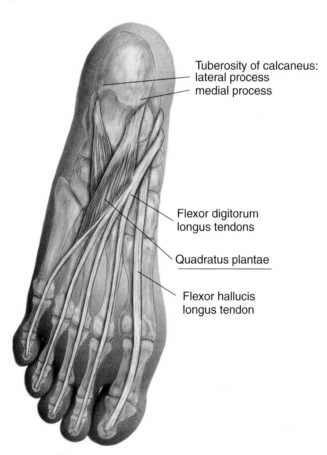

Tuberosity of calcaneus:
lateral process
medial process

Flexor digitorum longus tendons

Quadratus plantae

Flexor hallucis longus tendon

Figure 10-35 Anatomy of quadratus plantae

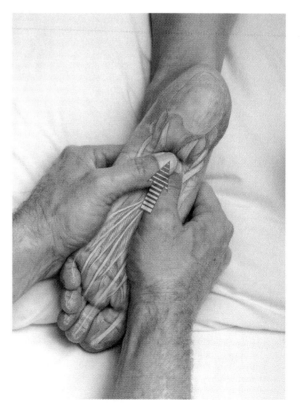

Figure 10-36 Compression of quadratus plantae trigger point

Flexor Digiti Minimi Brevis (Fig. 10-37)

FLEX-er DIDGE-I-tee MIN-I-mee BREV-is

Etymology Latin *flexor,* flexor + *digiti,* of the digit + *minimi,* smallest + *brevis,* short

Attachments

- Proximally, to the base of the fifth metatarsal bone and the sheath of peroneus longus tendon
- Distally, to the lateral surface of the base of the proximal phalanx of the little toe

Action

Flexes the proximal phalanx of the little toe

Referral Area

No isolated pain pattern

Other Muscles to Examine

Not applicable

Manual Therapy

See Toe Flexors, below.

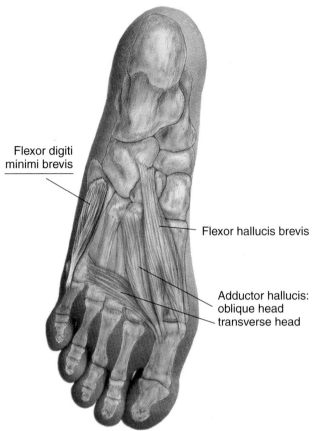

Figure 10-37 Anatomy of flexor digiti minimi brevis

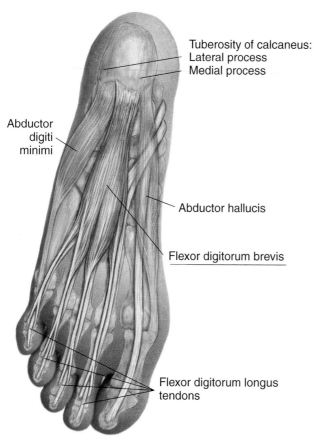

Tuberosity of calcaneus:
Lateral process
Medial process

Abductor
digiti
minimi

Abductor hallucis

Flexor digitorum brevis

Flexor digitorum longus
tendons

Figure 10-38 Anatomy of flexor digitorum brevis

Flexor digitorum brevis muscle (Fig. 10-38)

FLEX-er DIDGE-i-TORE-um BREV-is

Etymology Latin *flexor,* flexor + *digitorum,* of the digits + *brevis,* short

Attachments

- Proximally, to the medial process of the tuberosity of the calcaneus and the central portion of the plantar fascia
- Distally, to the middle phalanges of the four lateral toes by tendons perforated by those of flexor longus

Action

Flexes lateral four toes

Referral Area

Across the plantar foot just proximal to the toes

Other Muscles to Examine

Other intrinsic muscles of the foot

Manual Therapy

See Toe Flexors, below.

Flexor Hallucis Brevis (Fig. 10-39)

FLEX-er hal-LOOSE-is, HALL-loose-is BREV-is

Etymology   Latin *flexor,* flexor + *hallucis* (from *hallux,* great toe), of the great toe + *brevis,* short

Attachments

- Proximally, to the medial surface of cuboid and middle and lateral cuneiform bones
- Distally, by two tendons, embracing that of the flexor longus hallucis, into the sides of the base of the proximal phalanx of the great toe

Action

Flexes great toe

Referral Area

To the ball of the foot and the great toe on both plantar and dorsal aspects

Other Muscles to Examine

Flexor hallucis longus

Manual Therapy for Toe Flexors

STRETCH
- The client may lie either supine or prone.
- Holding the foot in one hand, place the heel of the other hand on the plantar surface of the toes, and slowly and gently press them into extension (Fig. 10-40).

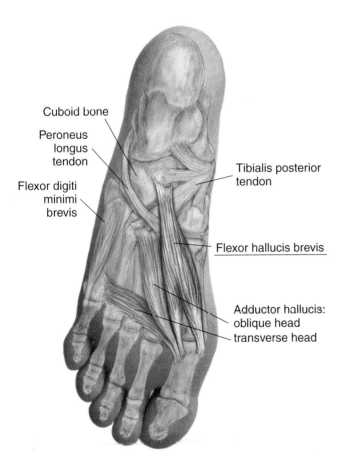

Figure 10-39   Anatomy of flexor hallucis brevis

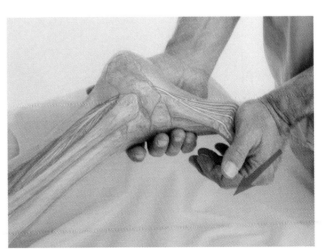

Figure 10-40   Stretch of the toe flexors

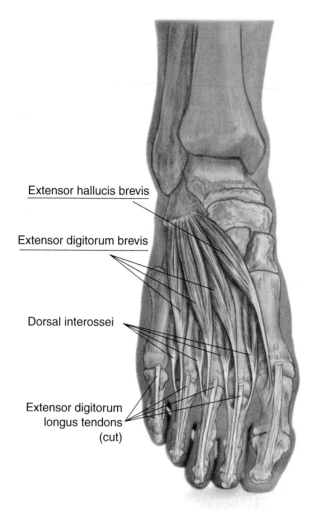

Extensor hallucis brevis

Extensor digitorum brevis

Dorsal interossei

Extensor digitorum
longus tendons
(cut)

Figure 10-41 Anatomy of extensor digitorum brevis

Extensor Digitorum Brevis (Fig. 10-41)

ex-TENSE-er didge-i-TORE-um BREV-is

Etymology Latin *extensor,* extender + *digitorum,* of the digits + *brevis,* short

Overview

Extensor hallucis brevis is the medial belly of extensor digitorum brevis, the tendon of which is inserted into the base of the proximal phalanx of the great toe.

Attachments

- Proximally, to the dorsal surface of the calcaneus
- Distally, by four tendons fusing with those of extensor digitorum longus, and by a slip attached independently to the base of the proximal phalanx of the great toe

Action

Extends toes

Referral Area

Over the dorsal aspect of the foot near the ankle

Other Muscles to Examine

- Extensor digitorum longus
- Extensor hallucis brevis

Manual Therapy

See General Manual Therapy for the Foot, below.

Abductor Hallucis (Fig. 10-42)

ab-DUCK-ter hal-LOOSE-is,
HALL-loose-is

Etymology   Latin *abductor* (from *ab,* away from + *ducere,* to lead or draw) + *hallucis* (from *hallux,* great toe), of the great toe

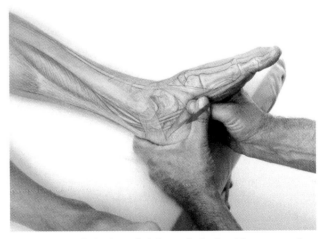

Figure 10-42   Anatomy of abductor hallucis

Attachments

■ Proximally, to the medial process of the calcaneal tuberosity, the flexor retinaculum, and the plantar aponeurosis
■ Distally, to the medial side of the proximal phalanx of the great toe

Action

Abducts great toe

Referral Area

Medial aspect of heel and foot (arch)

Other Muscles to Examine

Gastrocnemius

Manual Therapy

STRIPPING
■ The client lies supine.
■ The therapist stands at the client's feet.
■ Holding the foot in both hands, place the supported thumb on abductor hallucis at its distal end, just proximal to the base of the big toe.
■ Pressing firmly into the tissue, slide the thumb along the muscle as far as the heel (Fig. 10-43).

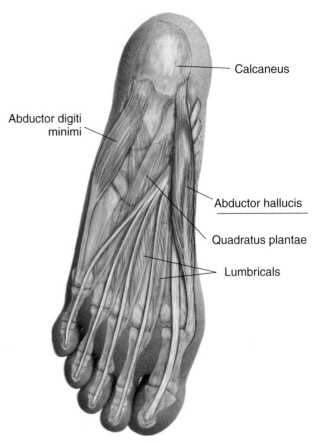

Figure 10-43   Stripping of abductor hallucis with supported thumb

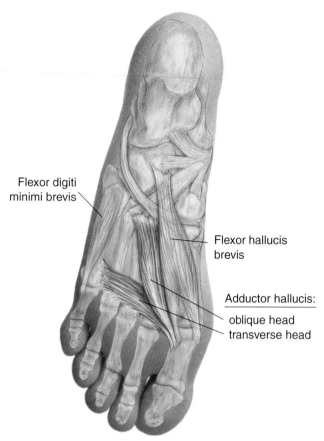

Flexor digiti
minimi brevis

Flexor hallucis
brevis

Adductor hallucis:

oblique head
transverse head

Figure 10-44 Anatomy of adductor hallucis

Adductor Hallucis (Fig. 10-44)

ad-DUCK-ter hal-LOOSE-is,
HALL-loose-is

Etymology Latin *adductor* (from *ad,* to or towards +
ducere, to lead or draw) + *hallucis* (from *hallux,* great toe),
of the great toe

 Attachments

- Proximally, by two heads, the transverse head from the capsules of the lateral four metatarsophalangeal joints
  and the oblique head from the lateral
  cuneiform and bases of the third and
  fourth metatarsal bones
- Distally, to the lateral side of the base
  of the proximal phalanx of the great
  toe

 Action

Adducts great toe

 Referral Area

To the distal plantar aspect of the foot
just proximal to the toes

 Other Muscles to Examine

Flexor digitorum brevis

 Manual Therapy

See General Manual Therapy for the
Foot, below.

Abductor Digiti Minimi (Fig. 10-45)

ab-DUCK-ter DIJ-I-tee MIN-I-mee

Etymology   Latin *abductor (ab,* away from + *ducere,* to lead), that which draws away + *digiti,* of the digit + *minimi,* smallest

Attachments

- Proximally, to the lateral and medial processes of calcaneal tuberosity
- Distally, to the lateral side of proximal phalanx of fifth toe

Action

Abducts and flexes little toe

Referral Area

To the outer edge of the distal aspect of the plantar foot

Other Muscles to Examine

Interossei

Manual Therapy

See General Manual Therapy for the Foot, below.

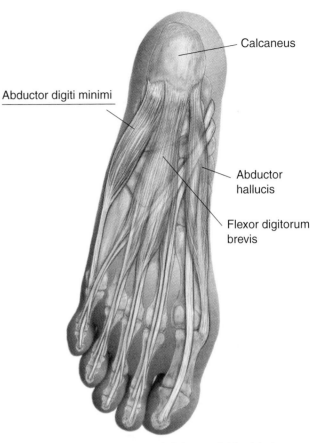

Figure 10-45   Anatomy of abductor digiti minimi

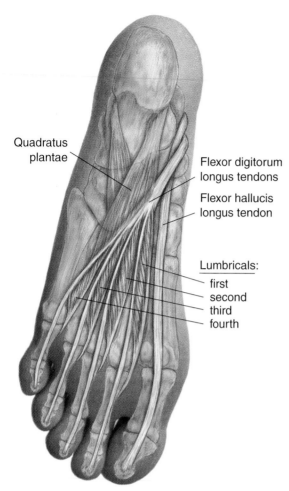

Quadratus plantae

Flexor digitorum longus tendons

Flexor hallucis longus tendon

Lumbricals:
first
second
third
fourth

Figure 10-46 Anatomy of lumbrical muscles

Lumbrical Muscles of the Foot (Fig. 10-46)

LUM-brick-al

Etymology Latin *lumbricus,* earthworm

 Attachments

Proximal:
- First: from the tibial side of the flexor digitorum longus tendon to the second toe
- Second, third, and fourth: from adjacent sides of all four tendons of this muscle

Distal:
- To the tibial side of the extensor tendon on the dorsum of each of the four lateral toes

 Action

Flex the proximal and extend the middle and distal phalanges

 Referral Area

No isolated pain patterns identified

 Other Muscles to Examine

Not applicable

 Manual Therapy

See General Manual Therapy for the Foot, below.

Interosseus Muscles of the Foot (Interossei) (Fig. 10-47)

IN-ter-OSS-ee-us (IN-ter-OSS-eh-ee)

Etymology   Latin *inter,* between + *os,* bone

Comment

Therapy is restricted to the dorsal interossei, as the plantar interossei cannot be accessed.

Attachments

Dorsal:
- Proximally, from the sides of adjacent metatarsal bones
- Distally, first into the medial, second into the lateral side of the proximal phalanx of second toe, the third and fourth into the lateral side of the proximal phalanx of the third and fourth toes

Plantar:
- Proximally, to the medial side of the third, fourth, and fifth metatarsal bones
- Distally, to the corresponding side of the proximal phalanx of the same toes

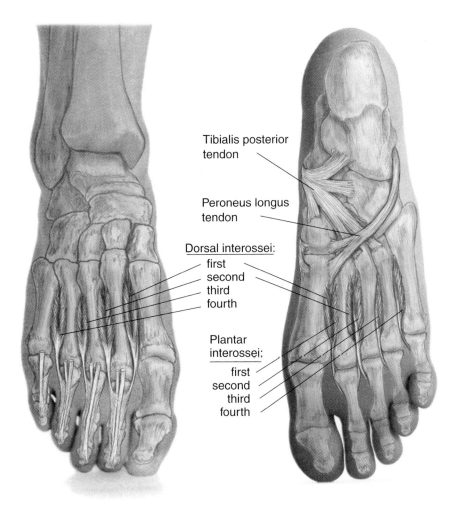

Tibialis posterior tendon

Peroneus longus tendon

Dorsal interossei:
first
second
third
fourth

Plantar interossei:
first
second
third
fourth

Dorsal view   Plantar view

Figure 10-47   Anatomy of interosseus muscles (interossei)

Action

- Dorsal: abduct toes 2-4 from an axis through the second toe
- Plantar: adducts the three lateral toes

Referral Area

Over the dorsal or plantar aspects of the corresponding phalanges

Other Muscles to Examine

Flexor and extensor muscles of the toes

Manual Therapy for the Dorsal Interosseous Muscles

STRIPPING
- The client lies supine.
- The therapist stands beside the client's legs facing the feet.
- Place the thumb on the dorsum of the foot in the space between the most lateral phalanges.
- Pressing firmly into the tissue, slide the thumb along this space to the toes (Fig. 10-48A).
- Repeat this procedure between each pair of phalanges until the whole foot has been treated (10-48B).
- This same procedure can be carried out standing at the client's feet and either pushing the thumb from distal to proximal, or pulling the thumb from proximal to distal (Fig. 10-49).

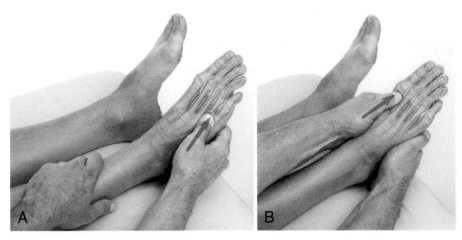

Figure 10-48   Stripping of dorsal interossei (therapist at client's legs)

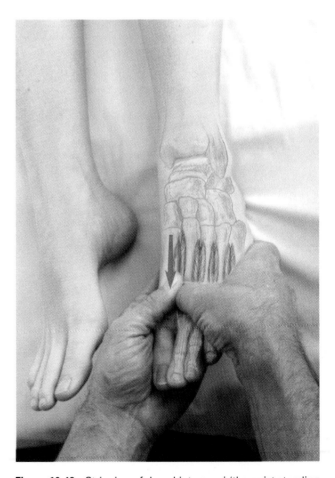

Figure 10-49   Stripping of dorsal interossei (therapist standing at client's feet)

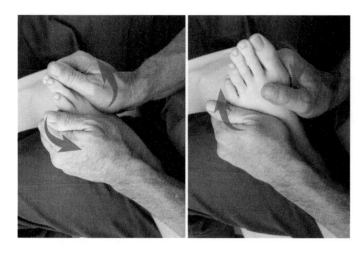

Figure 10-50 Shuckling the foot

General Manual Therapy of the Foot

These are general techniques for loosening the intrinsic muscles of the foot.

SHUCKLING

- Hold the foot in your lap with both hands grasping it on both sides, and move the hands back and forth in opposite directions.
- Do this over the entire breadth of the foot (Fig. 10-50).

SQUEEZING

Hold the foot in your lap in both hands and squeeze it, letting your hands slide gradually away from you until they slide off the toes (Fig. 10-51).

TOE-PULLING

Standing at the client's feet, hold the foot with one hand and pull each toe firmly toward yourself (Fig. 10-52).

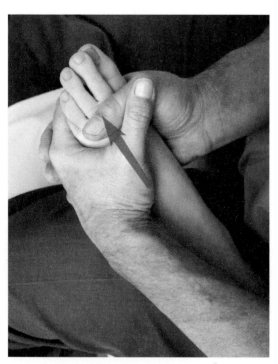

Figure 10-51 Squeezing the foot

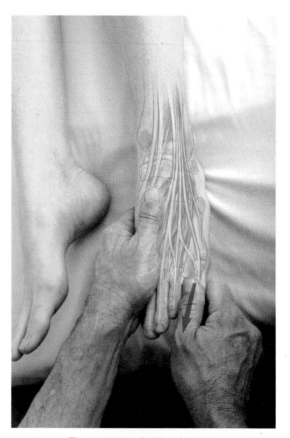

Figure 10-52 Pulling the toes

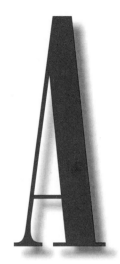

Anatomical Prefixes and Suffixes

GREEK AND LATIN PREFIXES

a-	not, without	bi-	two, both
ab-	away from	brady-	slow
ad-	to, toward	carcin(o)-	relating to cancer
ambi-	both	cardi(o)-	relating to the heart
an-	not, without	ccphal(o)-	relating to the head
ante-	before	circum-	around
anti-	against	con-	together, with

contra-	against	neo-	new
cyt(o)-	relating to cells	olig(o)-	few
de-	from, down from	or(o)-	relating to the mouth
dextr(o)-	relating to the right side	orth(o)-	straight
dia-	through, across	pachy-	thick
dis-	apart, separate	pan-	all
dys-	painful, faulty	para-	beside or abnormal
e-	out or away from	path(o)-	relating to disease
ec-	out or away from	ped(o)-	relating to children (or sometimes feet)
ecto-	outside		
en-	inside	phob(o)-	relating to excessive fear
endo-	inside	phon(o)-	relating to speech
epi-	over	pod(o)-	relating to feet
erythr(o)-	red	poly-	many
eu-	good or normal	post-	after
ex-	out or away from	pre-	before
exo-	outside	pro-	before
extra-	outside	psych(o)-	relating to mental function
fibr(o)-	relating to fiber	py(o)-	relating to pus
gastr(o)-	relating to the stomach	re-	again or back
hem(o)-	relating to blood	retro-	back or behind
hemat(o)-	relating to blood	scler(o)	hard
hemi-	half	sinistr(o)-	relating to the left side
hydr(o)-	relating to water	semi-	half
hyper-	excessive	son(o)-	relating to sound
hypo-	deficient	sten(o)-	narrow
infra-	below	sub-	under
inter-	between or among	super-	above
intra-	inside	supra-	above
lip(o)-	relating to fat	sym-	with or together
lith(o)-	relating to stone	syn-	with or together
macr(o)-	large	tachy-	fast
melan(o)-	black	tox(o)-	relating to poison
meso-	middle	trans-	across or through
meta-	beyond, after, or changed	tri-	three
micro-	small	troph(o)-	relating to nourishment
mono-	one	ultra-	beyond or excessive
morph(o)-	form	uni-	one
multi-	many	ur(o)-	relating to urine
necr(o)-	relating to death	vas(o)-	relating to vessels

GREEK AND LATIN SUFFIXES

-algia	pain	-gram	record
-cele	pouch or hernia	-graph	instrument for recording
-centesis	puncture	-ia	condition
-desis	binding	-iasis	presence or formation
-dynia	pain	-iatric(s), iatry	treatment
-ectasis	expansion	-icle	diminutive form
-ectomy	removal	-ism	condition
-emia	blood	-itis	inflammation
-genesis	origin	-ium	tissue or structure
-genic	originating	-logy, logist	study, one who studies

-lysis	dissolution	-ptosis	falling
-malacia	softening	-rrhage	burst out
-megaly	enlargement	-rrhagia	burst out
-meter, metry	measuring device, measurement	-rrhaphy	suture
-oid	resembling	-rrhea	flow
-ole	diminutive form	-rrhexis	rupture
-oma	tumor	-scope, scopy	instrument for examination, examination
-osis	condition		
-penia	abnormal reduction	-spasm	involuntary contraction
-pexy	fixation	-stasis	stop
-phil	attraction	-stomy	creation of an opening
-philia	attraction	-tomy	incision
-plasia	formation	-tripsy	crushing
-plasty	surgical repair	-ula	diminutive form
-poiesis	formation	-ule	diminutive form

LATIN NOUN ENDINGS

If the nominative singular is –a, then the possessive and the plural are –ae.

Examples: spina (spine), spinae

scapula, scapulae

fascia (bandage), fasciae

vertebra, vertebrae

Others: tibia, fibula, ulna, fossa, axilla, patella

If the nominative singular is –us, then the possessive and the plural are usually –i.

Examples: digitus (digit), digiti

humerus, humeri

radius, radii

Others: tarsus, carpus, peroneus, ramus

If the nominative singular is –um, then the possessive is –i and the plural is –a.

Examples: sacrum, sacri, sacra

sternum, sterni, sterna

cranium, cranii, crania

Others: infundibulum, acetabulum, tectum, cerebrum, pericardium

Some nouns and adjectives are in a different category, where the nominative singular is unpredictable.

Examples: pectus (chest), pectoris (of the chest), pectora

femur (thigh), femoris, femores

pelvis, pelvis, pelves

pubis, pubis, pubes

nates (buttock), natis, nates

corpus (body), corporis, corpora

latus (side), lateris, latera (not to be confused with the adjective latus = wide)

foramen, foraminis, foramina (aperture)

larynx, laryngis, larynges

coccyx, coccygis, coccyges

mater (mother), matris, matres

Note that adjectives based on these nouns are based not on the nominative, but on the possessive.

Examples: coccygeal, lateral, pectoral, laryngeal, femoral

Directional and Kinetic Terminology

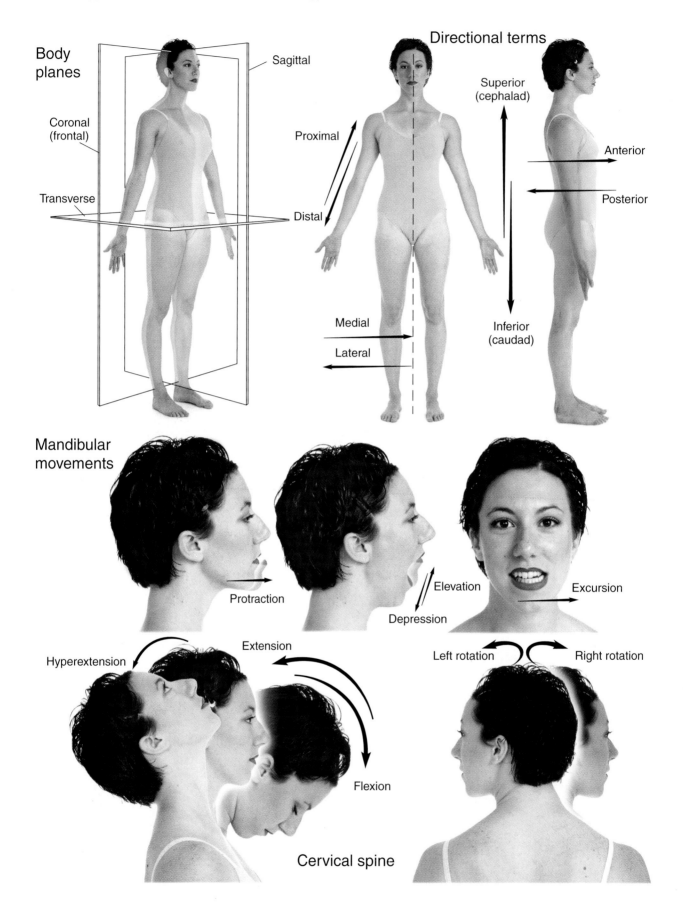

Body planes

Coronal (frontal)

Sagittal

Transverse

Directional terms

Superior (cephalad)

Proximal

Distal

Medial

Lateral

Inferior (caudad)

Anterior

Posterior

Mandibular movements

Protraction

Elevation

Depression

Excursion

Hyperextension

Extension

Flexion

Left rotation

Right rotation

Cervical spine

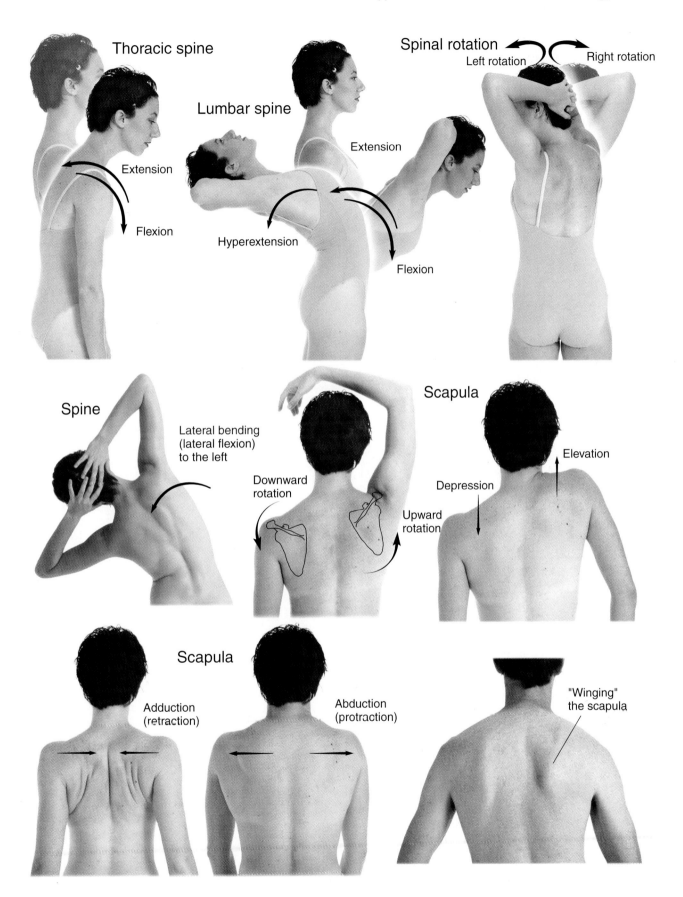

Thoracic spine

Extension

Flexion

Lumbar spine

Extension

Hyperextension

Flexion

Spinal rotation

Left rotation

Right rotation

Spine

Lateral bending
(lateral flexion)
to the left

Scapula

Downward
rotation

Upward
rotation

Depression

Elevation

Scapula

Adduction
(retraction)

Abduction
(protraction)

"Winging"
the scapula

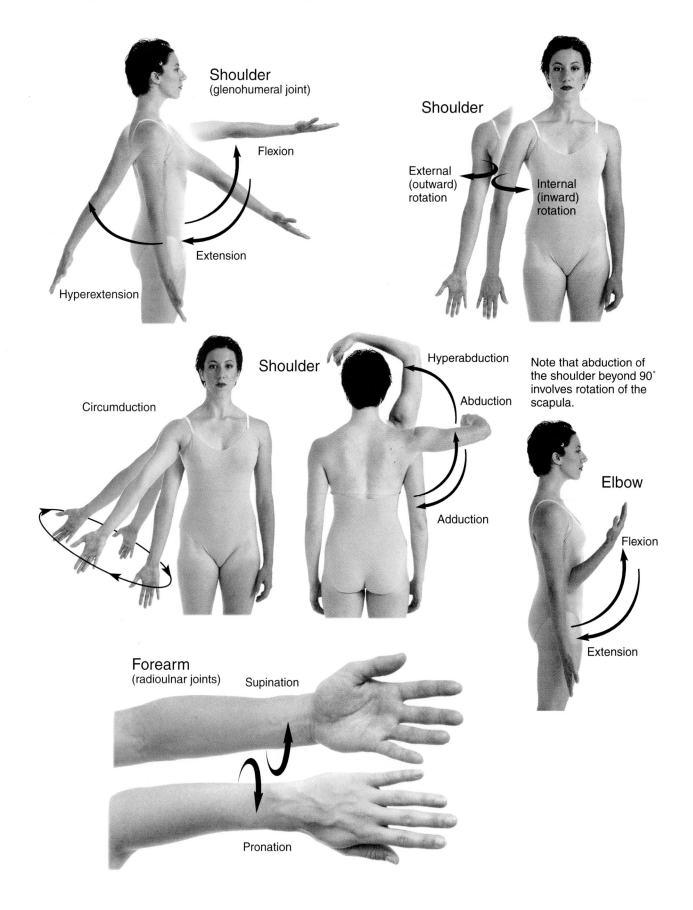

Shoulder
(glenohumeral joint)

Flexion

Extension

Hyperextension

Shoulder

External
(outward)
rotation

Internal
(inward)
rotation

Circumduction

Shoulder

Hyperabduction

Abduction

Adduction

Note that abduction of
the shoulder beyond 90°
involves rotation of the
scapula.

Elbow

Flexion

Extension

Forearm
(radioulnar joints)

Supination

Pronation

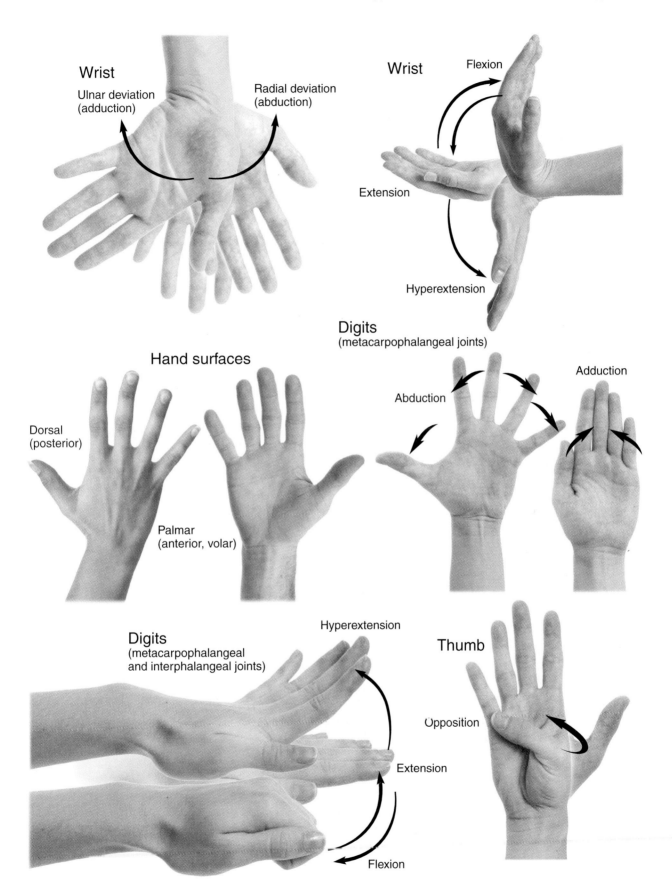

Wrist
Ulnar deviation (adduction)
Radial deviation (abduction)

Wrist
Flexion
Extension
Hyperextension

Digits
(metacarpophalangeal joints)
Abduction
Adduction

Hand surfaces
Dorsal (posterior)
Palmar (anterior, volar)

Digits
(metacarpophalangeal and interphalangeal joints)
Hyperextension
Extension
Flexion

Thumb
Opposition

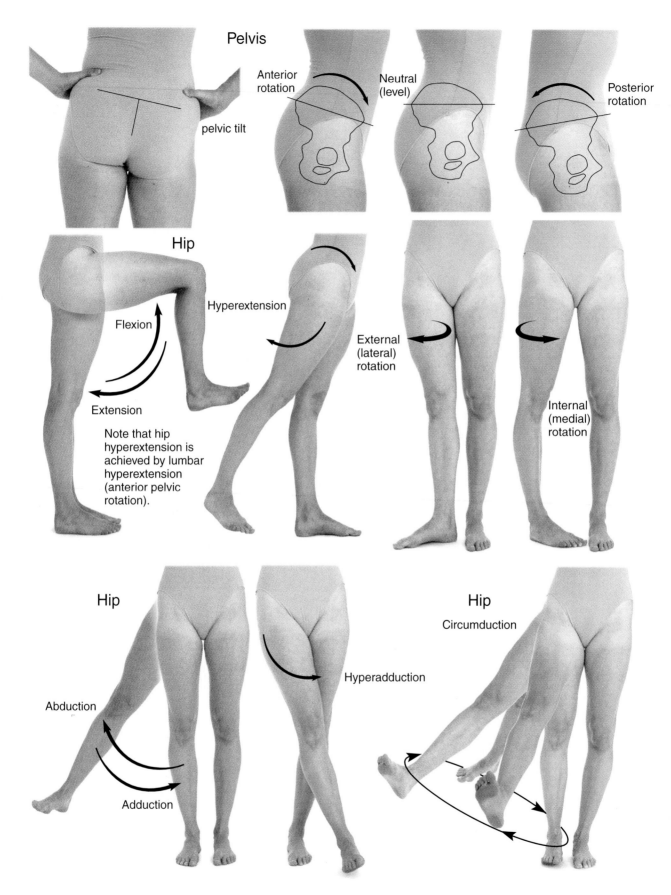

Pelvis

pelvic tilt

Anterior rotation

Neutral (level)

Posterior rotation

Hip

Flexion

Extension

Hyperextension

External (lateral) rotation

Internal (medial) rotation

Note that hip hyperextension is achieved by lumbar hyperextension (anterior pelvic rotation).

Hip

Abduction

Adduction

Hyperadduction

Hip

Circumduction

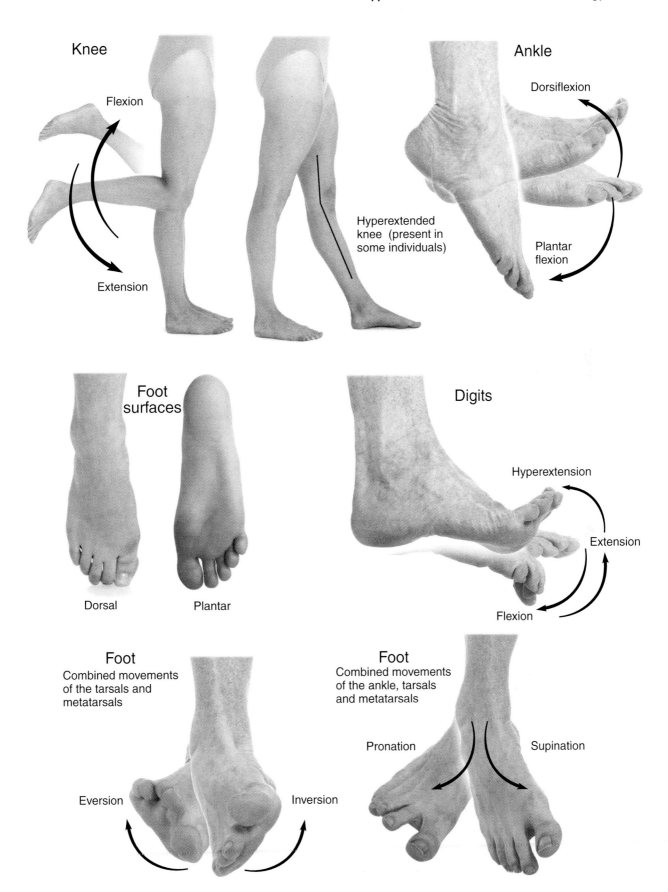

Knee

Flexion

Extension

Hyperextended knee (present in some individuals)

Ankle

Dorsiflexion

Plantar flexion

Foot surfaces

Dorsal

Plantar

Digits

Hyperextension

Extension

Flexion

Foot

Combined movements of the tarsals and metatarsals

Eversion

Inversion

Foot

Combined movements of the ankle, tarsals and metatarsals

Pronation

Supination

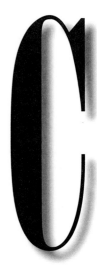

Muscles by Pain Referral Zone

This is an outline of muscles organized by pain referral zones. Each heading indicates an area in which pain might be experienced; under it is a list of muscles that typically refer pain to that area.

Head and neck
   Head
      Top of head (vertex)
         Sternocleidomastoid
         Splenius capitis

Back of head
   Trapezius
   Sternocleidomastoid
   Semispinalis capitis
   Semispinalis cervicis
   Splenius cervicis
   Suboccipital group
   Occipitalis
   Digastric
   Temporalis

Temporal (side of head)
    Trapezius
    Sternocleidomastoid
    Temporalis
    Splenius cervicis
    Suboccipital group
    Semispinalis capitis
Frontal (forehead)
    Sternocleidomastoid
    Semispinalis capitis
    Frontalis
    Zygomaticus major
Ear and temporomandibular joint (TMJ)
    Lateral
    Pterygoid
    Masseter
    Sternocleidomastoid (clavicular)
    Medial pterygoid
Eye and eyebrow
    Sternocleidomastoid (sternal)
    Temporalis
    Splenius cervicis
    Masseter
    Suboccipital group
    Occipitalis
    Orbicularis oculi
    Trapezius
Cheek and jaw
    Sternocleidomastoid (sternal)
    Masseter
    Lateral pterygoid
    Trapezius
    Digastric
    Medial pterygoid
    Platysma
    Orbicularis oculi
    Zygomaticus major
Toothache
    Temporalis
    Masseter
    Digastric
Neck
  Back of neck
    Trapezius
    Multifidi
    Levator scapulae
    Splenius cervicis
    Infraspinatus
  Throat and front of neck
    Sternocleidomastoid
    Digastric
    Medial pterygoid
Upper back, shoulder, and arm
  Upper back and shoulder

Upper thoracic back
    Scalenes
    Levator scapulae
    Supraspinatus
    Trapezius
    Multifidi
    Rhomboids
    Splenius cervicis
    Triceps brachii
    Biceps brachii
Back of shoulder
    Deltoids
    Levator scapulae
    Scalenes
    Supraspinatus
    Teres major
    Teres minor
    Subscapularis
    Serratus posterior superior
    Latissimus dorsi
    Triceps brachii
    Trapezius
    Iliocostalis thoracis
Front of shoulder
    Infraspinatus
    Deltoids
    Scalenes
    Supraspinatus
    Pectoralis major
    Pectoralis minor
    Biceps brachii
    Coracobrachialis
Arm, forearm, wrist, and hand
  Back of arm
    Scalenes
    Triceps
    Brachii
    Deltoid
    Subscapularis
    Supraspinatus
    Teres major
    Teres minor
    Latissimus dorsi
    Serratus posterior superior
    Coracobrachialis
    Scalenus minimus
  Front of arm
    Scalenes
    Infraspinatus
    Biceps brachii
    Brachialis
    Triceps brachii
    Supraspinatus
    Deltoids

Sternalis
Scalenus minimus
Subclavius
Elbow to finger
    Outside of the elbow (lateral epicondyle)
        Supinator
        Brachioradialis
        Extensor carpi radialis longus
        Triceps brachii
        Supraspinatus
        Fourth and fifth finger extensors
        Anconeus
    Inside of the elbow (medial epicondyle)
        Triceps brachii
        Pectoralis major
        Pectoralis minor
    Front, or inner (antecubital) surface,
        of the elbow
        Brachialis
        Biceps brachii
    Back of (dorsal) forearm
        Triceps brachii
        Teres major
        Extensores carpi radialis longus and
          brevis
    Point of the elbow (olecranon)
        Triceps brachii
        Serratus posterior superior
    Radial forearm
        Infraspinatus
        Scalenes
        Brachioradialis
        Supraspinatus
        Subclavius
    Inner (volar) forearm
        Palmaris longus
        Pronator teres
        Serratus anterior
        Triceps brachii
    Ulnar forearm
        Latissimus dorsi
        Pectoralis major
        Pectoralis minor
        Serratus posterior superior
    Inner (volar) wrist and palmar
        Flexor carpi radialis
        Flexor carpi ulnaris
        Opponens pollicis
        Pectoralis major
        Pectoralis minor
        Latissimus dorsi
        Palmaris longus
        Pronator teres
        Serratus anterior

Back of (dorsal) wrist and hand
    Extensor carpi radialis brevis
    Extensor carpi radialis longus
    Index to little finger extensors
    Extensor indicis
    Extensor carpi ulnaris
    Subscapularis
    Coracobrachialis
    Scalenus minimus
    Latissimus dorsi
    Serratus posterior superior
    First dorsal interosseous
Base of thumb and radial hand
    Supinator
    Scalenes
    Brachialis
    Infraspinatus
    Extensor carpi radialis longus
    Brachioradialis
    Opponens pollicis
    Adductor pollicis
    First dorsal interosseous
    Flexor pollicis longus
Volar finger (palm side)
    Flexores digitorum sublimis and
      profundus
    Interossei
    Latissimus dorsi
    Serratus anterior
    Abductor digiti minimi
    Subclavius
Back of (dorsal) finger
    Extensor digitorum
    Interossei
    Scalenes
    Abductor digiti minimi
    Pectoralis major
    Pectoralis minor
    Latissimus dorsi
    Subclavius
Torso
  Upper torso
    Side of chest
      Serratus anterior
      Latissimus dorsi
      Front of chest
      Pectoralis major
      Pectoralis minor
      Scalenes
      Sternocleidomastoid (sternal)
      Sternalis
      Illocostalis cervicis
      Subclavius
      External abdominal oblique

Mid-thoracic (middle of the back)
  Scalenes
  Latissimus dorsi
  Levator scapulae
  Iliocostalis thoracis
  Multifidi
  Rhomboids
  Serratus posterior superior
  Infraspinatus
  Trapezius
  Serratus anterior
Lower torso
  Low thoracic back
    Diaphragm
    Iliocostalis thoracis
    Multifidi
    Serratus posterior inferior
    Rectus abdominis
    Latissimus dorsi
  Lumbar (lower back)
    Longissimus thoracis
    Iliocostalis lumborum
    Iliocostalis thoracis
    Multifidi
    Rectus abdominis
    Gluteus medius
    Iliopsoas
  Buttock
    Gluteus medius
    Quadratus lumborum
    Gluteus maximus
    Semitendinosus
    Semimembranosus
    Piriformis
    Gluteus minimus
    Rectus abdominis
    Soleus
    Iliocostalis lumborum
    Longissimus thoracis
  Iliosacral (base of spine and upper edge
    of pelvis)
    Gluteus medius
    Quadratus lumborum
    Gluteus maximus
    Levator ani
    Coccygeus
    Rectus abdominis
    Soleus
    Multifidi
  Pelvis
    Levator ani
    Coccygeus
    Obturator internus
    Adductor magnus

Piriformis
Internal abdominal oblique
  Abdomen
    Rectus abdominis
    Abdominal obliques
    Iliocostalis thoracis
    Multifidi
    Quadratus lumborum
    Pyramidalis
    Transversus abdominis
Hip, leg and foot
  Hip and thigh
    Side of (lateral) hip and thigh
      Gluteus minimus
      Vastus lateralis
      Piriformis
      Quadratus lumborum
      Tensor fasciae latae
      Vastus intermedius
      Gluteus maximus
      Rectus femoris
    Front of (anterior) thigh
      Adductor longus
      Adductor brevis
      Iliopsoas
      Adductor magnus
      Vastus intermedius
      Pectineus
      Sartorius
      Quadratus lumborum
      Rectus femoris
    Mid-front of (medial) thigh
      Pectineus
      Vastus medialis
      Gracilis
      Adductor magnus
      Sartorius
    Back of (posterior) thigh
      Gluteus minimus
      Semitendinosus
      Semimembranosus
      Biceps femoris
      Piriformis
      Obturator internus
  Knee
    Front of (anterior) knee
      Rectus femoris
      Vastus medialis
      Adductor longus
      Adductor brevis
    Inner surface, toward the front of
      (anteromedial) knee
      Vastus medialis
      Gracilis

Rectus femoris
Sartorius
Adductor longus
Adductor brevis
Side of (lateral) knee
Vastus lateralis
Back of (posterior) knee
Gastrocnemius
Biceps femoris
Popliteus
Semitendinosus
Semimembranosus
Soleus
Plantaris
Leg, ankle and foot
Front of calf (anterior leg)
Tibialis anterior
Adductor longus
Adductor brevis
Outside of calf (lateral leg)
Gastrocnemius
Gluteus minimus
Peroneus longus
Peroneus brevis
Vastus lateralis
Back of calf (posterior leg)
Soleus
Gluteus minimus
Gastrocnemius
Semitendinosus
Semimembranosus
Soleus
Flexor digitorum longus
Tibialis posterior
Plantaris
Front of (anterior) ankle
Tibialis anterior
Peroneus tertius
Extensor digitorum longus
Extensor hallucis longus
Outside of (lateral) ankle
Peroneus longus
Peroneus brevis
Pcroncus tertius
Inner (medial) ankle
Abductor hallucis
Flexor digitorum longus

Back of (posterior) ankle
Soleus
Tibialis posterior
Heel
Soleus
Quadratus plantae
Abductor hallucis
Tibialis posterior
Back of (dorsal) forefoot
Extensor digitorum brevis
Extensor hallucis brevis
Extensor digitorum longus
Flexor hallucis brevis
Interossei of foot
Tibialis anterior
Bottom surface of (plantar) midfoot
Gastrocnemius
Flexor digitorum longus
Adductor hallucis
Soleus
Interossei of foot
Abductor hallucis
Tibialis posterior
Ball of the foot (metatarsal head)
Flexor hallucis brevis
Flexor digitorum brevis
Adductor hallucis
Flexor hallucis longus
Interossei of foot
Abductor digiti minimi
Flexor digitorum longus
Tibialis posterior
Back of (dorsal) great toe
Tibialis anterior
Extensor hallucis longus
Flexor hallucis brevis
Back of (dorsal) lesser toe
Interossei of foot
Extensor digitorum longus
Bottom surface of (plantar) great toe
Flexor hallucis longus
Flexor hallucis brevis
Tibialis posterior
Bottom surface of (plantar) lesser toe
Flexor digitorum longus
Tibialis posterior

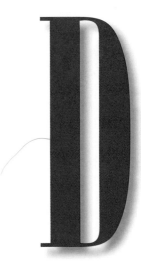

Suggested Readings

Clemente CD. Anatomy: A Regional Atlas of the Human Body, Ed. 3. Urban & Schwarzenberg, Baltimore, 1987.

Hammer WI. Functional Soft Tissue Examination and Treatment by Manual Methods, Ed. 2. Aspen, Gaithersburg, 1999.

Kendall FP, McCreary EK, Provance PG. Muscles: Testing and Function, Ed. 4. Williams & Wilkins, Baltimore, 1993.

Lieber RL. Skeletal Muscle Structure and Function: Implications for Rehabilitation and Sports Medicine. Williams & Wilkins, Baltimore, 1992.

Lowe W. Functional Assessment in Massage Therapy, Ed. 3. Orthopedic Massage Education & Research Institute, Bend, 1997.

Mense S, Simons DG, Russell IJ. Muscle Pain: Its Nature, Diagnosis, and Treatment. Lippincott Williams & Wilkins, Philadelphia, 2001.

Simons DG, Travell JG, Simons LS. Travell & Simons' Myofascial Pain and Dysfunction: The Trigger Point Manual, Vol.1, Ed. 2. Williams & Wilkins, Baltimore, 1999.

Travell JG, Simons DG. Myofascial Pain and Dysfunction: The Trigger Point Manual, Vol. 2. Williams & Wilkins, Baltimore, 1992.

Glossary

Actin filament The protein filament in a sarcomere that is pulled inward by the heads on the myosin filament to effect contraction

Active trigger point A trigger point that actively causes referred pain or related sensations without being directly stimulated

Agonists A muscle that is contracting to perform an action, opposed by an antagonist

Antagonists A muscle that opposes the action of an agonist

Articular process A small flat projection found on the surfaces of the arches of the vertebrae on either side incorporating an articular surface

Articular facet A small articular surface of a bone, especially a vertebra

Atlas First cervical vertebra, articulating with the occipital bone and rotating around the odontoid process of the axis
(Greek *Atlas,* in Greek mythology a Titan who supported the earth on his shoulders)

Axis The second cervical vertebra

Bindegewebsmassage German for *connective tissue massage,* a therapeutic approach developed by Elisabeth Dicke

Body mechanics The use of the therapist's body to perform effective work with minimum strain or injury

Bodywork Any holistic approach to examination and manual manipulation of the soft tissues of the body for therapeutic purposes

Cartilaginous joint A joint in which two bony surfaces are united by cartilage. The two types of cartilaginous joints are **synchondroses** and **symphyses.**

Caudad Toward the tail (coccyx)

Cephalad Toward the head

Chiropractic A health discipline that primarily deals with the joints of the vertebrae and their proper adjustment for health purposes

Clinical massage therapy Manual manipulation of the soft tissues to resolve specific problems of pain or dysfunction

Compression The application of pressure to the body using the hand, fist, elbow, knuckles, fingertips, or thumb

Concentric contraction Muscular contraction that results in shortening of the muscle

Condyle A rounded articular surface at the extremity of a bone

Connective tissue The supportive tissues of the body, made of a ground substance and fibrous tissues, taking a wide variety of forms. Although bone, blood, and lymph are technically connective tissues, the term is normally used in massage therapy and bodywork to refer to tendons, ligaments, and fascia

Core™ Myofascial Therapy A systematic approach to structure through the fascia that works along Langer's lines

Coronal A vertical plane perpendicular to the sagittal plane dividing the body into anterior and posterior portions, also called the frontal plane

Cross-fiber friction Deep stroking perpendicular to the fiber of a muscle, tendon, or ligament with the fingertips, thumb, or elbow

Deep Away from the surface of the body; the opposite of superficial (e.g., pectoralis minor lies deep to pectoralis major)

Distal Away from the center of the body or from the origin

Dorsal Relating to the back; posterior

Eccentric contraction Muscular contraction during lengthening of the muscle, helping to control movement

Exhaustion The state of muscle cells in which the energy source, ATP, is temporarily depleted

Facet A small surface, especially of bone. A facet joint is a joint comprised of two surfaces in contact

Fascia Fibrous connective tissue continuously enveloping the whole body, individual muscles, and parts of muscles

Fascicle A bundle of muscle fibers

Frontal A vertical plane perpendicular to the sagittal plane dividing the body into anterior and posterior portions; also called the coronal plane

Hellerwork™ A type of structural bodywork emphasizing fascial manipulation developed by Joseph Heller, MD, based on the work of Ida Rolf

Horizontal A plane perpendicular to the gravitational force

Idiopathic scoliosis A type of scoliosis of unknown origin that may commence in infancy (infantile scoliosis), childhood (juvenile scoliosis), or adolescence (adolescent scoliosis)

Ischemic compression Compression of a point in muscle tissue, usually of a trigger point, that obstructs the flow of blood in the tissue

Kyphosis Excessive flexion (convex curvature) of the spine

Langer's lines (lines of cleavage) Lines indicating the principal axis of orientation of the subcutaneous connective tissue fibers. These lines vary in direction with the region of the body surface

Latent trigger point A trigger point that refers pain or other sensations only when compressed; however, it may limit lengthening of the muscle in which it resides, or cause muscle shortening in its referral zone

Lateral Away from the sagittal midline of the body. The opposite of medial

Lordosis Excessive extension (concave curvature) of the spine

Mandible The lower jaw bone, which articulates with the temporal bone on either side

Massage therapy Manual manipulation of the soft tissues for relaxation, pain relief, or other healthful purposes

Medial Toward the sagittal midline of the body. The opposite of lateral

Motor unit A single motor neuron and the group of muscle fibers that it innervates

Muscle architecture The structure of a muscle in terms of the directions of its fibers

Muscle cell, skeletal A single cell of muscle tissue, containing several nuclei and many myofibrils, innervated along with other cells in the same motor unit by a single neuron

Muscle fiber Synonym for *muscle cell*

Myofascial release A system of fascial work intended to release, stretch, and influence the orientation of the fascia

Myofibril A sequential strand of sarcomeres within a muscle cell

Myofilament A filament of either myosin or actin, which together form the contractile element of muscle tissue

Myosin The protein filament in a sarcomere from which molecular "heads" extend to pull the actin filament inward to effect contraction

National Certification Board for Therapeutic Massage and Bodywork A national organization that tests and certifies qualified massage therapists and bodyworkers. Many states are requiring national certification (NCTMB) as a qualification for licensure

Neuromuscular junction The synaptic connection of the axon of the motor neuron with a muscle fiber

Neuromuscular therapy A systematic approach to myofascial treatment that attempts to interrupt the neuromuscular feedback that maintains pain or dysfunction. The two types are British (Leon Chaitow) and American (Judith Walker Delaney, Paul St. John)

Occipital condyles An elongated oval facet on the undersurface of the occipital bone on either side of the foramen magnum, which articulate with the atlas vertebra

Odontoid process A process projecting upward from the body of the axis vertebra around which the atlas rotates

Osteopathy A type of medicine that combines conventional medical diagnostic and treatment techniques with physical manipulation

Palmar Relating to the palm, the anterior surface of the hand in anatomical position

Passive shortening Reduction in the length of a muscle without contraction

Passive stretching Stretching or lengthening of a muscle by another person

Pennate Any muscle architecture in which the fibers lie at angles to the force-generating axis

Physical therapy A type of medical therapy in which passive movement and exercise are the primary means of treatment

Primary trigger point The original trigger point from an injury, which may generate other satellite trigger points

Process A projection or outgrowth from a bone

Proximal Nearer to the center of the body or origin

Reciprocal inhibition The relaxation of a muscle in response to the contraction of its antagonist

Recruitment The activation of motor units by motor neurons

Release Palpable relaxation and softening of myofascial tissue. In myofascial stretching, the therapist experiences release as a lengthening of the tissue. In compression of tender or trigger points, the therapist feels a softening in the tissue, and the client reports a lessening or cessation of pain

Rib hump A symptomatic elevation of the posterior ribs on one side during forward bending in idiopathic scoliosis

Rolfing™ A type of structural bodywork, originally called structural integration, developed by Ida Rolf, PhD, which focuses on manipulation of the fascia

Sagittal plane A vertical plane perpendicular to the frontal (coronal) plane, dividing the body into left and right sides (Latin *sagitta*, arrow)

Sarcomere A group of myofilaments forming the unit of contraction in a muscle

Sarcoplasmic reticulum The complex of vesicles and tubules that form a continuous structure around myofibrils and carry the chemical trigger, calcium, necessary to initiate muscle contraction at the molecular level

Satellite trigger point A secondary trigger point activated by a primary trigger point. Satellite trigger points will not respond to treatment without resolution of the primary trigger point

Scoliosis Any lateral curvature of the spine. The most common types are postural, idiopathic, neuromuscular, and congenital

Skin rolling A fascial treatment technique in which the therapist picks up folds of skin and superficial fascia with the fingertips using alternating hands

Stripping, stripping massage Moving pressure, usually along the fiber of a muscle from origin to insertion, using thumb(s), fingertips, the heel of the hand, the knuckles, the elbow, or the forearm

Superficial Nearer to the surface of the body; the opposite of deep (e.g., pectoralis major is superficial to pectoralis minor)

Swedish massage A general term for relaxation massage, derived from the type of massage taught by Per Henrik Ling

Synapse The point of contact of a nerve cell with another nerve cell, a muscle or gland cell, or a sensory receptor cell, across which chemical neurotransmitters move to transmit nerve impulses

Synchondrosis A union between two bones formed either by hyaline cartilage or fibrocartilage

Symphysis A union between two bones formed by fibrocartilage

Tender point Any point on the body that is tender; more specifically, one of a number of specific points posited by the osteopath Ernest Jones as indicating by myofascial lesions treatable by the strain-counterstrain (positional release) technique

Traditional western medicine The anatomically and physiologically based approach to diagnosing and treating disease and injury that predominates health care in Western cultures; also known as allopathic medicine

Transverse tubules Microscopic tubes surrounding and penetrating myofibrils that connect the sarcoplasmic reticulum to the muscle cell membrane

Trigger point A point in muscle or connective tissue that is painful in response to pressure and that refers or radiates pain to some other area of the body. Trigger points in muscle are found in taut bands in the tissue

Ventral A synonym for anterior, usually applied to the torso, from Latin *venter*, belly

Volar Referring to the palm of the hand (or, less often, the sole of the foot), usually used in reference to the anterior forearm

Index